Neurotic Disorders in the Elderly

Edited by
James Lindesay
University of Leicester, UK

Oxford   New York   Tokyo
OXFORD UNIVERSITY PRESS
1995

Oxford University Press, Walton Street, Oxford OX2 6DP
Oxford   New York
Athens   Auckland   Bangkok   Bombay
Calcutta   Cape Town   Dar es Salaam   Delhi
Florence   Hong Kong   Istanbul   Karachi
Kuala Lumpur   Madras   Madrid   Melbourne
Mexico City   Nairobi   Paris   Singapore
Taipei   Tokyo   Toronto
and associated companies in
Berlin   Ibadan

Oxford is a trade mark of Oxford University Press

Published in the United States
by Oxford University Press Inc., New York

© James Lindesay and the contributors listed on p. ix, 1995

A catalogue record for this book is available from the British Library

Library of Congress Cataloging in Publication Data
(Data available on request)

ISBN 0 19 262396 6

Typeset by
The Electronic Book Factory Ltd, Scotland
Printed in Great Britain on acid-free paper by
Biddles Ltd, Guildford & King's Lynn

Preface

The purpose of this book is to give health professionals working with elderly people a practical up-to-date review of what is known about neurotic disorders in this age group. Until relatively recently, clinical interest in these conditions has been limited by the more urgent demands made upon the mental health services by dementia and depression. However, the development of comprehensive community psychogeriatric services is increasingly bringing neurotic disorders in elderly people to professional notice, and there is a need for those who work in this setting to become more skilled in their diagnosis and management.

While recognizing that it is currently rather heretical to be using words such as 'neurosis' and 'neurotic' in a professional psychiatric context, the authors of this book take the view that there is more to be learned from taking a broad, dimensional view of neurotic disorders in the elderly than by adopting the narrow, categorical approach of the modern taxonomies. Accordingly, the subject matter is organized not by diagnosis but by areas of interest as follows: epidemiology; clinical assessment and diagnosis; the relationship with physical ill health; psychosocial factors; biological factors; psychological treatments, both behavioural and dynamic; and physical treatments. In addition, there are chapters on personality, alcohol and drug abuse, eating disorders, sex, and sleep in the elderly. Disturbances and disorders in these areas frequently aggravate and complicate neurotic disorders in old age, and it is important that they are considered in this context.

There is still much to be learned about neurotic disorders in late life, about their origins, course, and outcome, about their impact upon other disorders and upon health services generally, and about the effectiveness of different treatment strategies. It is our hope that readers of this book will be persuaded of the clinical importance of these conditions, and will be encouraged to contribute to the small but growing body of knowledge.

Leicester   J. E. B. L.
January 1995

Contents

Contributors

Robert C. Abrams
Associate Professor of Clinical Psychiatry, Cornell University Medical College, The New York Hospital, Westchester Division, New York, USA.

Klaus Bergmann
Consultant Psychiatrist, The Bethlem Royal and Maudsley Hospitals, London, UK.

Clare Bowler
Lecturer in Psychiatry for the Elderly, Department of Psychiatry, University of Leicester, Leicester, UK.

David Bramble
Senior Lecturer in Child and Adolescent Psychiatry, University of Nottingham, Nottingham, UK.

M. Robin Eastwood
Professor of Psychiatry and Preventative Medicine and Biostatistics, The University of Toronto, Ontario, Canada.

Sandra Evans
Consultant and Senior Lecturer in Psychiatry of Old Age, St Bartholomew's Hospital, London, UK.

Robin Jacoby
Clinical Reader in Old Age Psychiatry, Department of Psychiatry, University of Oxford, Oxford, UK.

John Kellett
Senior Lecturer in Old Age Psychiatry, St George's Hospital, London, UK.

James Lindesay
Professor of Psychiatry for the Elderly, Department of Psychiatry, University of Leicester, Leicester, UK.

Brian Martindale
Consultant Psychotherapist, Parkside Clinic, London, UK.

Michael P. Philpot
Consultant and Senior Lecturer in Psychogeriatrics, The Bethlem Royal and Maudsley Hospitals, London, UK.

Brice Pitt
Professor of Old Age Psychiatry, St Mary's Hospital Medical School, London, UK.

Stephen Ticehurst
Director, Psychogeriatric Unit, Hunter Area Mental Health Services, Newcastle, New South Wales, Australia.

R. T. Woods
Senior Lecturer in Psychology, University College, London, UK.

Introduction: The concept of neurosis
JAMES LINDESAY

The concept of neurosis is going through troubled times, and its use in this book as an organizing principle needs some justification and defence. So far as classifications of disease are concerned, we live in an age of splitters rather than lumpers, with modern psychiatric practice and research dominated by taxonomies that emphasize discontinuities and differences rather than continuities and similarities. Clinicians have been identifying discrete disorders within the broad church of neurosis for over a century, but it is only recently that the usefulness of this term as a major taxonomic category has been called into question. The publication of the third edition of the *Diagnostic and statistical manual of mental disorders* (DSM-III) in the United States in 1980 (American Psychiatric Association 1980) was a landmark in this respect. By adopting a purely descriptive and non-theoretical approach to psychiatric classification, it abandoned the notion of neurosis as a unifying category on the grounds that it was a redundant term with unwarranted aetiological assumptions that grouped together conditions that would be more appropriately classified elsewhere. As a result, the old neurotic disorders were dispersed and rearranged under a new set of categories, an approach that has been maintained in subsequent versions of this classification (Table 0.1). Other nosological systems, notably the World Health Organization's *International classification of diseases* (ICD), have been less extreme in this respect, and the concept of psychological causation is still used in the tenth edition of ICD (ICD-10) to group a wide range of conditions in its chapter on 'neurotic, stress-related and somatoform disorders' (World Health Organization 1992) (Table 0.1). However, here also the emphasis is upon difference rather than relatedness. These classifications currently determine how patients are diagnosed and treated, how health statistics are collected and how the funding for health care and research is allocated, so it is not surprising that alternative approaches to these conditions currently have some difficulty in making their way in the world.

A historical perspective is helpful here, since professional disagreement over the classification of neurotic symptomatology is not new (Hare 1991). From antiquity until the Reformation, the argument was in effect a turf dispute between physicians and theologians, centring around whether they were the result of bodily disorders, or the manifestation of possession by evil spirits. By the seventeenth century it was accepted that these conditions had natural causes, and the debate then turned to the precise mechanism by which disease in one particular organ (the womb, the spleen) could produce the wide range of physical and psychological symptoms observed. In the eighteenth century,

Table 0.1. Modern classifications of neurotic disorders.

ICD-10	DSM-III	DSM-III-R	DSM-IV
Mood disorders	*Affective disorders*	*Mood disorders*	*Mood disorders*
F34: Persistent mood disorders	Other specific affective disorders	Depressive disorders	Depressive disorders
Dysthymia	Dysthymia	Dysthymia	Dysthymic disorder
Neurotic, stress-related, and somatoform disorders			
F40: Phobic anxiety disorders	*Anxiety disorders*	*Anxiety disorders*	*Anxiety disorders*
Agoraphobia	Agoraphobia with panic attacks	Panic disorder with agoraphobia	Panic disorder without agoraphobia
Social phobias	Agoraphobia without panic attacks	Panic disorder without agoraphobia	Panic disorder with agoraphobia
Specific phobias	Social phobia	Agoraphobia without history of panic disorder	Agoraphobia without history of panic disorder
F41: Other anxiety disorders	Simple phobia	Social phobia	Specific phobia
Panic disorder	Panic disorder	Simple phobia	Social phobia
Generalized anxiety disorder	Generalized anxiety disorder	Obsessive–compulsive disorder	Obsessive–compulsive disorder
Mixed anxiety and depressive disorder	Obsessive–compulsive disorder	Post-traumatic stress disorder	Post-traumatic stress disorder
F42: Obsessive–compulsive disorder	Post-traumatic stress disorder	Generalized anxiety disorder	Acute stress disorder
F43: Reaction to severe stress, and adjustment disorders			Generalized anxiety disorder
			Anxiety disorder due to a general medical condition
Acute stress reaction			Substance-induced anxiety disorder
Post-traumatic stress disorder			
Adjustment disorders			

Table 0.1. (cont.)

ICD-10	DSM-III	DSM-III-R	DSM-IV
F44: Dissociative disorders	*Dissociative disorders*	*Dissociative disorders*	*Dissociative disorders*
Dissociative amnesia	Psychogenic amnesia	Multiple personality disorder	Dissociative amnesia
Dissociative fugue	Psychogenic fugue	Psychogenic fugue	Dissociative fugue
Dissociative stupor	Multiple personality	Psychogenic amnesia	Dissociative identity disorder
Trance and possession disorders	Depersonalization disorder	Depersonalization disorder	Depersonalization disorder
Dissociative disorders of movement and sensation			
F45: Somatoform disorders	*Somatoform disorders*	*Somatoform disorders*	*Somatoform disorders*
Somatization disorder	Somatization disorder	Body dysmorphic disorder	Somatization disorder
Undifferentiated somatoform disorder	Conversion disorder	Conversion disorder	Conversion disorder
Hypochondriacal disorder	Psychogenic pain disorder	Hypochondriasis	Hypochondriasis
Somatoform autonomic dysfunction	Hypochondriasis	Somatization disorder	Body dysmorphic disorder
Persistent somatoform pain disorder		Somatoform pain disorder	Pain disorder associated with psychological factors
		Undifferentiated somatoform disorder	Pain disorder associated with both psychological factors and a general medical condition
F48: Other neurotic disorders			Undifferentiated somatoform disorder
Neurasthenia			
Depersonalization–derealization syndrome			

the debate became more reminiscent of modern concerns, with disagreement over whether hysteria and hypochondriasis were specific disorders, or different forms of the same disorder. There was eventually a consensus that these disorders were indeed related and that they were ultimately caused by disturbances of the peripheral nervous system—so-called 'nervous disorders'. The term 'neurosis' was coined at this time by Cullen (1784), and it embraced within its subclassification a wide range of conditions including epilepsy, hysteria, and melancholia. By the mid-nineteenth century, however, attempts to find the cause of these disorders in the physiology and pathology of the peripheral nerves had been largely abandoned, and attention moved to factors such as constitution and environment, with neurosis being seen as the result of adverse external agents impacting on weak, 'degenerate', and 'nervous' temperaments.

Most of our modern ideas concerning these disorders relate in some way to this general explanatory model, although different aspects of the interaction between constitution and environment have been emphasized by different disciplines. Biological psychiatry focuses on the brain, social psychiatry and sociology on the external agents, and psychology—broadly defined—on the interaction between them, as expressed in terms of conditioning, cognitions, personality, psychodynamics and so on. Until the end of the Second World War, the biological, social and psychological formulations of the neuroses all accepted their fundamental interrelatedness, and their continuity with the normal emotions of anxiety and sadness (Klerman and Weissman 1989). The last twenty years have seen a breakdown in this consensus; while social and psychological models of neurotic disorders continue to regard them as related, the rapid growth of biological psychiatry has focused attention instead on the differences between them, with researchers dissecting out specific conditions from the body of neurosis on the basis of particular physiological characteristics, responses to drugs, genetic heritability, and even neuropathology. In the United States, this change in thinking, enshrined in DSM-III, was encouraged by clinical psychiatrists' dissatisfaction with the psychoanalytic approach to these disorders.

THE CATEGORICAL APPROACH

The modern practice of medicine involves decision making, problem solving, and service planning; all these activities are more straightforward if the information is ordered categorically. As clinicians, managers and researchers, we are all more comfortable with 'cases', so it is not surprising that our classifications of disease tend to reflect this. Is the broad, unifying concept of neurosis therefore obsolete? Is there still any sense in which conditions as apparently diverse as phobia, hypochondriasis, hysterical dissociation, somatization and the rest can be regarded as related to each other in ways that are useful to our understanding of their aetiology and management? There is a quite a lot of evidence to suggest that the answers to these questions are 'no' and 'yes' respectively: as Tyrer (1989) says:

Aubrey Lewis (1975) referred to 'hysteria' as a tough old word that would tend to outlive its obituarists. 'Neurosis' is even tougher: it predates psychoanalysis by 150 years, although Freud and his followers added a great number of aetiological implications to the term, they did not alter its basic description. It will not be discarded easily and it has sufficient unifying characteristics for its advocates to be confident in its defence.

Tyrer (1989, 1990) has reviewed the evidence in favour of a general neurotic syndrome. As he and others point out, the usefulness of any clinical classification depends upon its ability to identify distinct populations, to remain stable over time, to guide treatment, and to predict long-term outcome. In these respects, the current classifications of neurotic disorders in systems such as DSM-III-R, DSM-IV, and ICD-10 (Table 0.1) are for the most part not satisfactory.

In the first place, at all ages there is considerable overlap between the specific neurotic disorders, and between them and other psychiatric disorders, notably depression. This is particularly true of non-psychiatric populations; in community surveys of both younger adults and the elderly, there is high co-morbidity between anxiety disorders, with about one-third of those who are anxious being also depressed, and vice versa (Boyd *et al*. 1984; Angust and Dobler-Mikola 1985; Lindesay *et al*. 1989). Modern taxonomies manage the problem of co-morbidity by establishing hierarchies of disorders in which one diagnosis trumps another if both are present. Within the neuroses it is by no means clear how such a hierarchy should be organised, and the existing conventions are arbitrary and often misleading.

A second difficulty with the current classifications is that they are unstable over time. Retrospective studies show that the lifetime experience of more than one neurotic diagnosis is more frequent than would be expected by coincidence (Andrews *et al*. 1990; Lindesay 1991), and in prospective studies there are substantial shifts over time between categories such as anxiety and depression, usually in the direction of depression (Tyrer *et al*. 1987; Angst 1990; Larkin *et al*. 1992). In the case of panic disorder, its association with subsequent agoraphobia is such that there has been some revisionist recombining of the two diagnoses into a single entity in DSM-III-R and DSM-IV.

Third, the modern classifications are not very helpful in predicting patient response to particular forms of treatment. So-called 'antidepressant' drugs are more effective in the treatment of generalized anxiety than are the so-called 'anxiolytics', and the response to non-pharmacological treatments, such as cognitive therapy, also appears to be relatively independent of diagnosis (Quality Assurance Project 1985; Andrews and Moran 1988; Mattick *et al*. 1990).

The modern classifications are most successful in their delineation of phobic disorders and obsessive–compulsive disorder (OCD). In particular, OCD differs from other neurotic disorders in being a relatively stable diagnosis over time, in showing an early and specific response to treatment with serotonergic drugs, and in having a placebo response rate to drug treatment which is much lower than that seen in depression and anxiety. Its classification by the DSM system as an anxiety disorder is anomalous, and in the future it may find its place alongside other neurodevelopmental conditions such as Gilles de la Tourette's syndrome.

THE DIMENSIONAL APPROACH

One reason why categorical classifications are inefficient when applied to non-psychotic mental disorders is that much neurotic disturbance, particularly the more minor and transient forms seen in primary care settings and in non-clinical populations, is more appropriately modelled in terms of dimensions rather than categories. Several dimensional models for neurotic symptoms and disorders have been proposed. Tyrer's general neurotic syndrome places generalized anxiety, dysthymia, panic and agoraphobia in a hierarchy of severity and impairment, with patients ascending and descending this hierarchy over time, depending upon the levels of external stress that they are experiencing. In this model, the nature of these stresses, together with constitutional factors such as gender and personality, are important in determining the predominant pattern of symptoms in individual cases (Tyrer 1985).

Another more comprehensive dimensional model of common mental disorders has recently been expounded by Goldberg and Huxley (1992). They point out that research into the dimensionality of these conditions has its difficulties: studies differ in the size and type of population studied, the number and definition of symptoms identified, and the statistical techniques employed. However, while there is disagreement over detail, the multivariate modelling of neurotic symptomatology in both clinical and non-clinical populations usually results in dimensions that are strongly related to the separate constructs of depression and anxiety. The model described by Goldberg and Huxley (1992) is based on latent trait analysis of General Health Questionnaire data from primary-care populations, which identifies two distinct but associated dimensions of depression and anxiety underlying the manifest symptomatology. These dimensions reflect the activity of cerebral neuronal systems in response to reward and punishment. Various factors influence the acquisition and loss of these symptoms, and these are classified by Goldberg and Huxley (1992) according to whether they determine vulnerability, destabilization or restitution.

Vulnerability factors are those that determine an individual's liability to develop psychological symptoms. Genetic and family studies of patients with neurotic disorders indicate that genetic factors have a non-specific effect in increasing the risk of disorder, possibly by their effect on emotional reactivity (Kendler *et al.* 1987; Andrews *et al.* 1990). Environmental factors, such as early parental loss, poor social support and physical illness and disability have also been shown to increase vulnerability to neurotic disorders.

Destabilization factors are the provoking factors that determine the acquisition of psychological symptoms in those vulnerable to developing them. Evidence from studies of both younger adults and the elderly point to the experience of life events, particularly those involving loss or threat, as being important in this respect.

Restitution factors determine the duration of psychological symptoms and recovery from them. Restitution can be uncomplicated (i.e. patients recover fully from their episodes of depression or anxiety either with or without treatment) or it can be complicated by the development of inappropriate distress-management strategies such as phobic avoidance, dissociation, depersonalization, obsessionality and somatization, which if persistent lead to the relatively stable clusters of symptoms and behaviour that we call neuroses. Presumably personality factors such as 'defence style' (Pollock and Andrews 1989) have their effect on the course of neurotic disorders by predisposing individuals to particular responses to distress. Other conditions not traditionally classified as neuroses, such as substance abuse and eating disorders, can also be understood as neurotic restitutions. As Goldberg and Huxley (1992) put it:

Viewed from a dimensional standpoint, a categorical diagnosis is merely a hypothetical construct, or a way of labelling an individual who has spent more than a specified time in a deviant position in two-dimensional symptom space. In terms of our model, the individual has destabilised, and has been unable to restitute spontaneously. Sometimes the categorical label will just reflect the general position of the individual (e.g. 'major depressive episode', 'dysthymic disorder', 'anxiety state' or 'anxious depression') but at other times the label will reflect the way in which the individual is attempting to reduce their symptoms, as in 'obsessive–compulsive disorder', 'conversion hysteria' or 'somatisation disorder'.

The great advantage of dimensional models such as this is that they remind us that neurotic disorders are *processes*, and not merely the constrained symptomatic snapshots described in the categorical classifications. This is particularly important when considering elderly patients, who often come with lifelong histories of illness experience which cannot be understood except as a process in which individual vulnerability, the force of circumstances, the chosen responses to distress and the consequences of these have all played their part. Another advantage of this model is that it incorporates the depressive component of many neurotic processes. The milder forms of depression encountered in clinical practice have never been well served by the psychiatric classifications; early categories such as 'neurotic' and 'reactive' depression have not been found to be particularly discriminating or predictive, and modern equivalents such as 'dysthymia' are no better (Snaith 1991). Depressive symptoms are particularly common as a component of neurotic disorders in elderly patients—indeed, some have gone so far as to state that depression is the neurosis of old age—and no account of these conditions in this age group can afford to ignore this.

The evidence concerning the various vulnerability, destabilization, and restitution factors involved in the aetiology and outcome of neurotic disorders in the elderly is reviewed in the chapters that follow. To date, research into these conditions in this age group has been limited, and many inferences still have to be drawn from work with younger adults. In fact, elderly people are a very useful population in which to study neurotic disorders: as a group, they are very diverse, and are exposed to a wide range of relevant physical, environmental and psychosocial factors; it is possible to study, albeit retrospectively, the full life course of the illness; genetic studies are more efficient because the greater age of the probands and their first-degree relatives means that they have had a greater opportunity to express their vulnerability; and it is also possible to study the impact of acquired organic cerebral impairments on onset, course, and outcome. It is likely that any research into neurotic disorders in this age group will improve our understanding of these conditions at all ages.

THE CLINICAL IMPORTANCE OF NEUROTIC DISORDERS

To what extent is it justifiable for health services to interest themselves in neurotic disorders at the present time, when resources are scarce and the unmet needs of those with more severe conditions such as schizophrenia and dementia are still so great? Decisions about the clinical importance of disorders are based on judgements about factors such as frequency, severity, distress, treatability and cost in terms of service utilization and welfare expenditure, and to date these judgements have been rather arbitrary and ill-informed where neurotic disorders are concerned (Kreitman 1989). This is particularly true for the elderly population, and the evidence reviewed in this book makes it clear that neurotic disorders in the elderly are worthy of more clinical attention than they currently enjoy. Whatever the size of the health budget allotted to the management of these conditions in the years to come, it is essential that the elderly population receive their fair share.

Frequency

It is evident from the review of the epidemiology of neurotic disorders in the elderly in Chapter 1 that they are relatively common, particularly in the community and at the level of primary care. Their scarcity at the secondary-care level is due to non-presentation, non-recognition and non-referral rather than to non-existence.

Severity

As with younger adults, neurotic disorders in the elderly have a broad spectrum of severity, with a significant minority of cases being mild and transient and requiring little in the way of medical intervention. However, a significant proportion are substantially distressed and disabled, and a small minority are among the most difficult and demanding cases that health and social services have to deal with. As well as causing distress in their own right, neurotic disorders in old age also commonly aggravate and complicate the presentation and course of other physical and psychiatric disorders (see Chapters 2 and 3), and need to be recognized and managed as part of the overall programme of treatment.

Treatability

Another important reason why clinicians should be alert to the existence of neurotic disorders in their elderly patients is that many are treatable by existing physical and psychological means (see Chapter 6, 7, and 8). Early identification and treatment in at-risk groups such as the physically ill elderly has the potential to prevent much of the chronic distress and disability associated with these conditions.

Cost

Analysis of burden of disease shows that health-service expenditure on neurotic disorders in the general population is considerable, at about 6 per cent of total National Health Service (NHS) costs in the United Kingdom. While this proportion will be lower in the elderly as a result of non-recognition and non-treatment of these disorders, there is likely to be a compensating increase in indirect costs due to repeated attendances at GP surgeries, excessive use of non-psychiatric health services, prescription of unnecessary and inappropriate medication, and the provision of inappropriate domiciliary services supporting individuals at home. In addition to these direct and indirect service costs, there is also the cost of informal care that is borne by families and friends.

CONCLUSIONS

One consequence of the development of specialized comprehensive psychiatric services for the elderly population in recent years is that neurotic disorders are increasingly being referred for assessment and treatment. This, together with the projected increase in the numbers of elderly people and the probability that this age group will in future be much more demanding of the full range of health care than it is at present, means that primary care and psychogeriatric services need to plan together how the needs of those with neurotic disorders can best be met. It is likely that, as with younger adults, the primary care team will be responsible for the identification and treatment in most cases, supported as necessary by specialist services. In order to be in a position to provide this support, however, psychogeriatric teams will themselves have to become more experienced in recognizing and managing these conditions, particularly those that are severe and complicated. To this end, this book aims to provide those working with the elderly with a review of what is currently known about neurotic disorders in the elderly population, together with some practical guidance concerning their treatment.

REFERENCES

American Psychiatric Association (1980). *Diagnostic and statistical manual of mental disorders* (3rd edn). American Psychiatric Association, Washington.

Andrews, G., and Moran, C. (1988). The treatment of agoraphobia with panic attacks: are drugs essential? In *Panic and phobias II. Treatments and variables affecting course and outcome* (ed. I. Hand and H.-U. Wittchen), Springer-Verlag, Heidelberg.

Andrews, G., Stewart, G., Morris-Yates, A., Holt, P., and Henderson, S. (1990). Evidence for a general neurotic syndrome. *British Journal of Psychiatry*, **157**, 6–12.

Angst, J. (1990). Depression and anxiety: a review of studies in the community and in primary care. In *Psychological disorders in general medical settings* (ed. N. Sartorius, D. Goldberg, G. de Girolamo, J. Costa e Silva, Y. Le Crubier, and H.-U. Wittchen). Huber-Hogrefe, Bern.

Angst, J., and Dobler-Mikola, A. (1985). The Zürich Study VI. A continuum from depression to anxiety disorders? *European Archives of Psychiatry and Neurological Science*, **235**, 179–86.

Boyd, J. H., Burke, J. D., Gruenberg, E., Holzer, C. E., Rae, D. S., George, L. K., *et al.* (1984). Exclusion criteria of DSM-III: a study of co-occurrence of hierarchy-free syndromes. *Archives of General Psychiatry*, **41**, 983–9.

Cullen, W. (1784). *First lines of the practice of physic.* Reid and Bathgate, Edinburgh.

Goldberg, D., and Huxley, P. (1992). *Common mental disorders: a bio-social model.* Tavistock/Routledge, London.

Hare, E. (1991). The history of 'nervous disorders' from 1600 to 1840, and a comparison with modern views. *British Journal of Psychiatry*, **159**, 37–45.

Kendler, K. S., Heath, A. C., Martin, N. G., *et al.* (1987). Symptoms of anxiety and symptoms of depression. Same genes, different environment? *Archives of General Psychiatry*, **122**, 451–7.

Kreitman, N. (1989). Mental health for all? *British Medical Journal*, **299**, 1292–1293.

Klerman, G., and Weissman, M. (1989). Continuities and discontinuities in anxiety disorders. In *The scope of epidemiological psychiatry* (ed. P. Williams, G. Wilkinson, and K. Rawnsley), pp. 181–195. Routledge, London.

Larkin, A. B., Copeland, J. R. M., Dewey, M. E., Davidson, I. A., Saunders, P. A., Sharma, V. K., *et al.* (1992). The natural history of neurotic disorder in an elderly urban population. Findings from the Liverpool Longitudinal Study of Continuing Health in the Community. *British Journal of Psychiatry*, **160**, 681–6.

Lewis, A. (1975). The survival of hysteria. *Psychological Medicine*, **5**, 9–12.

Lindesay, J. (1991). Phobic disorders in the elderly. *British Journal of Psychiatry*, **159**, 531–41.

Lindesay, J., Briggs, K., and Murphy, E. (1989). The Guy's / Age Concern Survey: prevalence rates of cognitive impairment, depression and anxiety in an urban elderly community. *British Journal of Psychiatry*, **155**, 317–29.

Mattick, R., Andrews, G., Hadzi-Pavlovic, D., and Christenses, H. (1990). Treatment of panic and agoraphobia: an integrative review. *Journal of Nervous and Mental Diseases*, **178**, 567–76.

Pollock, C., and Andrews, G. (1989). The defense style associated with specific anxiety disorders. *American Journal of Psychiatry*, **146**, 455–60.

Quality Assurance Project. (1985). Treatment outlines for the management of anxiety states. *Australian and New Zealand Journal of Psychiatry*, **19**, 138–51.

Snaith, P. (1991). *Clinical neurosis* (2nd edn), pp. 73–103. Oxford University Press, Oxford.

Tyrer, P. (1985). Neurosis divisible? *Lancet*, **i**, 685–8.

Tyrer, P. (1989). *Classification of neurosis.* John Wiley, Chichester.

Tyrer, P. (1990). The division of neurosis: a failed classification. *Journal of the Royal Society of Medicine*, **83**, 614–16.

Tyrer, P., Alexander, J., Remington, M., and Riley, P. (1987). Relationship between neurotic symptoms and neurotic diagnosis: a longitudinal study. *Journal of Affective Disorders*, **13**, 13–21.

World Health Organization (1992). *International classification of diseases* (10th revision). World Health Organization, Geneva.

1

Epidemiology

M. ROBIN EASTWOOD and JAMES LINDESAY

INTRODUCTION

Epidemiology is the study of the distribution of disorders in populations, and of the several factors which influence that distribution. In the relatively short history of epidemiological psychiatry, there have been many changes in the conceptualization and classification of its disorders, particularly in the case of the neuroses where there has been a profound shift away from a broad single category towards the notion of specific discrete disorders (see Introduction). As a result, the findings from early studies using broad, idiosynchratic diagnoses are not directly comparable with modern epidemiological efforts.

The development of standardized methods and operationalized diagnostic criteria was a considerable advance in psychiatric epidemiology, leading as it did to great improvement in the reliability and comparability of results. However, the validity of these criteria remains open to question, and there are currently several distinct and different diagnostic systems for the epidemiologist to choose from when studying neurotic disorders. Nosologies such as the *International classification of diseases* (ICD) (World Health Organization 1977) and the American *Diagnostic and statistical manual of mental disorders* (DSM) (American Psychiatric Association 1980) have different histories and purposes, and while there has been considerable convergence in their most recent manifestations (ICD-10 and DSM-IV), there are still some glaring differences. All this makes it difficult for the reviewer to compare the evidence and draw meaningful conclusions; rather than take sides, this chapter will review all the available evidence concerning the distribution and associations of neurotic disorders in the elderly, from both the early and the more modern studies.

EARLY STUDIES

A good place to start looking at the epidemiology of neurotic disorders in the elderly is *The handbook of mental health and aging* edited by Birren and Sloane (1980), which contains a chapter on 'Epidemiology of mental disorders among the aged in the community' by Kay and Bergmann (1980) and a separate review of the neuroses by Simon (1980). These authors review the evidence concerning the prevalence and incidence of neuroses in elderly populations from various clinical and field studies carried out for the most part in Great Britain and Scandinavia (Table 1.1). There was considerable variation in the scope, purpose, and design of these early studies. Some were of general adult populations, and included only a small number of elderly subjects (Bremer 1951). Others (e.g. Sheldon (1948); Parsons (1965)) were confined to the elderly population, but covered both their mental and physical health. The investigation by Kay *et al.* (1964*a*, *b*) was the first to concern itself primarily with determining the prevalence of mental disorders in an elderly population. In some studies, the authors were particularly interested in specific conditions, such as neuroses (Primrose 1962) or personality types (Essen-Møller 1956). Bergmann (1971) excluded subjects with organic brain syndromes and functional psychosis from his study sample. The process of data collection in these studies was also highly variable. In some cases the interviews were performed by one or more psychiatrists (Essen-Møller 1956; Kay *et al.* 1964*a*, *b*; Parsons 1965), in others by a general practitioner (Bremer 1951; Primrose 1962) or a physician (Sheldon 1948). Sometimes indirect interviews were used, with a psychiatrist interviewing the general practitioner or other informant in some cases (Nielsen 1962; Jensen 1963). In some studies a structured interview was used; in others data collection was a flexible process involving multiple unstructured interviews supplemented by information from informants and case records.

These studies were carried out before the development of specific explicit criteria for psychiatric disorders, and the recorded diagnoses were based on the individual clinical judgements of the interviewers. These varied considerably, and the descriptions of the categories used are not always sufficiently detailed to permit comparisons. Three broad categories of mental disorder were recognized (personality disorders, neuroses, and psychoses), but the thresholds separating them evidently varied, particularly with regard to neuroses and personality disorders. The diagnostic categories used in these surveys also reflect different national and local approaches to the classification of psychiatric disorders. For example, a condition defined as a psychogenic psychosis in Scandinavia would have been identified by a British psychiatrist as either schizophrenia or a neurosis (Nielsen 1962). Where cases of neurosis were further classified as 'mild' or 'severe', the severity criteria used also varied, with some authors basing their judgement on symptomatology and disability, and others defining it in terms of the use of services. 'Mild' cases identified in these studies were probably subclinical; in one study, the rate of mild neurosis alone was 26 per cent (Bergmann 1971). Finally, it should be borne in mind that a proportion of cases will have been classified either as personality disorders (if chronic) or affective disorders (if depressed), and that some mild and non-problematic disorders, such as specific phobias, will have escaped detection altogether.

In view of these difficulties, it is not possible to deduce a great deal about the epidemiology of neurotic disorders in the elderly from the early studies.

Table 1.1. Pre-1975 studies of neurosis and personality disorder in elderly community populations.

Study	Survey Period	Location	Type	Age (years)	n	Prevalence period	Neurosis (%)	Personality disorder (%)	Total %	95% CI
Sheldon (1948)	1945	Wolverhampton, UK	P	60/65+	477	Point	9.4	3.2	12.6	3.0
Bremer (1951)	1939–44	Northern Norway	D	60+	119	5y	5.0	12.6	17.6	6.9
Busse & Dovenmohle. (1960)	1959	Durham, USA	P	60+	222	Point	11.3	—	—	
Essen-Møller (1956)	1947	Scania, Sweden	D	60+	443	Point	1.4	10.6	12.0	3.0
Nielsen (1962)	1961	Samso, Denmark	P	65+	978	6m	4.0	4.8	8.8	1.8
Primrose (1962)	1959–60	Scotland	D	65+	222	1y	10.4	2.2	12.6	4.4
Jensen (1963)	1961–62	Denmark	D	65+	546	Point	1.4	—	—	
Kay et al. (1964a)	1960	Newcastle, UK	P	65+	517	Point	8.9	3.6	12.5	2.9
Parsons (1965)	1961	Swansea, UK	P	65+	228	Point	4.8	—	—	
Bergmann (1971)	1964–66	Newcastle, UK	P	65–80	300	Point	18.3	6.3	24.6	4.9

P = Population sample; D = delimited population

However, some general conclusions may be drawn. Simon (1980) considers on the basis of this evidence that 5–10 per cent of the elderly have definite neuroses, and 8–17 per cent if personality disorders are included. When neurosis and personality disorder are combined into a single category the agreement between the various studies is, in the words of Kay *et al.* (1964*a*), 'rather striking'. The most common symptom patterns were depression, anxiety states, hypochondriacal concerns and chronic fatigue states. Specifically, it appears that depression, rather than anxiety, is the neurosis of the elderly. Bergmann (1971) found that depression supplanted anxiety neurosis in old age with rates of 4 per cent for males and 11 per cent for females, for neurosis of significant severity.

Another consistent finding of the early surveys is that these disorders were more prevalent in elderly women than in elderly men, although the sex difference was less than that found in younger age groups where these were also studied. Neurosis tended to be diagnosed more often in women, and personality disorder more often in men (Neugebauer 1980), a finding that may reflect diagnostic bias rather than a real sex difference. In a detailed examination of the factors associated with neurosis in the elderly, Bergmann (1971) found that the features distinguishing late-onset cases from non-cases were: female sex, physical disability, and abnormally 'insecure/rigid' and 'anxious/hysterical' personalities. By contrast, the only feature distinguishing non-cases from subjects with chronic neurotic symptoms was hypochondriasis—as Bergmann comments, 'they enjoyed the best of ill-health without having to suffer a significantly greater amount of it than the normal subjects' (Bergmann 1971). Compared with late-onset cases, chronic cases were less physically disabled and less depressed; they also reported more childhood neurotic traits and poor relationships with their parents.

Few of the earlier studies report incidence rates, but the evidence available suggests that these are low, and that neurosis, like most psychiatric disorders, starts in young people and falls off during lifetime; Hagnell (1970), a critical source of data, wondered whether things get better with age. Kay *et al.* (1964*a*) estimated that only 5% of the neuroses in their sample were of late onset and with no previous history of disorder; in Bergmann's sample (1971) however, about half of the anxiety states (both mild and moderate) were of late onset.

Neuroses and personality disorders were, taken together, the commonest psychiatric disorders present in the elderly community populations studied. This is in stark contrast to hospital and out-patient populations at that time, where neuroses and personality disorders formed only a small proportion of the elderly caseload. The prevalence rates of neurotic disorders in hospital populations declined sharply with age. Early studies of the incidence and prevalence of neuroses in psychiatric in-patients showed a peak onset of neurosis in early maturity followed by a decline in prevalence thereafter (Shepherd and Gruenberg 1957).

General practice studies of the prevalence of minor psychiatric morbidity show consultation rates to be relatively consistent through life, with a declining rate of new consultations being more than offset by a steady accumulation of chronic cases (Shepherd *et al.* 1981). The difference between the rates of neuroses in hospital and general practice populations was well demonstrated by Kessel and Shepherd (1962), who found that although the prevalence of cases of neurosis in psychiatric hospital and out-patient populations peaked at about 30 years of age and fell in higher age groups, the rates diagnosed by general practitioners remained constant with increasing age. As Shepherd and Gruenberg (1957) have pointed out, the fall in the prevalence of neurotic disorders in elderly age groups in psychiatric populations is due not only to a fall in their prevalence in the general population, but also to a lessening of severity and complaint in these groups, and to reduced awareness by doctors of these disorders. The selection process that determines who is identified as a psychiatric case and so receives treatment has been described by Goldberg and Huxley (1980) in their 'filter' model of the pathway to psychiatric care. An individual's passage through the four filters (the subject's decision to consult, detection of disorder, psychiatric referral, admission to a hospital bed) is determined by various factors, notably the age and sex of the subject, the severity of the disorder, and the doctor's attitudes. The evidence suggests that anxiety disorders in the elderly do not pass readily through these filters; as Bergmann (1978) has pointed out, elderly neurotic patients do not have sufficient 'nuisance value' to be clinically conspicuous. However, they may be inappropriately using other non-psychiatric health services; in a succinct age-specific analysis of the neuroses, McDonald (1973) showed that referrals to psychiatry declined with age, with older neurotic patients being referred instead to internal medicine.

In summary, then, up until 1980 the epidemiology of psychiatry of old age had largely been carried out in northern Europe. Prevalence data from case register, survey, and general practitioner sources indicated that rates increased throughout life, suggesting an accumulation of chronic cases. In contrast, incidence rates fell off with age. Referrals to psychiatry also fell with increasing age, due to non-presentation, non-identification and misdiagnosis. Patients were thought to be physically ill and were referred to specialties other than psychiatry. Elderly females were more neurotic than males, and were so for different reasons: males through physical illness and females through personality. There was some evidence that psychosocial variables may play a part in the aetiology and maintenance of these disorders.

MODERN STUDIES

Epidemiological studies of neurosis since 1980 have expanded and developed these themes in the context of the operationalised specific disorders defined in DSM, ICD, and other diagnostic systems. These systems operate similar constructs for these disorders, but their criteria for 'caseness' appear to differ, at least in the elderly, as their very different prevalence estimates demonstrate.

The Epidemiologic Catchment Area study

It was in 1980 that the Americans harnessed the contemporary wisdom of DSM-III for use in what came to be called the Epidemiologic Catchment Area (ECA) study. Under the patronage of Rosalind Carter, wife of the then President, the Americans wanted to look at standard diagnoses from the DSM-III series (American Psychiatric Association 1980), defined by Research Diagnostic Criteria (RDC), in a number of sites across the United States. Previous epidemiological studies in the United States, such as the Midtown Manhattan Study (Srole *et al.* 1962) and the Stirling County Study (Leighton *et al.* 1963), had employed dimensions of mental impairment, and their findings were not useful to health service planners who required information on the rates of treated and untreated specific psychiatric disorders in the population. It was also thought that American psychiatry would be dignified by having its own prevalence rates.

This immense, complicated, and sophisticated exercise has so far resulted in many journal articles, and in the book entitled *Psychiatric disorders in America* (Robins and Regier 1991). In their words, the ECA study was:

a major collaborative, multicentre research project (which) from the time of inception and refinement of the concept at the National Institute of Mental Health (NIMH) in 1977, through the completion of data collection from 20,000 people in five sites, data analysis, and finally data presentation, every imaginable scientific, administrative and political problem has arisen and been addressed . . . we now have a data base to define the prevalence of mental disorders, syndromes and symptoms in this country—matched by a parallel description of how our mental health, general medical and other human services respond to individuals with these disorders.

Wave 1 of the ECA study was essentially a cross-sectional study with highly structured interviews administered by lay people (the Diagnostic Interview Schedule (DIS) and a Health Services Questionnaire), and sampling techniques that allowed the results to be generalized to the United States population as a whole. It made considerable use of the notion of lifetime prevalence, for which it was subsequently criticized on technical grounds, to offset the difficulty of dealing with duration of illness. What light has this enormous exercise thrown on the neuroses of the elderly? They were not dealt with in detail at all ECA sites, although the elderly population was over-sampled in North Carolina and New Haven. The total study will therefore be discussed in order that the elderly may be compared and contrasted with younger age groups.

In *Psychiatric disorders in America* (Robins and Regier 1991), there are ten chapters dealing with specific conditions, followed by an overview. Since the concept of neurosis was abandoned in DSM-III, and its contents dismembered and dispersed, we must search for the remains. They appear to be in Chapter

4 ('Affective disorders'), Chapter 7 ('Panic and phobia disorders'), Chapter 8 ('Generalized anxiety disorder'), Chapter 9 ('Obsessive compulsive disorder') and Chapter 10 ('Somatization disorder'). As with a whodunit, it is possible to get the gist of the story by reading the end first. Overall, 20 per cent of American adults had a current disorder and 32 per cent had experienced a disorder at some time in their lives. Most disorders, apart obviously from cognitive impairment, started early in life. Men had a greater lifetime prevalence but, for period prevalences, there was no gender difference. Those over 65 years had had less disorder (21 per cent) than those aged 18–44 years (39 per cent), particularly in white populations. A possible explanation for this was that the elderly were survivors, with the psychiatrically ill having died prematurely; and, conversely, the young being more prone to alcohol and drug abuse, antisocial personality and depression.

Coming to specific disorders, there was a ranking of 14 conditions in terms of prevalence. The former neurotic conditions came: phobia (first), generalized anxiety (third), dysthymia (seventh), obsessive–compulsive disorder (ninth), panic (tenth), and somatization disorder (fourteenth). Remission showed a different ranking: generalized anxiety (first), panic disorder (second), phobic disorder (third), obsessive–compulsive disorder (fourth), and somatization disorder (fifth). Dysthymia is omitted as its active status is unknown.

Using the criterion of 90 per cent of all cases revealed, all the neurotic disorders had occurred by the early fifties of the subjects. Those with a propensity to later onset were depression, obsessive–compulsive disorder, phobic disorder and panic disorder. While younger people had more lifetime prevalence than their elders, there was no substantial excess for somatization disorders, generalized anxiety disorder, phobic disorder, or panic disorder. Women had more lifetime prevalence of disorder for somatization and obsessive–compulsive disorder; and more period prevalence for somatization disorder, generalized anxiety disorder, panic disorder, and phobic disorder (Table 1.2). Most neurotic conditions showed co-morbidity, particularly between panic, phobic, anxiety, and somatization disorders.

Dysthymia

Dysthymia is defined in DSM-III as: 'a chronic disturbance of mood involving either depressed mood or loss of interest or pleasure in all, or almost all, usual activities . . .' Respondents meet criteria for dysthymia if their depressed mood lasts over two years but they have too few associated symptoms to meet criteria for major depression and if they have no psychotic symptoms such as delusions or hallucinations. An obvious question raised by this definition is whether DSM-III dysthymia and the older category of neurotic depression are synonymous.

In terms of frequency, dysthymic disorder (3 per cent lifetime prevalence) came second to major affective disorder (5 per cent); and, while other affective disorders (changed to mood disorders in DSM-III-R (American Psychiatric Association 1987)) predominated in the young, dysthymia remained the same

Table 1.2. Prevalence and incidence rates of specific DSM-III mental disorders (ECA study).

		Males	Females	Total
One-month prevalence (%) (Regier *et al.* 1988)				
Dysthymia	65+	1.0	2.3	1.8
	All ages	2.2	4.2	3.3
Phobic disorder	65+	2.9	6.1	4.8
	All ages	3.8	8.4	6.2
Panic disorder	65+	0.0	0.2	0.1
	All ages	0.3	0.7	0.5
Obsessive–compulsive disorder	65+	0.7	0.9	0.8
	All ages	1.1	1.5	1.3
Somatization	65+	0.0	0.2	0.1
	All ages	0.0	0.2	0.1

		Males	Females	Total
Annual incidence per 100 person-years of risk (Eaton *et al.* 1989)				
Phobic disorder	65+	2.66	5.52	4.29
	All ages	2.33	5.38	3.98
Panic disorder	65+	0.00	0.07	0.04
	All ages	0.30	0.76	0.56
Obsessive–compulsive disorder	65+	0.12	1.00	0.64
	All ages	0.39	0.92	0.69

between 18 and 64 years and then declined. Women had double the rate of men and more occurred in Whites and Hispanics than Blacks. Dysthymia was extensively co-morbid with major depression (the so-called double depression), and with Bipolar I and II disorders.

Generalized anxiety disorder

The core feature of generalized anxiety in DSM-III is persistence of 'unrealistic or excessive' anxiety symptoms of at least one month's duration (this was altered to six months in DSM-III-R in 1987). It is a sign of the lowly status of generalized anxiety disorder as a residual category in DSM-III that this condition was not enquired about at all in Wave 1 of the ECA study, and the available data comes from the Wave 2 re-interview of subjects one year later.

For all ages the rate was 3.8 per cent one-year prevalence (2.4 per cent of males and 4.95 of females), including cases co-morbid with other disorders, with half this rate of anxiety exclusively. Women, Blacks, and the young predominated. While the rate was lowest in the elderly, there was a peak in middle age (45–64 years overall), particularly in Black males and Hispanic females. The lifetime prevalence range was between 4.0 and 6.6 per cent in three centres for all ages and 2.6–4.6 per cent in those over 65 years. For both sexes the condition tended to be chronic. Onset was at any age, with about 3 per cent starting after 65 years. In the North Carolina elderly sample (the Piedmont Health Survey), generalized anxiety was associated with increased use of both general and mental health services (Blazer *et al.* 1991).

Panic disorder

Panic attacks are sudden feelings of apprehension or fear during which symptoms occur that are related to the nervous system, cardiovascular system, or to psychosensory functioning; when three or more attacks occur within a three week period, are associated with four or more concomitant psychophysiological sysmptoms, and are not associated with a phobic stimulus, then they meet DSM-III criteria for panic disorder

Panic disorder had a low rate, namely 1.5 per cent for lifetime and 0.9 per cent for annual prevalence in all age groups, particularly those aged over 65 years, where it was often absent. However, as Von Korff and Eaton (1989) have pointed out, panic disorder is a chronic episodic disorder, and is therefore likely to be under-represented in cross-sectional surveys. Interestingly, in Hispanic women, there was a linear increase in the prevalence of panic with age, with those over 65 years having the highest rate of all age, sex, and ethnic groups.

Phobic disorders

A phobia is 'an unreasonable fear of a particular situation'. To meet the ECA criteria for severity, the fear had to have led to help seeking, medication, or severe interference with activities due to exposure or avoidance. The three types defined were simple, social, and agoraphobia.

The one-year and lifetime prevalence rates of phobic disorder (all types) were 9.7 per cent and 14.3 per cent respectively for all age groups. For specific types, the order was simple phobia, agoraphobia, and social phobia. In contrast to panic disorder, phobic disorders certainly occurred in the elderly, and there was much less discrepancy between age groups. Looking at those over 65 years, rates for men were 7.8 per cent for lifetime and 4.9 per cent for annual prevalence; the corresponding figures for women were 13.7 per cent and 8.8 per cent. There was some overlap between the panic and phobic disorder groups.

Obsessive–compulsive disorder

Obsessions are described in DSM-III as 'recurrent, persistent ideas, thoughts, images or impulses that are egodystonic . . . Attempts are made to ignore or repress them.' Compulsions 'are repetitive and seemingly purposeful behaviours that are performed according to certain rules or in a stereotyped fashion'. To qualify as a disorder, they must either be a significant source of stress or interfere significantly with personal and social life.

The lifetime prevalence proved to be unexpectedly high at 2.6 per cent, with an annual prevalence of 1.6 per cent. Most cases had started by 30 years and pretty well all by 50 years of age. The disorder was found to be chronic. As with other anxiety disorders, women had more than men. Persons over 65 years had the least disorder. Co-morbidity, especially major depression, and alcohol and drug abuse were found in a majority of cases overall.

Somatization disorder

DSM-III somatization disorder is 'the presentation of multiple physical complaints in multiple organ systems for which no organic cause can be found'. To some extent, therefore, it is hysteria reborn. To qualify, women had to have had 14 of 37 somatization symptoms and men 12 of 33. There is now gender equality in DSM-III-R. It was thought that somatization disorder in some way resembled hypochondriasis which is 'an exaggerated attention to physical problems or the belief that normal physical signs or sensations are abnormal'. To this end a hypochondriasis/subsomatization concept was developed and named 'somatization syndrome'.

The lifetime prevalence of somatization disorder was found to be rare at 0.13 per cent (men 0.02 per cent and women 0.23 per cent). Black women were exceptional at 0.78 per cent, still a low rate. Nevertheless, it was a chronic condition; lifetime and period prevalence were about the same. The majority had started by the teenage years, and age had no bearing on prevalence rates.

The concept of somatization syndrome (four symptoms in men and six in women) was much more common, albeit just as chronic. The lifetime prevalence was 11.5 per cent and period prevalence 4 per cent. Blacks, especially women, were again particularly prone, and age bore little relation to rates. Both disorder and syndrome had extensive co-morbidity, disorder especially with phobic disorder, major depression, panic, and obsessive–compulsive disorder; syndrome with phobic disorder, major depression, and dysthymia.

Following the second wave of the ECA study, it was possible to calculate incidence rates for DSM-III disorders, and the relationship between incidence and age for some of these is explored by Eaton *et al.* (1989). For most disorders, first incidence fell with age in both sexes (Table 1.2), but among the neurotic conditions this effect was least pronounced for phobic disorder and obsessive–compulsive disorder; in the latter condition there was a non-significant upturn in the first incidence rate after 65 years in women.

In summary, the findings from the ECA study suggest that, by and large, lifetime prevalence rates of psychiatric disorder decrease with age, leaving the elderly with the least psychiatric illness experience. However, it is interesting that this differential appeared to be insubstantial in two of the six neurotic conditions, i.e. phobic disorders and somatization. Between 18 and 29 years and above 65 years the rates for dysthymia, general anxiety disorder, and obsessive–compulsive disorder dropped by approximately half while panic disorder fell markedly to about 15 per cent.

The findings of the ECA study leave many questions unanswered. Is mental illness (or some specific syndromes) increasing with successive cohorts? Did psychiatric patients from the older cohorts die prematurely, leaving relatively well survivors? Did the ECA investigators miss cases by asking the wrong questions? The only direct evidence to answer these questions is from a few longitudinal studies (Murphy *et al.* 1987; Rorsman *et al.* 1982), where it was found that depression was a risk factor for premature death. Given that dysthymia is the most common of the neurotic conditions, how many cases would be lost to studies of the elderly if it does cause early death?

Studies using GMS/AGECAT

British interest in the epidemiology of psychiatric disorders in the elderly has also developed considerably since 1980. Although the Geriatric Mental State (GMS) was developed and described in the 1970s (Copeland *et al.* 1976), it only became complete as an epidemiological tool when the computerized AGECAT diagnostic system was incorporated (Copeland *et al.* 1986). This groups the GMS items into 157 symptom components which are then assigned to eight diagnostic clusters and sorted according to their importance to establish the level of certainty of diagnosis for each cluster. There are five levels of confidence, 1 and 2 being subcase and 3, 4, and 5 being syndrome case. Researchers armed with GMS/AGECAT first looked at the distribution of dementia, depression, and neurosis in men and women over 65 in New York and London (Copeland *et al.* 1986). The data from London and New York have been merged to look at age and gender differences in the elderly population. Males had rates of 13.1 per cent for depression and 1.6 per cent for neurosis; females 20.5 per cent for depression and 1.7 per cent for neurosis. Depression was made up of psychotic (DP) and neurotic (DN) types, which Copeland *et al.* (1987*a*) considered to be not dissimilar to the distributions of DSM-III major affective disorder and dysthymic disorder. Women had more of both types of depression, but not to a significant degree. Most depression was DN. Interestingly, diagnostic syndrome cases of depression seemed to decline with age in women, but not men.

AGECAT neurosis is subclassified as hypochondriacal, obsessional, phobic, and anxiety. AGECAT identified very few cases of neurosis, but a significant minority had symptoms at the subcase levels of phobic, anxiety, and obsessional categories, suggesting that the differences between these studies and those using other diagnostic criteria such as DSM-III are for the most part the result of AGECAT operating more stringent severity criteria (Lindesay and Banerjee 1993). The rates of case and subcase AGECAT neurosis were similar in both sexes; there were no consistent age–sex differences, and project psychiatrists diagnosed illness in women more often than did AGECAT. The authors considered that the low rates for neurosis supported the view of Kay and Bergmann (1980) that depression is the dominant neurosis in the elderly.

Epidemiological data using GMS/AGECAT are also available from samples of elderly people in Liverpool (Copeland *et al.* 1987*b*) and Hobart (Kay 1988), and from a cohort of Icelandic octagenarians (Magnussen 1989). The findings of these studies with regard to neurotic categories are comparable with those of the New York and London surveys. The Liverpool Longitudinal Study of Continuing Health in the Community has continued to study the epidemiology of psychiatric disorders in the elderly using GMS/AGECAT, and in 1992 they reported on the natural history of neurosis in this sample (Larkin *et al.* 1992). In this succinct paper the group discussed the utility of the term 'neurosis' and whether there was a general neurotic syndrome or distinct subtypes. The paper describes a three year follow-up wherein a typical epidemiological two-thirds was re-interviewed. The results were akin to those in the group's 1987(*a*) paper, with 10.9 per cent prevalence for all neuroses and 2.4 per cent for non-depressive neuroses. These were at the 3–5 confidence levels (based on interfering with lifestyle or being a problem) while the majority were at level 2. A critical feature of AGECAT is that it is hierarchical, such that for example depression supersedes and therefore eliminates anxiety. There was an excess of females at the outset but, due to a fall in female rates, this discrepancy narrowed over the three years. While prevalence was constant, cases varied in severity so that, cross-sectionally, different people had caseness and subcaseness during this study. Interestingly, 19 per cent recovered spontaneously. The calculated incidence rate was 4.4/1000 per year. Depression apart, the order of frequency of the neuroses was anxiety, phobias, hypochondriasis, and, much less frequently, obsessional neurosis. The authors thought that Tyrer's 'general neurotic syndrome' (Tyrer 1989) was supported by their work since it 'can be seen as a single syndrome with a prolonged course and variation in predominance of different symptoms over time . . . he [Tyrer] suggested that anxiety and depressive symptoms are the predominant mix in the syndrome, as in fact was the case here.'

The Guy's / Age Concern Survey

This study by Lindesay *et al.* (1989) was carried out in an inner London health district using an interview schedule made up of a *mélange* of standard instruments. All of the anxiety disorders, except for post-traumatic stress disorder and obsessive–compulsive disorder, were rated. For lesser depression (8+ on the depression (D) scale of the Comprehensive Assessment and Referral Evaluation (CARE) Schedule) women had significantly higher rates (13.5 per cent) than men (8.4 per cent), but this was not true for greater depression (13+ on the D scale). Lesser depression rose smoothly with age in women, but was hectic in men, possibly varying with physical illness and mortality. For anxiety there was no significant gender difference. General anxiety disorder and depression, especially lesser depression, were significantly associated. Panic disorder was not found. Phobic disorders were more common in women (13.9 per cent) than men (4.2 per cent); the reported fears were similar to those found in younger adults, that is, going out alone, travelling, enclosed spaces, insects and animals, and being alone at home. Age within this elderly sample did not have a bearing. Agoraphobia was the most common, followed by specific and social phobia.

In the discussion, the results were stated to be in accord with other American and British studies, i.e. Blazer and Williams (1980), Gurland *et al.* (1983) and Copeland *et al.* (1987*b*). With regard to anxiety, the old do not panic, but they do have specific and situational fears. Rates of generalized anxiety at 3.7 per cent and phobias at 10 per cent were higher than reported by other studies, but these figures included depressed subjects who are excluded by hierarchical diagnostic systems such as DSM-III and AGECAT. Depression, generalized anxiety, and agoraphobia were associated with higher rates of physical ill health in this sample (Lindesay 1990).

Phobic disorders in this urban elderly sample have been examined in a detailed case–control study by Lindesay (1991). Cases generally had more neurotic symptoms than controls and a greater likelihood of a past psychiatric history. One-third were of late onset, and these cases tended to be agoraphobic in nature.

The Gospel Oak Study

In this survey (Livingston *et al.* 1990), elderly residents of an electoral ward in London were screened with the depression scale of the CARE Schedule, and 15.9 per cent were found to be depressed. Depression was associated with disordered sleep and somatic complaints, and depressed subjects were more likely to be in contact with health services.

CROSS-CULTURAL COMPARISONS

Henderson *et al.* (1992) in Australia write that:

The epidemiology of depression in later life is a subject that calls for close attention. This is because there is such uncertainty about its true prevalence both nationally and internationally; and its recognition by health professionals may be markedly incomplete . . . The reality is that age is frequently accompanied by many undesirable events such as bereavement, chronic physical illness, disability and loss of independence. It is therefore intuitively reasonable to believe that the elderly are often the victims of depressing circumstances. One likely consequence is that depression is the most frequent psychiatric disorder in daily clinical practice with elderly persons.

He pointed out that the findings from prevalence studies on depression or depressive symptoms range from 10 per cent to 45 per cent. He felt that this variation was due to including somatic symptoms. Studies restricted to depressive illness or major depression have a range of 2–20 per cent. Henderson *et al.* (1993), using the Canberra Interview for the Elderly (Social Psychiatry Research Unit 1992), looked at depression in Australians over 70 years of age in and around Canberra. The response rate in this community sample was 69 per cent. Using ICD-10 criteria, the point prevalence for depressive episodes was 3.3 per cent. For DSM-III-R criteria, the same rate was 1 per cent for major depressive episodes and 0.6 per cent for dysthymia. Nevertheless, the kappa statistic for agreement between classifications was only 0.4. Looking at depressive symptoms alone, only 29 per cent had none, but the symptoms tended to aggregate in a few people. Symptoms were related to a past history of depression and current general physical health, but not to age. The most important influence on variation in these symptoms was, however, neuroticism. All in all, the elderly had depressive symptoms rather than disorders and the rates in Australia were akin to North American findings. Separately, Jorm *et al.* (in press) have found that neuroticism was correlated with health, and what mattered was perception rather than objective measures, especially among women. This was reflected in a modest association in use of health services. Earlier, Henderson *et al.* (1986) found that the elderly were more satisfied and less socially connected than younger people. As might be expected, the depressed were even less connected but did not complain about it.

Henderson (1992) has also presented data from three Japanese studies which showed depression to have a low prevalence (around 1 per cent), and what was called neurosis was somewhere between 1.2 per cent and 4.7 per cent. He argued that the different generations in Japan still live together and that this prevents loneliness. Moreover the elderly Japanese seem to keep busy. He sees these socio-cultural structures as preventing depression in the elderly, and argues that there is a considerable need for further cross-cultural studies.

Busse (1992), from the USA, quotes Blazer *et al.* (1987) from a North Carolina study to the effect that 0.7 per cent had major depression, 2.1 per cent neurotic depression (dysthymia), and 1.2 per cent depression with anxiety. While 73 per cent of the sample were well, a further 23 per cent had varying degrees of depressive symptoms. Thus, he saw that reduced quality of life due to ageing, disease and disability, loss, and impoverishment were associated with depression. He pointed out that, in the USA, women were more socially isolated, had more chronic disease and disabilities, and were poorer than men; this helped explain their higher rate of depression.

In a Swedish study (Enzell 1983) about 80 per cent of sixty-nine-year-olds attending for health check-ups had depressive symptoms and 44 per cent had neurotic disorders. In South Africa Ben Arie *et al.* (1987) found a prevalence rate for depression of 13 per cent in a community sample of Black people, but with much hypochondriasis. In the USA, however, Costa and McCrae (1985) thought that the stereotype of elderly men and women as hypochondriacal was unfounded. This view was confirmed by Barsky *et al.* (1991). In the USA Stallones *et al.* (1990) looked at a community-based probability sample using telephone interviews. Depressive symptoms were found in 9.9 per cent; risk factors were being female (especially Black), being single, having poor subjective health, and having limited social matrices. Palinkas *et al.* (1990) also found that depressive symptoms were inversely associated with the size of social networks. Again in the USA, Gatz and Hurwicz (1990) asked whether old people were more depressed and, from applying the 20-item CES-D scale, found that the old did not have more depressive symptoms but were more pessimistic. In the UK Bowling (1990) showed that, in those over 85 years, 27 per cent were probable psychiatric cases, based upon psychometric examination. While they complained of somatic problems, variables such as age, sex, social matrices, and loneliness did not count. They tended not to contact their general practitioners. In Singapore, Kua (1990) showed that among elderly Chinese the prevalence of depression was 4.6 per cent; it was mild and occurred more in younger old people and females. Again in the USA. In Finland, Kivel *et al.* (1988) looked at Finns over sixty years of age. Rates for dysthymic disorder were 17.2 per cent for men and 22.9 per cent for women.

CONCLUSIONS

In summary, the early European studies of neurosis in the elderly found that period prevalence was in the region of 4–9 per cent, with most cases being of depression. Prevalence tended to accumulate with age, incidence waned, and specialist psychiatric referrals declined, with cases being referred to general health services instead. Risk factors were female gender, physical illness, abnormal personality traits, loneliness, marital difficulties, and bereavement. Modern studies using standardized measures have found rather higher rates of neurotic disorders in the elderly, with depression and anxiety most prominent. The ECA study showed a decline in prevalence rates with age, though not consistently across the neurotic disorders. Being female was less of a risk factor and gender differences varied by study. Other variable risk factors for neurotic disorders were ethnic group, reduced quality of life, loneliness, poor physical health, and personality type. The impact of factors such as loneliness and hypochondriasis were not consistent across cultures, and it may be that in societies where the elderly are cherished, depression, and anxiety are less common.

REFERENCES

American Psychiatric Association (1980). *Diagnostic and statistical manual of mental disorders* (3rd edn). Division of Public Affairs, American Psychiatric Association, Washington.
American Psychiatric Association (1987). *Diagnostic and statistical manual of mental disorders* (3rd edn, revised). Division of Public Affairs, American Psychiatric Association, Washington.
Barsky, A. J., Frank, C. B., Cleary, P. D., Wyshak, and Klerman, G. (1991). The relation between hypochondriasis and age. *American Journal of Psychiatry*, **148**, 923–8.
Ben Arie, O., Swartz, L., and Dickman, B. J. (1987). Depression in the elderly living in the community: its presentation and features. *British Journal of Psychiatry*, **150**, 169–74.

Bergmann, K. (1971). The neuroses of old age. In *Recent developments in psychogeriatrics* (ed. D. W. K. Kay and A. Walk), pp. 39–50. Headley Bros, Ashford.

Bergmann, K. (1978). Neurosis and personality disorder in old age. In *Studies in geriatric psychiatry* (ed. A. D. Isaacs and F. Post), pp. 41–75. Wiley, London.

Birren, S. E., and Sloane, R. B. (1980). *The handbook of mental health and aging.* Prentice-Hall Inc., New Jersey.

Blazer, D. G., and Williams, C. D. (1980). Epidemiology of depression and dysphoria in an elderly population. *American Journal of Psychiatry*, **137**, 439–44.

Blazer, D. G., Hughes, D. C., and George, L. K. (1987). The epidemiology of depression in an elderly community population. *Gerontologist*, **36**, 699–706.

Blazer, D. G., George, L. K., and Hughes, D. (1991). The epidemiology of anxiety disorders: an age comparison. In *Anxiety in the elderly* (ed. C. Salzman and B. D. Lebowitz), pp. 17–30. Springer Publishing Co., New York.

Bowling, A. (1990). The prevalence of psychiatric morbidity among people aged 85 and over living at home: associations with reported somatic symptoms and with consulting behaviour. *Social Psychiatry and Psychiatric Epidemiology*, **25**, 132–40.

Bremer, J. (1951). A social psychiatric investigation of a small community in northern Norway. *Acta Psychiatrica Scandinavica*, Supp. 62.

Busse, E. W., and Dovenmuhle, R. H. (1960). Neurotic symptoms and predisposition in ageing people. *Journal of the American Geriatrics Society*, **8**, 328–336.

Busse, E. W. (1992). Quality of life: affect and mood in late life. In *Aging and mental disorders: international perspectives* (ed. M. Bergener, K. Hasegawa, S. I. Finkel, and T. Nishimura), pp. 38–55. Springer Publishing Co., New York.

Copeland, J. R. M., Kelleher, M. J., Kellett, J. M., Gourlay, A. J., Gurland B. J., Fleiss, J. L., *et al.* (1976). A semi-structured clinical interview for the assessment of diagnosis and mental state in the elderly. The Geriatric Mental Status Schedule, development and reliability. *Psychological Medicine*, **6**, 439–49.

Copeland, J. R. M., Dewey, M. E., and Griffiths-Jones, H. M. (1986). Computerized psychiatric diagnostic system and case nomenclature for elderly subjects: GMS and AGECAT. *Psychological Medicine*, **16**, 89–99.

Copeland, J. R. M., Gurland, B. J., Dewey, M. E., Kelleher, M. J., Smith, A. M. R., and Davidson, I. A. (1987a). Is there more dementia, depression and neurosis in New York? a comparative study of the elderly in New York and London using the computer diagnosis AGECAT. *British Journal of Psychiatry*, **151**, 466–73.

Copeland, J. R. M., Gurland, B. J., Dewey, M. E., Kelleher, M. J., Smith, A. M. R., and Davidson, I. A. (1987b). The distribution of dementia, depression and neurosis in elderly men and women in an urban community: assessed using the GMS-AGECAT. *International Journal of Geriatric Psychiatry*, **2**, 177–84.

Costa, P. T., and McCrae, R. R. (1985). Hypochondriasis, neuroticism and aging: when are somatic complaints unfounded? *American Psychologist*, **40**, 19–28.

Eaton, W. W., Kramer, M., Anthony, J. C., Dryman, A., Shapiro, S., and Locke, B. Z. (1989) The incidence of specific DIS/DSM-III mental disorders: data from the NIMH Epidemiologic Catchment Area program. *Acta Psychiatria Scandinavica*, **79**, 163–178.

Enzell, K. (1983). Psychiatric study of 69-year-old health examinees in Stockholm: factors of possible importance for the mental health of the elderly. *Acta Psychiatrica Scandinavica*, **67**, 414–28.

Essen-Møller, E. (1956). Individual traits and morbidity in a Swedish rural population. *Acta Psychiatrica et Neurologica Scandinavica*, Supp. 100.

Gatz, M., and Hurwicz, M. C. (1990). Are old people more depressed? Cross-sectional data on Center For Epidemiological Studies Depression Scale factors. *Psychology and Aging*, **5**, 284–90.

Goldberg, D., and Huxley, P. (1980) *Mental illness in the community.* Tavistock, London.

Gurland, B., Copeland, J., Kuriansky, J., Simon, R., Stiller, P., and Birckett, P. (1983). *The mind and mood of aging.* Croom Helm, London.

Hagnell, O. (1970). The incidence and duration of episodes of mental illness in a general population. In *Proceedings of the Aberdeen Symposium on Epidemiology* (ed. E. H. Hare and J. K. Wing), pp. 213–224. Oxford University Press, London.

Henderson, A. S., Grayson, D. A., Scott, R., Wilson, J., Rickwood, D., and Kay, D. W. K. (1986). Social support, dementia and depression among the elderly living in the Hobart community. *Psychological Medicine*, **16**, 379–90.

Henderson, A. S., Hasegawa, K., *et al.* (1992). The epidemiology of dementia and depression in late life. In *Aging and mental disorders: International perspectives* (ed. M. Bergener, K. Hasegawa, S. I. Finkel, and T. Nishimura). Springer Publishing Co., New York.

Henderson, A. S., Jorm, A. F., MacKinnon A., Christensen, H., Scott, L. R., Korten, R. E., *et al.* (1993). The prevalence of depressive disorders and the distribution of depressive symptoms in later life: a survey using draft ICD-10 and DSM-III-R. *Psychological Medicine*, **23**, 719–729.

Jensen, K. (1963). Psychiatric problems in four Danish old age homes. *Acta Psychiatrica Scandinavica*, Supp. 169.

Jorm, A. F., Christensen, H., Henderson, S., Korten A. E., MacKinnon, A. J., Scott, R., *et al.* Neuroticism and self-reported health in an elderly community sample. *Personality and Individual Differences.* (In press.)

Kay, D. W. K. (1988). Anxiety in the elderly. In *Handbook of anxiety. Vol. 2: Classification, etiological factors, and associated disturbances* (ed. R. Noyes, M. Roth and G. D. Burrows), pp. 289–310. Elsevier, Amsterdam.

Kay, D. W. K., and Bergmann, K. (1980). Epidemiology of mental disorders among the aged in the community. In *Handbook of mental health and ageing* (ed. J. E. Birren and R. B. Sloane), pp. 34–56. Prentice-Hall Inc., New Jersey.

Kay, D. W. K., Beamish, P., and Roth, M. (1964*a*). Old age mental disorders in Newcastle-upon-Tyne. Part I: A study of prevalence. *British Journal of Psychiatry*, **110**, 146–58.

Kay, D. W. K., Beamish, P., and Roth, M. (1964*b*). Old age mental disorders in Newcastle-upon-Tyne. Part II: A study of possible social and medical causes. *British Journal of Psychiatry*, **110**, 668–82.

Kessel, W. N., and Shepherd, M. (1962). Neurosis in hospital and general practice. *Journal of Mental Science*, **108**, 159–66.

Kivel, S. L., Pahkala, K., and Laippala, P. (1988). Prevalence of depression in an elderly population in Finland. *Acta Psychiatrica Scandinavica*, **78**, 401–13.

Kua, E. H. (1990). Depressive disorder in elderly Chinese people. *Acta Psychiatrica Scandinavica*, **81**, 386–8.

Larkin, A. B., Copeland, J. R. M., Dewey, M. E., Davidson, I. A., Saunders, P. A., Sharma, V. K., *et al.* (1992). The natural history of neurotic disorder in an elderly urban population. Findings from the Liverpool Longitudinal Study of Continuing Health in the Community. *British Journal of Psychiatry*, **160**, 681–6.

Leighton, D. C., Harding, J. S., Macklin, D. B., Hughes, C. C., and Leighton, A.

H. (1963). Psychiatric findings of the Stirling County Study. *American Journal of Psychiatry*, **119**, 1021–6.

Lindesay, J. (1990). The Guy's / Age Concern Survey: physical health and psychiatric disorder in an urban elderly community. *International Journal of Geriatric Psychiatry*, **5**, 171–8.

Lindesay, J. (1991). Phobic disorders in the elderly. *British Journal of Psychiatry*, **159**, 531–41.

Lindesay, J., and Banerjee, S. (1993). Phobic disorders in the elderly: a comparison of three diagnostic systems. *International Journal of Geriatric Psychiatry*, **8**, 387–393.

Lindesay, J., Briggs, K., and Murphy, E. (1989). The Guy's / Age Concern Survey: prevalence rates of cognitive impairment, depression and anxiety in an urban elderly community. *British Journal of Psychiatry*, **155**, 317–29.

Livingston, G., Hawkins, A., Graham, N., Blizard, B., and Mann, A. (1990). The Gospel Oak Study: prevalence rates of dementia, depression and activity limitation among elderly residents in inner London. *Psychological Medicine*, **20**, 137–46.

McDonald, C. (1973). An age-specific analysis of the neuroses. *British Journal of Psychiatry*, **122**, 477–80.

Magnussen, H. (1989). Mental health of octagenarians in Iceland. *Acta Psychiatrica Scandinavica*, Supp. 349.

Murphy, J. M., Monson, R. R., Olivier, D. C., Sobol, A. M., and Leighton, A. H., (1987). Affective disorders and mortality. *Archives of General Psychiatry*, **44**, 473–80.

Neugebauer, R. (1980). Formulation of hypotheses about the true prevalence of functional and psychiatric disorders among the elderly in the United States. In *Mental illness in the United States: epidemiological estimates* (ed. B. P. Dohrenwend and B. S. Dohrenwend). Praeger, New York.

Nielsen, J. (1962). Geronto-psychiatric period-prevalence investigation in a geographically delimited population. *Acta Psychiatrica Scandinavica*, **38**, 307–30.

Parsons, P. L. (1965). Mental health of Swansea's old folk. *British Journal of Preventive and Social Medicine*, **19**, 43–7.

Primrose, E. R. J. (1962). *Psychological illness: a community study*. C. C. Thomas, Springfield, Ilinois.

Palinkas, L. A., Wingard, D. L., and Barrett-Connor, E. (1990). The biocultural context of social networks and depression among the elderly. *Social Science and Medicine*, **30**, 441–7.

Regier, D. A., Boyd, J. H., Burke, J. D., Rae, D. S., Myers, J. M., Krammer, M., *et al.* (1988). One-month prevalence of mental disorders in the United States. *Archives of General Psychiatry*, **45**, 977–986.

Robins, L., and Regier, D. (ed.) (1991). *Psychiatric disorders in America*. The Free Press, New York.

Rorsman, B., Hagnell, O., and Lanke, J. (1982). Violent death and mental disorders in the Lundby Study: Accidents and suicides in a total population during a 25 year period. *Neuropsychobiology*, **8**, 233–40.

Sheldon, J. H. (1948). *The social medicine of old age*. Oxford University Press, London.

Shepherd, M., and Gruenberg, E. M. (1957). The age for neurosis. *Millbank Memorial Fund*, **35**, 258–65.

Shepherd, M., Cooper, B., Brown, A. C., and Kalton, G. (1981). *Psychiatric illness in general practice*. Oxford University Press, London.

Simon, A. (1980). The neuroses, personality disorders, alcoholism, drug use and misuse and crime in the aged. In *Handbook of mental health and ageing* (ed. J. E. Birren and R. B. Sloane), pp. 653–670. Prentice-Hall Inc., New Jersey.

Social Psychiatry Research Unit (1992). The Canberra interview for the elderly: a new field instrument for the diagnosis of dementia and depression by ICD-10 and DSM-III-R. *Acta Psychiatrica Scandinavica*, **85**, 105–13.

Srole, L., Langner, T. S., Michael, S. T., Opler, M. K., and Rennie, T. A. C. (1962). *Mental health in the metropolis: the Midtown Manhattan Study*, Vol. 1. McGraw-Hill, New York.

Stallones, L., Marx, M. B., and Garrity, T. F. (1990). Prevalence and correlates of depressive symptoms among older U.S. adults. *American Journal of Preventive Medicine*, **6**, 295–303.

Tyrer, P. (1989). *Classification of neurosis*. Wiley, Bristol.

Von Korff, M. R., and Eaton, W. W. (1989). Epidemiologic findings on panic. In *Panic disorder: theory, research and therapy* (ed. R. Baker). Wiley, London.

World Health Organization (1977) *Manual of the international statistical classification of diseases, injuries and causes of death*. World Health Organization, Geneva.

2

Assessment and diagnosis
ROBIN JACOBY and KLAUS BERGMANN

SIMILARITIES AND DIFFERENCES BETWEEN OLDER AND YOUNGER PATIENTS

Dementia and depression, the two major psychiatric disorders of old age, are usually quite easily recognised by careful clinicians. Sometimes, however, diagnosis is difficult because of factors which are peculiar to older patients. In depression, for example, there may be masking of low mood with hypochondriacal symptoms that are mistaken for cancer. In dementia, a well preserved social facade allied to an evasive style ('I never took much notice of current affairs') may conceal cognitive deficits unless more penetrating enquiry is undertaken. So it is with neurotic disorders, that failure to appreciate the significance of a clinical presentation will lead to a wrong diagnosis or no diagnosis at all. Part of the reason for this failure lies in a misunderstanding of the differences between younger and older patients.

Failure of recognition

The great majority of neurotic illness presents not to psychiatrists but to primary-care physicians. Shepherd *et al.* (1981) for example found 63.4 per cent of neurotic as against 4.2 per cent of psychotic patients in a general practice survey. Incidence and prevalence data for psychiatric illness in general and neurotic disorders in particular from this and other studies (see Chapter 1) suggest that both rise in the third and fourth decades of life, with prevalence continuing to rise into the fifth, following which there is a steep decline (e.g. Shepherd and Gruenberg 1957; Shepherd *et al.* 1981). New psychiatric cases after the age of 65 years as a percentage of all psychiatric cases presenting in primary care in a London study (Shepherd *et al.* 1981) were found to be only about 10 per cent, which accords with more recent data from Germany (Cooper 1986). Even though the majority of these cases were suffering from neurotic disorders, this does not constitute a large proportion of the whole and contributes to a prevalent if certainly erroneous view that neurosis is the domain of the young and early middle-aged.

It is not merely incidence and prevalence data which lead to the conclusion that neurotic disorders in the elderly tend to be underestimated. When general practitioners do apply a psychiatric diagnosis to their older patients, the latter are less likely to be referred to a psychiatrist or to receive supportive psychotherapy from the general practitioner than younger patients. By contrast, they are more likely to be dulled into insensitivity and put at risk of falls and delirium by the prescription of sedatives and tranquillizers (Shepherd *et al.* 1981).

Why do elderly people presenting with neurotic symptoms to psychiatrists or general practitioners fail to gain recognition for what they are? Why, too, do they receive less appropriate treatment? To a great extent this has to do with ageist prejudice and lack of education on the part of professionals. More specific answers lie perhaps with the manner in which role expectations are conceived. Let us, for example, rephrase the questions as, 'Why do younger people with neurotic disorder get referred for psychotherapy?' The answer might be because they fail to meet role expectations in regard to relationships, application to work, sexuality, and so on. Role expectations for the elderly in our society are not only different, but can often be offensively low. To caricature the point, if the role expectations for younger persons were wandering, self-neglect, and incontinence they, too, would not be deemed neurotic.

The relative frequency of anxiety and depression

Anxiety symptoms are particularly common across the spectrum of old age psychiatry. Examples of phobic anxiety, diffuse tension, panic attacks, and autonomic anxiety have been clearly described (Lindesay *et al.* 1989; Lindesay 1991; Sheikh *et al.* 1991). Careful enquiry, however, reveals that depressive symptoms very often accompany anxiety in the elderly, which is not necessarily the case with younger patients. Bergmann *et al.* (1979) carried out a two-stage community survey of over 800 residents, employing the Geriatric Mental State Schedule on screen-positive subjects, and the prevalence of organic states was reported. Unpublished data from this survey revealed only one subject to be suffering from anxiety without depressive symptoms. This sort of finding has underpinned the oft-repeated statement to trainees that neurotic symptoms, especially anxiety, arising *de novo* in old age reflect a depressive illness until proved otherwise. The pathoplastic colouring of depression with anxiety in old age is well recognized (e.g. Post 1962, 1972) and was one of the defining characteristics of so-called 'involutional melancholia' (Rosenthal 1968), a concept now discredited as an entity separate from depressive illness. However, a contrary view that pure anxiety is in fact seen, i.e. separate from depression, has been eloquently put by Lindesay (1991), reopening debate of an idea that had perhaps become too fixed in classical teaching. The latter has been partly based upon the hierarchical ordering of symptoms on a scale where depression comes above anxiety. Lindesay's important contribution here has been to question the validity of this hierarchy and to seek to uncouple the link. The debate is fuelled on the one side by the fact that clinicians treating anxiety in older patients tend to avoid anxiolytic drugs in favour of antidepressants with sedative properties. Evidence on the other side is that some elderly patients respond well to psychological anxiety management without antidepressants. The debate continues.

In a community survey using relatively stringent criteria of caseness, Copeland *et al.* (1987) found low rates of phobic illness. This supports the traditional view that, apart from the 'space' type (Marks 1981), these conditions are rare in old age. It would be unwise to accept this contention without reservation since phobias are liable to be masked in a manner which is analogous to the masking of depression in old age. In particular, they may be concealed by physical illness which offers prima-facie justification for the restrictions that patients impose upon themselves. Closer investigation, however, often reveals a phobic element which is not accompanied by objective physical findings.

Case 1

A 73-year-old lady, always somewhat anxiety-prone, suffered a myocardial infarction, went through a brief hospital admission and was then discharged home. She was somewhat depressed for a few weeks after discharge, but this improved. At the time she was seen at home she was reasonably well but firmly convinced that her heart was in such a condition that she was not fit to go out of her house. When asked what was the evidence for her belief in her incapacity, she said that when she stood at the top of the stairs she felt so giddy and far away that she was afraid of pitching downstairs. She had to go downstairs and up again on all fours, which she demonstrated at great speed and with agility, giving a performance that required considerable fitness and cardiac reserve. Her fears and disability were explained both by herself and family as due to her weak heart.

The meaning of hysterical symptoms

Older people differ from younger patients in their modes of clinical presentation. For instance, dramatic primary hysterical disorders and acute obsessional neuroses which are seen in the young and middle-aged are only rarely observed in the elderly. Hysterical symptoms do occur, but more often in the context of a syndrome of abnormal illness behaviour in the manner of Briquet's syndrome (Perley and Guze 1962; Woodruff *et al.* 1982) than with classical conversion or dissociation reactions. Where conversion and/or dissociation symptoms do arise, they tend to represent an attempt by the patient to communicate underlying occult organic illness such as a carcinoma, an early awareness of organic cerebral dysfunction or an underlying functional illness such as depression. The following case is a brief example of such a patient.

Case 2

A 76-year-old lady presented to a psychiatric unit with histrionic acting-out behaviour, hurling herself about the bed and being so 'ataxic' that she would get jammed between the bed and the wall. There were episodes during which she burnt her bedclothes with lighted cigarettes and had no memory of having done so. Psychiatric examination did not reveal any evidence of a cognitive deficit and neurological examination was negative. However, a routine chest X-ray showed a large hilar shadow later confirmed as a carcinoma of the lung. At the patient's request, over a number of interviews the truth about her medical condition was made apparent to her. Her behaviour improved, she was able to use her remaining time seeing her family. She stayed calm and peaceful up to the time of her death.

PRESENTATIONS OF NEUROSIS IN OLD AGE

Primary care

The majority of neurotic illnesses are first manifest in primary-care settings. Perhaps the most typical is hypochondriacal elaboration concealing anxiety, depression, or phobic disorders.

Case 3

A 70-year-old woman told her general practitioner she had indigestion. He, as was proper, took a history related to the gastrointestinal tract, and examined her physically for that system. He also ordered some simple laboratory tests which proved normal and prescribed an antacid. The patient returned to his surgery a fortnight later, saying she was no better but worse. The doctor changed the prescription and prescribed an H_2 antagonist for a presumed peptic ulcer. Over the ensuing weeks the patient did not improve and was referred to the local hospital for endoscopy. No abnormality was detected. At this point, some three months after first presentation, a 'psychiatric' explanation for her symptoms was considered. A more detailed history revealed severe anxiety with depressive symptoms related to her daughter's recent separation and divorce.

This patient was suffering from a late-onset neurotic disorder, but it is mainly patients with chronic neurotic problems dating back to younger adult life who present to their general practitioners with hypochondriacal elaboration, and who are sometimes said to enjoy the best of ill health. For these patients containment and limit setting may be more beneficial than active intervention with drugs and/or psychotherapy. However, it is very important for primary-care physicians to be alert to the fact that the inefficacy of repeat prescriptions, the burden of repeat attendances at the surgery, the importunate demands for home visits, and frequent out-of-hours calls engendered by panic attacks with or without hyperventilation may all indicate the need for a psychiatric assessment. By contrast, those with late-onset neurotic disorders, especially phobias and anxiety states related to depression, may either not present to general practitioners at all or do so only at a late stage. Unfortunately, these patients suffer greater stress and disability than those with chronic disorders (Bergmann 1971; Lindesay 1991).

It should not be presumed that the so-called 'normal' elderly population are necessarily more hypochondriacal than those who are younger. Although this presumption is often made by lay people and professionals alike, Bergmann (1989) found that only 6 per cent of normal community residents over 65 years of age had hypochondriacal symptoms. There do not seem to be comparable data in younger people, but 6 per cent is not a high figure. The Epidemiologic Catchment Area studies in the United States found no relationship between rates of somatization and age (Swartz *et al.* 1991).

A particular difficulty in both community and hospital settings is that hypochondriacal symptoms may occur alongside organic disease, and care must be taken not to miss either. Furthermore, it is as well to remember that Occam's razor[1] becomes blunt where the elderly are concerned. The training and mental set of most doctors tend to make them consider it more important not to miss organic rather than psychiatric—especially neurotic—disorder. The way in which the general practitioner dealt with the woman with indigestion described above exemplifies the problem. The consequence, however, not only denies patients correct diagnosis, effective treatment, and prevention of excessive investigation, but also tends to obscure the possibility of both organic and neurotic disorders being present at the same time.

Hospital

There is an accumulating wealth of evidence that elderly patients admitted to non-psychiatric hospital wards show a high prevalence of psychiatric disorder. It should not be assumed that this is solely or even mainly dementia. Bergmann and Eastham (1974), in a survey of admissions to acute medical wards in Newcastle upon Tyne, found 14 per cent with neurotic depression and 8 per cent with an anxiety state, i.e. 22 per cent in total with neurotic symptoms. Compare this with 7 per cent with dementia. Other workers have also found high rates of depression in geriatric acute medical admissions (e.g. O'Riordan *et al.* 1989; Ramsay *et al.* 1991; Burn *et al.* 1993), whilst Turrina *et al.* (1992) discovered considerable DSM-III-R (*Diagnostic and statistical manual of mental disorders*, third edition, revised) mental disorder in elderly patients attending a medical day hospital in Verona. Of this Italian sample, 22 per cent suffered from dysthymic disorder, non-major depression, or anxiety disorder. In the study of Burn *et al.* (1993) 24 per cent suffered from depressive neurosis and/or anxiety by AGECAT (Copeland *et al.* 1987, 1988). Ramsay *et al.* (1991) used a variety of standardized and validated instruments on a consecutive series of acute geriatric medical admissions, and found that whilst 10 per cent could be assigned a formal diagnosis of depression a further 40 per cent suffered from depressive symptoms.

What is the significance of these data for the assessment of patients with

---

[1] Generally known as, 'Entities are not to be multiplied without necessity,' but more correctly as, 'It is vain to do with more what can be done with fewer.' (Russell 1961.)

neurotic disorder admitted to non-psychiatric hospital wards? The problem is first one of *awareness*. Research in this area, insofar as there is any, has tended to concentrate on major depression. Koenig *et al.* (1988) found that junior medical staff were not good at recognizing major depression in elderly medical inpatients. How much worse were they with neurotic disorders? The latter are not a group to endear themselves to medical and nursing staff on busy acute medical and surgical wards. Bergmann and Eastham (1974) touched on this issue when they subdivided the functionally ill—predominantly neurotic—according to variables that significantly differentiated them from the psychiatrically normal. Four major symptom groups emerged: anxiety and tension, depressive symptoms, depressive appearance, and irritability. Irritability also differentiated the functionally ill from those with organic brain syndromes. Clinical experience supports these findings. Most psychiatrists are aware that the querulous and complaining patient is the one who alienates the staff, making it difficult for the former to receive and the latter to give appropriate care. Indeed, as this sort of behaviour increases there is a decreasing likelihood of the patient not only obtaining appropriate investigation and management of their physical disorder, but also exploration of the psychological one. It is only too easy to label a genuinely physically ill patient as 'awkward' or 'neurotic' (a term of abuse to many health care professionals) with the resultant danger of missing diagnosis and treatment which are obscure and difficult respectively. The case of carcinoma bronchus already described (p. 33) is an example of this.

Residential care

Many of the points that apply to hospital or even general practice also apply to residential care. This particular setting varies in its focus from country to country (Mann 1991). For instance in the USA and Germany the emphasis has been more medical (nursing homes) whereas in the UK it was more social (local authority residential homes) until recent legislative changes, the full consequences of which have yet to become apparent. Whatever the ethos and whoever the provider, rates of mental illness and disability are considerable (Mann *et al.* 1984; Cooper 1986). The main problem is of course dementia with its implications for high dependency, but concentration on the recognition of organic cerebral impairment in residential settings can be at the expense of recognizing and therefore appropriately managing depression and neurotic disorder.

There is some evidence that many of those entering residential care, in the UK at least, are people with long-standing personality and relationship difficulties (Stout, quoted in Bergmann *et al.* 1983). It is not difficult to determine the psychopathological basis for this evidence. The lifestyle in residential care, which represents for most people a transfer from more or less complete independence to greater or lesser degrees of dependence, is likely to lead to the acquisition of learned helplessness (Seligman 1975). This in turn sets up a vicious cycle because of the tendency of those looking after the elderly to respond in maladaptive ways. At worst it is by aggression or even maltreatment. Morally preferable but in no way beneficial, is the unremitting, cloying sweetness displayed by some care staff, which bespeaks a refusal to take their clients' protests seriously. The vicious cycle is given another turn by those residents who unconsciously appreciate the danger of displaying their angry feelings and the need to introject them in order to avoid being labelled 'difficult', with all the negative consequences which that entails (Liberman and Raskin 1971).

That depression in residential homes leads to more than distress to the sufferer is clear. Mann *et al.* (1984) in a survey of residential homes in the London Borough of Camden found that nearly 40 per cent of those examined using the Brief Assessment Schedule scored high enough to be classed as depressed. It is fairly certain that the majority of these people would have been more likely to lie at the neurotic rather than psychotic end of the depressive spectrum. Of more practical importance, both for assessment and management, is that '. . . depression [was] shown to be associated with an increased rate of dependency and problem behaviour both for those residents with and without mild or moderate dementia. In most instances the presence of depression double[d] the rate of daily dependence or problem behaviours.'

ASSESSMENT AND SCREENING IN VARIOUS SETTINGS

Assessment and screening of patients for neurotic disorders depend upon the setting and purpose for which they are to be carried out. Formal research instruments are effective at determining group morbidity levels. But, as Lindesay (1992) has pointed out, whilst they allow for a certain degree of reliability and comparability, their validity is more open to question and rules for caseness differ between them. It is not appropriate to discuss a comprehensive list of such instruments here and only a few will be mentioned because they have been used in specifically relevant contexts. In the UK, GMS/AGECAT (Copeland *et al.* 1987) and in the US the Diagnostic Interview Schedule (DIS) allied to DSM-III have been widely used for community prevalence studies (see Chapter 1). In their study of strain on 150 carers of the demented elderly, Levin *et al.* (1989) used the General Health Questionnaire (GHQ) (Goldberg 1978), detecting high levels of depression (essentially of neurotic type) in a population whose mean age was 61.4 years and many of whom were much older.

Instruments such as the GHQ, the Geriatric Mental State (GMS), and the Diagnostic Interview Schedule (DIS) are research tools which were not designed and are not suitable for everyday use. In clinical practice other approaches are needed which amount in essence to the taking of a good history and making a proper examination of the mental state. In order for this to be achieved the first requirement is to raise the level of awareness among those who care for the elderly, and to do so not simply at the level of organic impairment. In some geriatric wards, for example, mental state assessment is considered complete if a cognitive screening instrument, such as the Mental Test Score (MTS) (Hodkinson 1973) or Mini Mental State Examination (MMSE) (Folstein *et al.*

1975), has been administered. This is not sufficient. The increased rates of psy-chiatric disorder in elderly medical in-patients provide a valuable opportunity for detection and treatment, and short screening tests may help the non-psychiatrist to consider the possibility that a patient is anxious or depressed. For depression, the Geriatric Depression Scale (Yesavage and Brink 1983) has been found of use, especially as it lacks somatic items which may make patients seem more depressed than they really are. Similarly, BASDEC (Brief Assessment Schedule Depression Cards—Adshead *et al.* 1992) is quick and user-friendly. The Hospital Anxiety and Depression Scale (Zigmond and Snaith 1983) has brief scales for each of those emotions, and also avoids somatic items.

Most physicians who qualified during or before the 1960s will have had little or no undergraduate training in old-age medicine or psychiatry. On the contrary, many will have been exposed to and will have absorbed the most negative concepts during this formative period. In order to set this right, the raising of levels of awareness of old age mental disorders should begin in the earliest stages of medical and nursing training. Medical students need to know that an early awareness of the health needs of the elderly is not simply a moral imperative but also a practical one. Demographic trends have dictated that much of their time as house officers (interns and residents) will be spent in dealing with elderly patients. Elderly neurotic patients on medical and surgical wards will prove to be among the most difficult, aggravating, and time consuming if they are not recognized for what they are (Bergmann and Eastham 1974). On medical and surgical wards the value of a good psychiatric liaison service is to be emphasized in both educating junior doctors and nurses and facilitating correct clinical and social management. Unfortunately, a good liaison service is still the exception. The rule for physicians, surgeons, and even some geriatricians tends to be *ad hoc* consultation for disposal.

The demographic trends affecting hospital practice apply also to the com-munity, and raising awareness of general practitioners is equally important. These primary-care physicians are also usually those who care for the elderly in residential homes. In the UK, efforts have been made to improve training through the qualifying membership examination of the Royal College of General Practitioners. In 1985 the Diploma in Geriatric Medicine of the Royal College of Physicians was instituted with the specific intention of increasing the interest and expertise of general practitioners in old-age medicine and psychiatry.

Raising awareness has to be coupled with reducing the resistance of many doctors to looking for mental illness, and neurotic disorders in particular—a resistance born of fear of therapeutic impotence. We are reminded here of the Max Beerbohm cartoon of a Knight of the Round Table who asks his colleagues what they intend to do with the Holy Grail when they find it. Thus, although this chapter deals with assessment and screening, possible interventions need to be mentioned as an incentive to diagnosis. Since neurotic disorders in the elderly are frequently co-morbid with depression, the standard pharmacological and psychotherapeutic treatments are available and should be used. Other interventions are less well known to non-psychiatrists.

Firstly there is focused problem-solving. Secondly, there is structured grief-and-loss work, which should not be confined simply to bereavement and separation. Many elderly patients express in neurotic symptoms their grief at the loss of social status and self-image (at work, within the family, etc.), a loss which is frequently complicated by concurrent physical illness. Physicians in both hospital and primary care tend unconsciously to deny their patients this experience by brushing it aside with remarks such as, 'It's your age'[1]. A third effective intervention is a cognitive approach on an individual or group basis (Yost *et al.* 1986). Fourthly, life review (Butler 1963) should be considered either as an adjunct to other treatment or as the main element of psychotherapy in patients for whom other methods have proved unsuitable or incompletely effective, in particular for those with long-standing neurotic symptoms that are not part of a depressive episode. Finally, what about psychoanalytic approaches to treatment of the elderly? These have not been popular since Freud himself was denigrating about the possibilities (Freud 1967 *a,b,c*). Karl Abraham (1920) did consider certain older patients suitable for analysis and he appeared to recognise neurotic reactions manifesting themselves in later life. However, closer examination of his work reveals that these patients of so-called 'advanced age' were only in their fifties. Paul Schilder (1940) has described in some detail analytic concepts that might be applicable to psychological processes connected with ageing, such as 'libidinous [*sic*] re-arrangement' in response to impaired bodily functions, and also abnormal reaction patterns of complaint—'giving up completely' and 'retreat into fantasy'. It is in fact only relatively recently that serious attempts have been made to reverse the negative attitude to dynamic, psychoanalytically based psychotherapy with older patients (see Chapter 7) (Radebold 1991).

CO-MORBIDITY

Many of the conditions co-morbid with neurotic disorders in the elderly have already been mentioned. In particular, we have discussed the relationship of neurotic symptoms, notably anxiety, to depression and physical illness. There is no need for repetition other than to summarize here that in addition to anxiety the three neurotic masks of depression in old age—hysterical, obsessional, and hypochondriacal respectively—are traps for the unwary clinician who is liable to miss the correct diagnosis and deny the patient appropriate treatment.

Dementia, too, may present with neurotic symptoms, especially anxiety and depression. Bergmann (1979*a*) showed higher levels of affective symptoms in a

---

[1] The distinguished Scottish geriatrician, Sir Ferguson Anderson, relates how a doctor said this once to a patient complaining of pain in one knee, the patient replying, 'That's funny because my other knee's the same age'.

less severely demented community sample as compared with hospital patients. Even in a hospital group, milder dementia was found to be associated with affective symptoms (Jacoby and Levy 1980). It is likely that this was related to insight, the less demented retaining more insight and therefore more likely to become depressed. However, in addition to affective symptoms it is our experience that dementia may present with anxiety, hysterical, and obsessional symptoms, either in addition to clear-cut cognitive impairment or masking it from the family if not indeed from the clinician. The neurotic and affective presentation of a dementing illness is illustrated by the following patient.

Case 4

A 58-year-old lady had been in the habit of knitting very complex Shetland sweaters for members of her family, free of charge for her labour but receiving payment for the wool. She began to make small errors and they reproached her for wasting the money they had spent on the wool. She began to be tearful, depressed, and frightened of facing her family. Formal testing of memory and orientation revealed no errors but her spatiovisual abilities were markedly impaired. A non-dominant parietal-lobe tumour was suspected but neuroimaging revealed no more than slight generalized cortical atrophy. In order to protect her from her punitive and rather vengeful family she was offered day hospital care and over the next 18 months she was gradually observed to develop an amnestic syndrome and increasing inability to cope with day to day life.

No assessment of an elderly patient with neurotic disorder can be complete without some evaluation of the pre-existing personality. Lifelong anxiety-prone traits and, to lesser extent, anankastic insecure traits seem to discriminate significantly between normal elderly subjects and those community residents who appear to develop neurotic disorder in later life (Bergmann 1971).

This does not necessary imply a causal relationship but does help to account for the strong anxiety and obsessional features which colour and even mask the less severe affective disorders. Conversely, depression in the elderly may affect the degree and the expression of maladaptive traits (Thompson *et al.* 1988; Zimmerman *et al.* 1990). The masking of a subtle affective disorder by maladaptive personality may lead to therapeutic nihilism. Bergmann (1991) has summarized the predominating evidence indicating the stability of personality traits with increasing age. Therefore a careful enquiry concerning personality in earlier life is mandatory for an adequate assessment of neurotic disorder in old age.

CLINICAL INVESTIGATION

A carefully elicited history and a mental-state examination taking account of the patient's age are the key to diagnosis and management. For full details of the assessment of the elderly psychiatric patient, see Oppenheimer and Jacoby (1991). With regard to neurotic disorders in particular, a search should be made for the possible precipitating causes of physical presentations. We have already alluded to this, especially in the case examples. Precipitating causes will include important life events (Murphy 1982) as well as more subtle changes in circumstances such as the evolution of family relationships beyond a level to which the patient has been able to adjust. Benbow *et al.* (1990) have underlined the therapeutic benefit from an exploration of family relationships and the way in which their psychopathological elements have been brought to bear on the development of symptoms.

The importance of maladaptive family relationships has been recognized for some time. Post (1958) described the stresses resulting in the role reversal in dependent daughters of dominant mothers when the daughters became the principal carers. Bergmann (1979*b*) has outlined some other descriptions of family interactions including the 'fallen dictator' and the 'power reversal situation'—or, in the vernacular, when the worm turns!

Such interactions could be analysed in terms of various dimensions, including dominance–submission, autonomy–dependence, and positive–negative reinforcement. These dimensions were studied empirically in an unselected group of elderly psychiatric day patients (Bergmann *et al.* 1984). The outcome measure employed was the global clinical rating after 3 months. The patients who rewarded their relatives with positive reinforcement were the only ones to show a significantly better outcome. When only demented patients were examined, then the submissive patients also showed a significantly better outcome. There is room for more sophisticated formulations of family interactions and prospective empirical outcome studies.

The social precipitants of neurotic illness need to be elicited (see Chapter 4). Poor housing, poor nutrition, poverty, and social isolation are all relevant factors. Many elderly people live in high-crime areas of inner-city deprivation, left behind by children who have moved out into the suburbs or to other towns. Older people are more in fear of crime than other age groups, although they are in fact less likely to become its victims (Hough and Mayhew 1983). Nevertheless, the fear of crime can precipitate neurotic symptoms, especially phobic anxiety and avoidance (Jacoby 1991).

The contribution of low intelligence to the genesis of neurosis in later life would appear to be likely on common-sense clinical grounds. This association was examined in a longitudinal study of randomly selected community-resident elderly (Nunn *et al.* 1974). Psychiatric and psychometric assessments were carried out on 178 subjects and repeated six years later. Evidence was found that below-average intelligence is one of several factors which independently contribute to the development or persistence of neurotic disorder in old age.

Finally, a physical examination and laboratory investigations should be carried out as clinically indicated. If a neurotic basis to physical symptoms is suspected a physical check-up must not be avoided because of co-morbidity, although it can be futile to pursue a seemingly endless course of physical investigation when the true cause of the complaint is psychological. It is therefore preferable to reach an understanding with the patient about laboratory tests and so forth at an early stage, that is to say, setting limits beyond which the doctor will not go unless the clinical circumstances have changed and further tests are warranted.

CONCLUSIONS

Epidemiological evidence points to much unrecognized and untreated neurotic illness in the community, in general hospital wards and in residential-care settings. The first step towards changing this situation is to raise the level of awareness among health professionals of several disciplines. There is also a need for improved training for primary-care and hospital physicians in the basic skills of psychiatric anamnesis and mental-state examination. More specifically, doctors need to be familiar with the masks and co-morbidity partners of neurosis in the elderly, such as hypochondriacal concealment of psychological distress or, conversely, neurotic concealment of physical illness. Attitude changes are required in all health care workers: first, to stop regarding neurosis as a pejorative term to apply to unlikeable patients; and second, to discard the prejudice that these conditions are untreatable. Many psychiatrists working with the elderly might argue that, in the presence of organic cerebral disease and functional psychosis, a preoccupation with neurotic disorder could be seen as a luxury. However, an understanding of emotional problems and a psychological approach to distress in this age group informs and colours all types of work with the elderly mentally ill. Being aware that the accurate diagnosis of neurotic disorders is necessary, difficult, and therapeutically worthwhile will help to avoid much needless suffering.

REFERENCES

Abraham, K. (1920). The applicability of psychoanalytic treatment to patients at an advanced age. In *Selected papers of Karl Abraham* (trans. D. Bryan and A. Strachey 1927), pp. 312–17. International Psychoanalytic Library 13, Hogarth, London.

Adshead, F., Day Cody, D., and Pitt, B. (1992). BASDEC: a novel screening instrument for depression in elderly medical in-patients. *British Medical Journal*, **305**, 397.

Benbow, S., Egan, D., Marriott, A., Tregay, K., Walsh, S., Wells, J., and Wood, J. (1990). Using the family life cycle with later life families. *Journal of Family Therapy*, **12**, 321–40.

Bergmann, K. (1971). The neuroses of old age. In *Recent developments in psychogeriatrics* (ed. D. W. K. Kay and A. Walk), pp. 39–50. Headley Brothers, Ashford.

Bergmann, K. (1979a). The problem of early diagnosis. In *Alzheimer's disease: early recognition of potentially reversible deficits* (ed. A. I. M. Glenn and L. J. Whalley), pp. 68–77. Churchill Livingstone, Edinburgh.

Bergmann, K. (1979 b). How to keep the family supportive. *Geriatric Medicine*, 53–57.

Bergmann, K. (1989). The normal elderly—the by product of a survey. In *Contemporary themes in psychiatry* (ed. K. Davison and A. Kerr), pp. 251–6. Gaskell, London.

Bergmann, K. (1991). Psychiatric aspects of personality in older patients. In *Psychiatry in the elderly* (ed. R. Jacoby and C. Oppenheimer), pp. 852–71. Oxford University Press, Oxford.

Bergmann, K., and Eastham, E. J. (1974). Psychogeriatric ascertainment and assessment for treatment in an acute medical ward setting. *Age and Ageing*, **3**, 174–88.

Bergmann, K., Proctor, S., and Prudham, D. (1979). Symptom profiles in hospital and community resident elderly persons with dementia. In *Brain function in old age* (ed. F. Hoffmeister and C. Muller), pp. 60–7. Bayer Symposium VII, Springer Verlag, Berlin.

Bergmann, K., Jacoby, R., Coleman, P., Jolley, D., and Levin, E. (1983). The limitation and possibilities of community care for the elderly demented. In *Elderly people in the community: their service needs*, pp. 141–67. DHSS/HMSO, London.

Bergmann, K., Manchee, V., and Woods, R. T. (1984). Effects of family relationships on psychogeriatric patients. *Journal of the Royal Society of Medicine*, **77**, 840–4.

Burn, W. K., Davies, K. N., McKenzie, F. R., Brothwell, J. A., and Wattis, J. P. (1993). The prevalence of psychiatric illness in acute geriatric admissions *International Journal of Geriatric Psychiatry*, **8**, 171–4.

Butler, R. N. (1963). The life review: an interpretation of reminiscence in the aged. *Psychiatry*, **26**, 65–76.

Cooper, B. (1986). Mental illness, disability and social conditions among old people in Mannheim. In *Mental health in the elderly* (ed. H. G. Häfner, N. Moschel, and N. Sartorius), pp. 35–45. Springer, Berlin.

Copeland, J. R. M., Dewey, M. E., Wood, N., Searle, R., Davidson, I. A., and McWilliam, C. (1987). Range of mental illness among the elderly in the community: prevalence in Liverpool using the GMS-AGECAT package. *British Journal of Psychiatry*, **150**, 815–23.

Copeland, J. R. M., Dewey, M. E., Henderson, A. S., Kay, D. W., Neal, C. D., Harrison, M. A. M., *et al.* (1988). The Geriatric Mental State (GMS) used in the community: replication studies of the computerised diagnosis, AGECAT. *Psychological Medicine*, **18**, 219–53.

Folstein, M. F., Folstein, S. E., and McHugh, P. R. (1975). 'Mini-mental state'. A practical method for grading the cognitive state of patients for the clinician. *Journal of Psychiatric Research*, **12**, 189–98.

Freud, S. (1967a). Die Sexualität in der Ätiologie der Neurosen. In *Gesammelte Werke* (Collected Works) Vol. I (5th edn). Fischer, Frankfurt/Main.

Freud, S. (1967b). Über Psychotherapie. In *Gesammelte Werke* (Collected Works) Vol. V (5th edn). Fischer, Frankfurt/Main.

Freud, S. (1967c). Die endliche and unendliche Analyse. In *Gesammelte Werke* (Collected Works) Vol. XVI (5th edn). Fischer, Frankfurt/Main.

Goldberg, D. (1978). *Manual of the general health questionnaire*. NFER Publishing Company, Windsor.

Hodkinson, H. M. (1973). Mental impairment in the elderly, *Journal of the Royal College of Physicians of London*, **7**, 305–17.

Hough, M., and Mayhew, P. (1983). The *British crime survey: first report*. Home Office Study No. 76, pp 22–27. HMSO, London.

Jacoby, R. (1991). Psychiatric aspects of crime and the elderly. In *Psychiatry in the elderly* (ed. R. Jacoby and C. Oppenheimer), pp. 915–23. Oxford University Press, Oxford.

Jacoby, R. J., and Levy, R. (1980). Computed tomography in the elderly: diagnosis and functional impairment. *British Journal of Psychiatry*, **136**, 256–69.

Koenig, H. G., Meador, K. G., Cohen, H. J., and Blazer, D. G. (1988). Detection and treatment of major depression in older medically ill hospitalised patients. *International Journal of Psychiatric Medicine*, **18**, 17–31.

Levin, E., Sinclair, J., and Gorbach, P. (1989). *Families, services and confusion in old age*, pp. 132–43. Avebury, Aldershot.

Liberman, P., and Raskin D. E. (1971). Depression: a behavioral formulation. *Archives of General Psychiatry*, **24**, 515–23.

Lindesay, J. (1991). Anxiety disorders in the elderly. In *Psychiatry in the elderly* (ed. R. Jacoby and C. Oppenheimer), pp. 735–57. Oxford University Press, Oxford.

Lindesay, J. (1992) Neurotic disorders. *Reviews in Clinical Gerontology*, **2**, 311–21.

Lindesay, J., Briggs, C., and Murphy, E. (1989). The Guy's / Age Concern Survey: prevalence rates of cognitive impairment, depression and anxiety in an urban elderly community. *British Journal of Psychiatry*, **155**, 317–29.

Mann, A. H. (1991). Epidemiology. In *Psychiatry in the Elderly* (ed. R. Jacoby and C. Oppenheimer) pp. 89–112. Oxford University Press, Oxford.

Mann, A. H., Graham, N., and Ashby, D. (1984). Psychiatric illness in residential homes for the elderly. A survey in one London borough. *Age and Ageing*, **13**, 257–65.

Marks, I. (1981). Space 'phobia': a pseudo-agoraphobic syndrome. *Journal of Neurology, Neurosurgery and Psychiatry*, **44**, 387–91.

Murphy, E. (1982). Social origins of depression in old age. *British Journal of Psychiatry*, **141**, 135–42.

Nunn, C., Bergmann, K., Britton, P. G., Foster, E. M., Hall, E. H., and Kay, D. W. K. (1974). Intelligence and neurosis in old age. *British Journal of Psychiatry*, **124**, 446–52.

Oppenheimer, C., and Jacoby, R. (1991). Assessment of the elderly patient: psychiatric examination. In *Psychiatry in the elderly* (ed. R. Jacoby and C. Oppenheimer), pp. 169–98. Oxford University Press, Oxford.

O' Riordan, T. G., Hayes, J. P., Shelley, R., O'Neill, D., Walsh, J. D., and Coakley, D. (1989). The prevalence of depression in an acute geriatric medical assessment unit. *International Journal of Geriatric Psychiatry*, **4**, 17–21.

Perley, M. J., and Guze, S. B. (1962). Hysteria: the stability and usefulness of clinical criteria. *New England Journal of Medicine*, **266**, 421–6.

Post. F. (1958). Social factors in old age psychiatry. *Geriatrics*, **13**, 576–80.

Post, F. (1962). *The significance of affective symptoms in old age*. Oxford University Press, Oxford.

Post, F., (1972). The management and nature of depressive illness in late life: a follow through study. *British Journal of Psychiatry*, **121**, 393–404.

Radebold, H. (1991). Individual psychotherapy. In *Psychiatry in the elderly* (ed. R. Jacoby and C. Oppenheimer), pp. 373–85. Oxford University Press, Oxford.

Ramsay, R., Wright, P., Katz, A., Bielawska, C., and Katona, C. (1991). The detection of psychiatric morbidity and its effects on outcome in acute elderly medical admissions. *International Journal of Geriatric Psychiatry* **6**, 861–6.

Rosenthal, S. H. (1968). The involutional depressive syndrome. *American Journal of Psychiatry*, **124** (supplement), 21–35.

Russell, B. (1961). *History of Western Philosophy*. George Allen and Unwin, London.

Schilder, P. (1940). Psychiatric aspects of old age and aging. *American Journal of Orthopsychiatry*, **10**, 62–72.

Seligman, M. E. P. (1975). *Helplessness: on depression, development and death*. Freeman, San Francisco.

Sheikh, J. I., King, R. J., and Taylor, C. B. (1991). Comparative phenomenology of early-onset versus late-onset panic attacks. *American Journal of Psychiatry*, **148**, 1231–1233.

Shepherd, M., and Gruenberg, E. M. (1957). The age for neuroses. *The Millbank Memorial Fund Quarterly*, **35**, 258–65.

Shepherd, M., Cooper, B., Brown, A. C., Kalton, G., and Clare, A. (1981). *Psychiatric illness in general practice* (2nd edn). Oxford University Press, Oxford.

Swartz, M., Landerman, R., George, L. K., Blazer, D. G., and Escobar, J. (1991). Somatization disorder. In *Psychiatric disorders in America* (ed. L. N. Robins and D. A. Regier), pp. 220–255. The Free Press, New York.

Thompson, L. W., Gallagher, D., and Czirr, R. (1988). Personality disorder and outcome in the treatment of late life depression. *Journal of Geriatric Psychiatry*, **21**, 133–53.

Turrina, C., Siciliani, O., Dewey, M. E., Fazzari, G., and Copeland, J. R. M. (1992). Psychiatric disorders among elderly patients attending a geriatric medical day hospital: prevalence according to clinical diagnosis (DSM-III-R) and AGECAT. *International Journal of Geriatric Psychiatry*, **7**, 499–504.

Woodruff, R. A., Goodwin, D. W., and Guze, S. B. (1982). Hysteria (Briquet's syndrome). In *Hysteria* (ed. A. Roy). John Wiley, Chichester.

Yost, E. B., Bleuler, L. E., Corbishley, M. A., and Allender, J. R. (1986). *Group cognitive therapy: a treatment approach for depressed older patients*. Pergamon Press, New York.

Zigmond, A. S., and Snaith, R. P. (1983) The Hospital anxiety and depression scale. *Acta Psychiatrica Scandinavica*, **67**, 361–70.

Zimmerman, M., Pfohl, B. M., Coryell, W., Corenthal, C., and Stangel, D. (1990). Major depression and personality disorder. Abstract NR667. In *Proceedings of 143rd Annual Meeting, American Psychiatric Association*. New York.

3

Neurotic disorders and physical illness
BRICE PITT

INTRODUCTION

Neurotic disorders in the elderly are associated with increased rates of mortality and physical morbidity. This association is apparent in community populations (Bergmann 1971; Kay and Bergmann 1966; Lindesay 1990), and is particularly marked in those known to health services; not only is physical illness more prevalent in elderly psychiatric patients (Kay and Roth 1955; Bergmann 1971; Murphy 1983), but elderly medical in-patients also have substantially higher rates of psychiatric disorders. Studies of elderly medical populations using standardized interview and diagnostic methods such as the Diagnostic Interview Schedule (DIS)/DSM-III and Geriatric Mental Sate (GMS)/AGECAT have reported rates of 9–23 per cent for depression (Koenig *et al.* 1988; O'Riordan *et al.* 1989; Burn *et al.* 1993) and 7 per cent for anxiety (Burn *et al.* 1993). Less is known about the relationship between neurotic disorders and physical illness in elderly people presenting to their general practitioners, but the evidence from studies of younger adults in primary-care settings indicates that neurotic disorders and physical illness often coexist in this population also (Bridges and Goldberg 1985).

The relationship between physical illness and psychiatric disorder is extremely complex, and separating cause from effect is difficult, even in well-designed prospective studies. The various ways in which they can be related to each other have been classified by Goldberg (1989) as follows:

1. Entirely physical illness where no psychiatric symptoms are present.

2. Physical illness with secondary psychiatric disorder where all the somatic symptoms can be attributed to the physical illness. The psychiatric illness would not have occurred without the physical illness, and treatment of it would not remove the somatic symptoms.

3. Physical illness with unrelated psychiatric illness where no aetiological link exists between the two. Treatment of one would not affect the other.

4. Somatized psychiatric illness where the patient presents with physical symptoms that are not attributed to a psychological cause. However, the patient's symptoms meet research criteria for psychiatric illness which if treated would alleviate or remove the physical symptoms.

5. Entirely psychiatric illness where either no somatic symptoms are present or the patient considers them to be part of a psychiatric illness.

To these five categories might be added a sixth, 'psychiatric illness with secondary physical illness', in which the physical illness is the result of unhealthy behaviours resulting from the psychiatric disorder, such as smoking and drinking, self-harm, self-starvation and self-neglect (see p.52). The long-term consequences of chronic neurotic disorder for physical health later in life are likely to be particularly important in the care and management of elderly people. A seventh category, 'psychologised somatic illness', is also occasionally encountered, in which the symptoms of physical illness are explained away by a frightened patient as, 'Just my nerves, doctor'.

THE IMPACT OF PHYSICAL ILLNESS

The physical ill health experienced by elderly people may be mild and transitory, or severe and a threat to life or continuing independence. It may afflict an individual who is all alone—by choice or circumstances—or in the bosom of a caring family, who has been healthy till now or has suffered frequent ill health—physical or mental or both. It may be treatable at home, or require a shorter or longer stay in hospital. The patient may be robust, extrovert, affluent, and resourceful—or the opposite of any or all of these qualities. The attitude to death may be one of acceptance, resignation, terror, or denial. All these factors may affect the person's response to the illness, as may the attitudes, empathy, and expertise of those who treat them.

Physical illness naturally evokes anxiety—about the diagnosis, pain, discomfort, disability, dependency, and death. The period of investigation, particularly in hospital, is especially fraught. It has to be an exceptionally stolid, stoical, or blasé patient who will not feel twinges of unease and intimations of mortality when bringing symptoms of a new and troublesome disorder, or symptoms that threaten the return of an old enemy (like cancer or angina), to medical attention. This anxiety may be deemed neurotic, however, when it is exaggerated, unduly prolonged, produces additional symptoms (e.g. the palpitations and chest pains of cardiac neurosis) or is in itself disabling. In relating anxiety and depression to physical illness the DSM-III (American Psychiatric Association 1980) concept of adjustment disorder (a maladaptive reaction to an identifiable psychosocial stress that occurs within the subsequent three months) may sometimes be a more appropriate label than any of the other categories of anxiety or depressive disorder. Some syndromes are common in association with physical ill health, yet are not to be found in standard classifications of psychiatric disorder. One such is an apathetic 'failure to thrive' (Braun *et al.* 1988), with listlessness, immobility, despondency, anorexia, and dysphoria, which doesn't quite match the prototype of depressive illness.

Factors that may contribute to a neurotic response to physical illness include:

an anxious, insecure, dependent personality (Bergmann 1971); low intelligence; a previous history of neurotic disorder; lack of current support; and, perhaps, maladroit management of the presenting disorder, with poor communication, inadequate, evasive, inconsistent information, and brusque insensitivity to the elderly patient's deep but tentatively expressed concerns.

NEUROSIS ARISING FROM PHYSICAL DISORDER

One of the common instances of neurotic disorders arising from physical disorder is cardiac neurosis, ranging from the mild, chronic anxiety symptoms that are quite frequent following myocardial infaction to severely disabling disorders in a minority of cases.

Case 1

Mr A. B., aged 68 years, who had been relieved of chronic, crippling anxiety 35 years previously by a leucotomy, relapsed after the second of two myocardial infarctions. He was convinced that a third was inevitable and would inevitably prove fatal, and having been admitted to a psychiatric ward in a general hospital he was terrified to leave lest he should be out of reach of cardiopulmonary resuscitation.

Case 2

Mr C. D., aged 76 years, having had two bypass operations for coronary artery insufficiency, was told, when he suffered further symptoms of angina and effort intolerance, that another bypass would be too risky, but that if he took care, exercise, and his tablets 'he should be all right'. He reacted with acute fear of dying, chest and back pain, insomnia, repeated emergency calls to his general practitioner (who told him there was 'nothing wrong' with his heart and lungs), and unwillingness to let his wife out of his sight: 'I might be dead when you get back.' When, despite this, she went to the hairdresser's he rang his daughter at work every ten minutes, saying he was dying, could not breathe, and was falling over. 'If I don't see you again, look after Mum!'

Isaacs (1992) has described the common fear of falling in old people with balance disorders: 'patients may be demoralized by fear. This may appear irrational, as when a man who is standing still and appears stable throws out his hands and announces, "I am falling." Staff often react to this by reassuring the patient and encouraging him to walk, but the patient is not easily reassured, and the extent of his fear has to be recognised.' The consequences may be the legacy of dizziness as well as giddiness, tripping, tumbling, and fractures, leading to a housebound existence. Marks (1981) has described a 'space phobia' in older adults, in association with disturbed balance and righting reflexes.

A frequent problem in hospital is the patient's failure to become mobile after a stroke, despite apparent reasonable physical recovery. This is often attributed to 'functional (or hysterical) overlay'—depression and dismay, dependency and fear of recurrence outside the safe environment of the ward, or angry impotence while awaiting a miracle recovery.

Case 3

Mr E. F., aged 77 years, had suffered a stroke causing a dense left hemiplegia four months previously. He was bland, passive, cognitively intact, and the despair of the physiotherapist and the nurses because he would make no effort at all to help himself. 'It came on all of a sudden,' he would say, 'and one day I'm sure that I'll wake up and find that it's gone in just the same way.'

However, failure to do as the medical team expect is sometimes due to subtle defects arising from lesions of the non-dominant hemisphere (Isaacs 1992).

Another common problem is the fear of being alone, often associated with continuing and distressing physical disability such as respiratory difficulty arising from chronic obstructive airways disease (COAD). COAD is associated with high levels of psychiatric morbidity, mainly depression (Kukull *et al.* 1986), frequently (and understandably) accompanied by anxiety and panic, though anxiety alone occurs in only 2 per cent of cases (Light *et al.* 1985).

The loss of sight, or a limb, or independence for any other physical cause is painful and demands major readjustment. Some people rise impressively to the challenge, but others are precipitated into extreme dependency and vulnerability. Unfortunately not all old people are prepared for death, and for some the awareness that they are dying or near to death is terrifying. In some individuals, the fears aroused by an episode of physical illness may result in disabling agoraphobia (Lindesay 1991).

Case 4

Mrs G. H., aged 69 years and suffering from Alzheimer's disease, had always feared her death. She would rub her wrist and exclaim, 'I hope I don't die!' Her daughter would reassure her, 'Of course you won't die, Mum.' Although she grew older and more demented, her fear remained and her daughter found it more difficult to reassure her.

A wide range of physical disorders may induce neurotic symptoms (Table 3.1), and these should always be considered if there is no history of any psychiatric disorder, or if there is nothing in the patient's circumstances to account for the neurosis. Hyperthyroidism is associated with high arousal (Kathol *et al.* 1986), and occasionally with depression—so-called 'apathetic hyperthyroidism'. The most usual manifestation of hypothyroidism (perhaps as a complication of thyroidectomy) is cognitive impairment, but sometimes others are anxiety, hypochondriasis, and panic attacks (Schiffer *et al.* 1988). Hypoglycaemia (most often drug or insulin induced) often causes anxiety symptoms. So-called 'hysteria' may herald cerebral tumour (Slater 1965), and malaise, unease, or frank depression may be prodromal manifestations of as yet undiagnosed malignancy

Table 3.1. Physical causes of neurotic symptoms in the elderly.

Cardiovascular	*Neurological*
Myocardial infarction	Head injury
Cardiac arrhythmias	Cerebral tumour
Orthostatic hypotension	Dementia
Mitral-valve prolapse	Delirium
	Epilepsy
Respiratory	Migraine
Pneumonia	Cerebral lupus erythematosus
Pulmonary embolism	Demyelinating disease
Emphysema	Vestibular disturbance
Asthma	Subarachnoid haemorrhage
Left-ventricular failure	CNS infections
Hypoxia	
Chronic obstructive airways disease	*Dietary and drug-related*
Bronchial carcinoma	Caffeine
	Vitamin deficiencies
Endocrine and metabolic	Anaemia
Hyperthyroidism	Sympathomimetics
Hypothyroidism	Dopamine agonists
Hypercalcaemia	Corticosteroids
Hypocalcaemia	Withdrawal syndromes
Cushing's disease	Akathisia
Carcinoid syndrome	Digoxin toxicity
Hypoglycaemia	Fluoxetine
Insulinoma	
Phaeochromocytoma	
Hyperkalaemia	
Hypokalaemia	
Hypothermia	

(Whitlock and Siskind 1979). Emotionalism following stroke is seen particularly in patients with lesions in the left frontal and temporal areas, and represents more than a psychologically understandable reaction to the stroke (House *et al.* 1989).

The withdrawal of hypnotics, sedatives, alcohol, and tobacco on admission to hospital may result in acute anxiety, and unease may result from the prescription of a wide variety of drugs, including beta blockers and other antihypertensives, corticosteroids, and antidepressants. It is important that the prescribing doctor accepts that patients may be describing unwelcome effects which are wholly related to the drug, even if they do not appear in the formulary, and may not be 'negative placebo reactors'. An eminent senior psychiatrist always made it his practice to try whatever drug he was contemplating giving his patients, and found that a single 25 mg dose of amitriptyline made him feel 'like a zombie' for 24 hours.

PHYSICAL SYMPTOMS ARISING FROM NEUROSIS

Neurosis may masquerade as physical illness or, more rarely, cause it. The tendency to somatize emotional disorder seems to increase with ageing (De Alarcon 1964; Blazer *et al.* 1986), although this clinical impression is no doubt reinforced by selection artefacts as a result of somatizing patients being more likely to consult their doctors. Feeling, perhaps, that they should not bother the doctor with anything other than physical complaints, anxious and depressed old people tend to express their feelings in bodily terms: 'I can't sleep'; 'I've got no energy'; 'I keep getting these palpitations'; 'My bowels are blocked'; 'I ache from head to toe'; 'I've got this funny pain over my eye'; 'I keep shaking'; 'I'm losing so much weight'. Consequently, they are liable to be treated symptomatically for their complaints —with hypnotics, analgesics, laxatives, and so on, or, especially when there is localized pain or weight loss, sent for laboratory and radiological investigation or referred to specialists. This may result in reassurance, bewilderment, or intensified hypochondria. The reassurance, 'I'm glad to tell you, Mrs Smith, that all the tests are completely normal and there's really nothing wrong with you!' is rarely therapeutic if Mrs Smith still feels unwell and suspects that the doctor has found something very wrong but will not disclose it, or that she is not being taken seriously, or that the doctors do not know what they are doing. To be effective, reassurance needs to be firm, informed, and to be part of taking the patient and the problem seriously: 'I'm glad to tell you that all the tests are negative, Mrs Smith, so it's most unlikely that you're suffering from cancer (or whatever dire disorder the patient may especially fear), but clearly there is something the matter and it may well be that my colleague Doctor Jones (the valued psychogeriatrician) can help you.' What seems trivial, irksome and time wasting to the hard-pressed doctor is, at the time, a matter of life and death to many patients.

'Pain is the commonest somatic symptom. It is a subjective experience which is not amenable to objective measurement and it can be communicated to another person only incompletely.' (Lloyd 1991.) It may give the diagnosis away, or obscure it. Ill-defined pain with no obvious or consistent precipitants, poorly localized, anatomically inexplicable and fluctuating unpredictably—often in a querulous, disgruntled patient who will not go away—makes even the stoutest medical heart sink. Such pain may be a manifestation of anxiety and explicable, at least in part, by tension, hypervigilance, or an over-active bowel. Psychogenic regional pain (Feinmann *et al.* 1984) is a well-established if atypical feature of depressive illness. Sometimes pain seems to express disaffection, the metaphor 'a pain in the neck' being expressed literally in a situation of, say, marital conflict.

Pain is often associated with hypochondriasis. One may cause the other, or both may derive from a state of anxiety or depression, or from a hypochondriacal personality (as in Molière's *La Malade Imaginaire*). Bergmann (1971) found hypochondriasis in 7 per cent of the otherwise normal elderly population, in 33 per cent of those with recent neurosis and in 36 per cent of those with chronic neurosis and personality disorder.

Fatigue syndromes are much less commonly diagnosed in old people than in younger. They might be just as prevalent, but more likely to be attributed to mild depression (understandable or not), to the 'failure to thrive' syndrome (see p. 47), to the effects of whatever mild abnormalities are found on examination or investigation (however irrelevant these probably are), to the latest prescription (often the best bet), or to the bored, lazy, ageist doctor's diagnostic catch-all: 'old age'.

True, uncomplicated hysterical conversion and dissociation are so very rare in old age that it is safer never to make the diagnosis. One is highly likely to find that the disorder turns out to be an atypical presentation of agitated depression, dementia or a serious neurological illness. In such cases, it may be that long-standing hysterical tendencies are being released by the primary disorder. By contrast, a 'functional overlay' to a physical illness, whereby the patient exaggerates disability in order to prolong the stay in the safety of hospital, is not at all unusual.

NEUROSIS AS A CAUSE OF PHYSICAL DISORDER AND MORTALITY

There are several explanations for the increased mortality in association with neurotic disorders in the elderly. This may be because of the association with serious physical illness, a possible effect of depression on the immune system, or the patient's loss of the will to live ('turning the face to the wall'). There is an association between bereavement and death from heart disease ('the broken heart' described by Parkes *et al.* (1969)), and the likeliest link between the two is depression (Murphy and Brown 1980). Connolly (1976) found that men admitted to intensive care with myocardial infarction had more life events in the previous three weeks than controls, but in the great majority the heart attack was not so precipitated. The immediate effects of anxiety on raising blood pressure are well known, and while the evidence that prolonged stress and tension result in lasting hypertension is unclear, relaxation techniques (yoga and biofeedback) have been shown to mitigate moderate hypertension (i.e. diastolic blood pressure around 100 mg Hg (Patel and North 1975)), and to reduce risk from coronary heart disease (Patel *et al.* 1985). Stroke sometimes follows rage or extreme grief, but whether it is significantly related to major life events and anxiety is not clear.

What is clearer is that those who smoke and drink to excess are more likely to be neurotic than those who do not (Haines *et al.* 1980), and that smoking is significantly related to lung, heart, and peripheral vascular disease, hypertension (Saunders 1987), stroke (Gill *et al.* 1986), dementia (Ron *et al.* 1982), and accidents. Haines *et al.* (1987) found that, although phobic anxiety was related to the development of ischaemic heart disease in middle-aged men, smoking history did not explain this association; they speculated that anxiety-related hyperventilation might cause coronary artery spasm, or that anxious individuals might have excessive hormonal responses to myocardial infarction.

THE MANAGEMENT OF NEUROSIS AND PHYSICAL ILLNESS

The view repeatedly expressed in this chapter is that neurosis related to physical disorder is not infrequently iatrogenic; it is nourished by haste, impatience, organ preoccupation, disregard of the patient as a person, ageism, leading questions, inconsistent and inadequate communication, and premature reassurance. Mishandled, a symptomless risk factor for later illness, like hypertension, may cause a patient to adopt a 'sick role', or an old person who has made a full recovery from a fracture or an infarction may become housebound. Respect for patients and their problems should be what draws most people to practise medicine in the first place, and it is much to be hoped that medical education will cherish this attitude and not drive it out of the young doctor's mind. Of course, overworked, rushed and weary doctors are less able to find the time in the first consultation which may save a great deal of time later.

House and Ebrahim (1991) remark that:

considering the impact of disease on the lifestyles of elderly patients has implications for the range of treatments that are relevant. Recognising that a patient has depressive symptoms should not lead automatically to the prescription of antidepressant drugs . . . Treatment may involve counselling the patient, modification of goals of physical therapy and discussion with carers, and will almost always require a multidisciplinary team approach.

Psychosocial approaches best suit neurotic disorders in the context of physical disorder, focusing on 'immediate' issues of dread, disability, the outlook, realistic plans, and empowering the patient as much as possible. Ideally, these will all be part of the therapeutic team's care plan (if the patient is in hospital), with appropriate advice and support from the liaison old-age psychiatrist or psychologist. Drugs are only useful for well-defined depression. Hypnotics and tranquillizers carry the danger of habituation, though this does not mean that they are never of short-term use. The patient who fails to make the recovery the team expect may have a different agenda, such as fear of regaining independence or anger at being afflicted, and such feelings need to be sought, exposed, discussed, and reckoned with. Specifics of the various treatments for neurotic disorders are given elsewhere in this book.

REFERENCES

American Psychiatric Association (1980). *Diagnostic and statistical manual of mental disorders* (3rd edn). American Psychiatric Association, Washington.

Bergmann, K. (1971). The neuroses of old age. In *Recent developments in psychogeriatrics* (ed. D. W. K. Kay and A. Walk), pp. 39–50. Headley Bros, Ashford.

Blazer, D., George, L., and Landerman, R. (1986). The phenomenology of late life depression. In *Psychiatric disorders in the elderly* (ed. P. Bebbington and R. Jacoby), pp. 143–52. Mental Health Foundation, London.

Braun, J. V., Wykle, M. H., and Cowling, W. R. (1988). Failure to thrive in older people: a concept derived. *Gerontologist*, **28**, 809–12.

Bridges, K. W., and Goldberg, D. P. (1985). Somatic presentations of DSM-III psychiatric disorders in primary care. *Journal of Psychosomatic Research*, **29**, 563–9.

Burn, W. K., Davies, K. N., McKenzie, F. R., Brothwell, J. A., and Wattis, J. P. (1993). The prevalence of psychiatric illness in acute geriatric admissions. *International Journal of Geriatric Psychiatry*, **8**, 175–80.

Connolly, J. (1976). Life events before myocardial infarction. *Journal of Human Stress*, **2**, 3–17.

De Alarcon, R. D. (1964). Hypochondriasis and depression in the aged. *Gerontology Clinic*, **6**, 266–77.

Feinmann, C., Harris, M., and Cawley, R. (1984). Psychological facial pain: presentation and treatment. *British Medical Journal*, **288**, 436–8.

Gill, J. S., Zezulka, A. V., Shipley, M. J., Gill S. K., and Beevers, D. G. (1986). Stroke and alcohol consumption. *New England Journal of Medicine*, **315**, 1041–6.

Goldberg, D. P. (1989). Discussion of Prof. Ottoson's paper. In *Interaction between mental and physical illness* (ed. R. Ohmann, H. L. Freeman, A. Franck Holmkvist, and S. Nielzen), p. 121. Springer-Verlag, Berlin/Heidelberg.

Haines, A. P., Imeson, J. D., and Meade, T. W. (1980). Psychoneurotic profiles of smokers and non-smokers. *British Medical Journal*, **280**, 1422.

Haines, A. P., Imeson, J. D., and Meade, T. W. (1987). Phobic anxiety and ischaemic heart disease. *British Medical Journal*, **295**, 297–9.

House, A., and Ebrahim, S. (1991) Psychological aspects of physical disease. In *Psychiatry in the elderly* (ed. R. Jacoby and C. Oppenheimer), pp 437–60. Oxford University Press, Oxford.

House, A., Dennis, M., Molyneux, A., Warlow, C., and Hawton, K. (1989). Emotionalism after stroke. *British Medical Journal*, **298**, 991–4.

Isaacs, B. (1992). *The challenge of geriatric medicine*, pp. 84–5. Oxford Medical Publications, Oxford.

Kathol, R. G., Turner, R., and Delahunt, J. (1986). Depression and anxiety associated with hyperthryoidism: response to antithyroid treatment. *Psychosomatics*, **27**, 501–5.

Kay, D. W. K., and Roth, M. (1955). Physical accompaniments of mental disorder in old age. *Lancet*, **ii**, 740–5.

Kay, D. W. K., and Bergmann, K. (1966). Physical disability and mental health in old age. *Journal of Psychosomatic Research*, **10**, 3–12.

Koenig, H. G., Meador, K. G., Cohen, H. J., and Blazer, D. G. (1988). Detection and treatment of major depression in older medically ill hospitalized patients. *International Journal of Psychiatry in Medicine*, **18**, 17–31.

Kukull, W. A., Koepsell, T. D., Inui, T. S., Borson, S., Okimoto, J., Raskind, M.A., *et al.* (1986). Depression and physical illness among elderly general medical clinic patients. *Journal of Affective Disorders*, **10**, 153–62.

Light, R. W., Merrill, E. J., Despars, J. A. Gordon, G. H. Matalipassi, L. R., *et al.* (1985). Prevalence of depression and anxiety in patients with COPD: relationship to functional capacity. *Chest*, **87**, 35–8.

Lindesay, J. (1990). The Guy's / Age Concern Survey: physical health and psychiatric disorder in an urban elderly community. *International Journal of Geriatric Psychiatry*, **5**, 171–8.

Lindesay, J. (1991). Phobic disorders in the elderly. *British Journal of Psychiatry*, **159**, 531–41.

Lloyd, G. L., (1991). *Textbook of general hospital psychiatry*. Churchill Livingstone, Edinburgh.

Marks, I. (1981). Space phobia: a pseudo-agoraphobic syndrome. *Journal of Neurology, Neurosurgery and Psychiatry*, **44**, 387–91.

Murphy, E. (1983). The prognosis of depression in old age. *British Journal of Psychiatry*, **142**, 111–19.

Murphy, E., and Brown, G. (1980). Life events, psychiatric disturbance and physical illness. *British Journal of Psychiatry*, **136**, 326–8.

O'Riordan, T. G., Hayes, J. P., Shelley, R., O'Neill, D., Walsh, J. B., and Coakley, D. (1989). The prevalence of depression in an acute geriatric medical assessment unit. *International Journal of Geriatric Psychiatry*, **4**, 17–21.

Parkes, C. M., Benjamin, B., and Fitzgerald, R. G. (1969). Broken heart: a statistical study of increased mortality among widowers. *British Medical Journal*, **i**, 740–3.

Patel, C., and North, W. R. S. (1975). Randomised control trial of yoga and biofeedback in the management of hypertension. *Lancet*, **ii**, 93–5.

Ron, M. A., Acker, W., Shaw, G. K., and Lishman, W. A. (1982). Computerised tomography of the brain in chronic alcoholism: a survey and a follow-up study. *Brain*, **105**, 497–514.

Saunders, J. B. (1987). Alcohol: an important cause of hypertension. *British Medical Journal*, **294**, 1819–21.

Schiffer, R. B., Klein, R. F., and Sider, R. G. (1988). *The medical evaluation of psychiatric patients*. Plenum Medical, New York.

Slater, E. (1965). Diagnosis of hysteria. *British Medical Journal*, **i**, 1395–9.

Whitlock, F. A., and Siskind, M. (1979). Depression and cancer: a follow-up study. *Psychological Medicine*, **9**, 747–52.

4

Psychosocial factors
JAMES LINDESAY

INTRODUCTION

In the 1950s and 1960s there was a great sense of optimism that the social sciences would revolutionize our understanding of the origins and course of mental illness, and that out of this understanding would come effective new means of treatment and prevention. To a large extent, this promise has not been fulfilled, and social psychiatry has been supplanted by biological psychiatry as the source of our hopes in this respect. This current neglect of the personal and the social is unfortunate, since there is a powerful body of evidence that psychosocial factors play a significant role in determining vulnerability to, onset of, and recovery from neurotic disorders at all ages. The impact of factors such as prolonged adversity, life events, early experiences, and social relationships upon the onset and course of these conditions needs to be properly appreciated and understood if they are to be effectively treated and prevented. This chapter reviews the evidence and the theories, particularly as they relate to elderly people with depression and other neurotic disorders.

SOCIAL ADVERSITY

There is a well-established relationship between adverse social circumstances and psychological ill health. Both epidemiological surveys of communities and studies of patient groups report associations between psychiatric symptomatology and indicators of adversity such as low occupational class, unemployment, poor housing, overcrowding, and restricted access to amenities such as transport (Harris 1988; Champion 1990). Elderly people in developed industrial societies are a particularly diverse group socio-economically; some enjoy the benefits of a lifetime of productive labour, including an occupational pension, and are comfortable by any standards, whereas others who have not accumulated this financial advantage endure some of the worst adversity of any age or social group. Importantly, it is the most elderly and physically vulnerable cohorts who are worst off in this respect. The financial disadvantage at the root of the social adversity experienced by many elderly people has its effect principally through their domestic environment. Elderly people spend a considerable amount of time at home, and rely upon this environment not only for their basic needs in terms of shelter, warmth, and sustinence, but also for their entertainment, social contacts, and intimate relationships (Grundy 1989). Data from sources such as the General Household Surveys (e.g. Office of Population Censuses and Surveys 1986) show that the elderly are less likely than younger age groups to be owner-occupiers and more likely to be tenants in the private rented sector; their housing is more likely to lack basic amenities such as central heating, telephones, refrigerators, and washing machines.

The evidence for an association between deprivation and psychopathology in the elderly is strongest in studies employing dimensional scales for characterizing depression and anxiety. For example, in a survey using self-report symptom scales, Himmelfarb and Murrell (1984) found that increased anxiety scores in a community sample of elderly people were associated with low socio-economic status, limited education, poor housing, rural domicile, and isolation. Similarly, Kennedy *et al.* (1989; 1990) found that low income was associated with increased risk of depression in their urban elderly sample. Conversely, in studies employing a categorical approach to the definition of depression and neurotic disorder, the evidence for association with social adversity is less clear. Blazer and Williams (1980) found a relationship between DSM-III (*Diagnostic and Statistical manual of mental disorders,* third edition) major depression and increased impairment of social and economic resources in the elderly, but in the later Epidemiologic Catchment Area (ECA) surveys in the United States, no relationship was found between DSM-III affective disorders and socio-economic variables such as occupation, household income, or education at any age, although there was some evidence of an association with urban residence (Weissman *et al.* 1991). Among neurotic conditions, generalized anxiety disorder was associated with low household income (Blazer *et al.* 1991), but otherwise the only associations were with increased financial dependency upon welfare and disability benefit. In the ECA study, phobic disorders in the elderly were associated with urban domicile, a finding supported by Walton *et al.* (1990) in their study of elderly women in New Zealand; it has been suggested that this is due to the poor quality of urban social networks (Blazer *et al.* 1985).

Separating cause from effect in these cross-sectional studies is difficult, as long-standing disorders can themselves have an adverse effect on occupation, income, and even educational attainment. For example, it is likely that much of the association between DSM-III disorders and financial dependency on the State found by the ECA study is due to the fact that psychiatric disorder is itself a qualifying disability for benefit. The association of adverse socio-economic status with increased levels of psychiatric symptoms rather than with with categorically defined cases of disorder suggests that it may be an indicator for factors that are important in the development of milder, subclinical forms of neurotic disturbance, but these factors are less relevent in the aetiology of more severe disorders.

How does prolonged social adversity cause psychiatric disorder in the elderly? Physical ill health is an important mediating factor in this age group, both as a vulnerability factor and a provoking agent (see Chapter 3). Socially and financially disadvantaged elderly people are more likely to become physically ill as a result of poor housing, poor diet, and the lack of basic amenities. The chronic stress imposed by prolonged adversity may also impair physical health through its impact on endocrine and immune systems (Khansari *et al.* 1990). Disadvantaged elderly people are also less able to compensate materially for any enduring disability caused by physical illness. The rates of other adverse life events experienced by individuals living in deprived circumstances are also increased (Prudo *et al.* 1981).

Poor self-esteem has been identified by Brown and Harris (1978) as a crucial mediator between vulnerability factors, including the 'structural vulnerability' of adverse social circumstances (Harris 1988), and psychiatric disorder. In their model, the low self-esteem created by vulnerability factors sensitizes individuals to the impact of adverse life events (see p.59). However, this model is derived from studies of relatively young women, and its role in the elderly is less clear. Self-esteem appears to be extremely resilient in late life, perhaps because individuals change their levels of aspiration and their reference groups of comparison as they age (Baltes and Baltes 1990), and so are able to adapt to changing circumstances. Longitudinal studies show that negative attitudes to ageing and dependency are predictive of declines in self-esteem in old age (Mertens and Wimmers 1987; Coleman *et al.* 1993).

Wheaton (1983) has suggested that prolonged social adversity and socio-economic disadvantage result in a sense of fatalism and impotence, associated with poor coping abilities in the face of adverse events. An interesting alternative hypothesis is that lifelong adversity may in fact be protective in some circumstances, since those with a lifetime's experience of hardship will have a wider repertoire of support and help-seeking skills both within and outside the family. The fact that suicide rates among elderly Blacks and Native Americans in the United States are lower than those of more prosperous Whites (Seiden 1981) supports this hypothesis, as does the finding by Fillenbaum *et al.* (1985) that it is men with marginal pre-retirement incomes whose well-being is more adversely affected by decline in economic status following retirement than those who were initially either poor or well-off.

LIFE EVENTS

It is apparent, at least in retrospective studies, that life events are a significant class of provoking agent which determine the timing of onset of some psychiatric disorders in vulnerable individuals. However, interpretation of the evidence is complicated by the existence of two distinct methodological and conceptual approaches to the subject. In the United States, most life-event research uses subject-rated check-lists to classify life events, and focuses on changes in behaviour following these events. By contrast, European studies use interviews and investigator-rated events, and the emphasis is upon the meaning of the event and the subject's emotional response to it. The check-list approach to identifying and classifying life events has been criticized on the grounds that it is vulnerable to recall bias and effort after meaning, particularly in subjects with mood disorders, and it has contributed relatively little to our understanding about the relationship between life events and illness. The firmest evidence that life events contribute to the onset and relapse of psychiatric disorders comes from studies employing investigator-rated events, notably those using the Life Events and Difficulties Schedule (LEDS) methodology developed by George Brown and his collaborators and followers (Brown and Harris 1978, 1989). Most of the evidence to date comes from studies of individuals aged below 65 years, although the study of Murphy (1982) demonstrates that severe adverse life events are also important in the onset of depression in the elderly. Elderly people report fewer life events, and the impact of events, in terms of unpleasantness and threat, seems to be less in older subjects (Brown and Harris 1978; Henderson *et al.* 1981), so it may be that only the most severe events are aetiologically significant in old age.

Brown considers that it is the meaning of events rather than their severity that is the most important factor determining whether or not they provoke onset of disorder. In particular, it is 'matching' events, in which specific individual commitments are frustrated by the event, that are more likely to cause disorder than others (Brown *et al.* 1987). Similarly, it is single events, or groups of events closely related in terms of their meaning for the individual, that are related to onset, rather than a general cumulative impact of a range of events (Brown and Harris 1989). Recent life-event research indicates that different types of life event, in terms of their meaning for the individual, may provoke the onset of different disorders; specifically, loss events are associated with depression and threatening events with anxiety (Brown 1993). Of course, the meaning of adverse events is not always clear-cut, with many being experienced by the individual as both a threat and a loss, and this may account for the frequent occurence of mixed anxiety/depression states.

An important limitation of the life-event research is that, however events and disorders are defined, only a proportion of the adverse events experienced by the population actually provoke disorders, and, conversely, only a proportion of the episodes of disorder that occur are preceded by events. As Murphy (1986) points out, this means that in the individual case it is not possible to be certain that a preceding event is causal, so the clinician must always pursue all aetiological possibilities, even when there is an apparently sufficient psychosocial explanation for the episode. Other physical and psychosocial vulnerabilities are important in determining whether or not an individual develops a disorder following an adverse event; for example, the lack of an intimate confiding relationship increases threefold the vulnerability of elderly people to the onset of depression following an adverse event (Murphy 1982) (see p.67).

It has recently been shown in women aged 18–60 years that life events also contribute to recovery from episodes of disorder (Brown *et al.* 1992). Here also, there appears to be a specificity effect, with recovery from depression being preceded by hopeful, fresh-start events, and recovery from anxiety being preceded by events that convey security or are anchoring. In depressed individuals, this effect of positive events on recovery is restricted to those not taking antidepressant medication (Brown 1993). Recovery in community populations is also associated, not surprisingly, with a decline in the rate of adverse events (Lin and Ensel 1984).

Bereavement

Bereavement is a relatively common severe adverse life event experienced by elderly people, but its impact on this age group is surprisingly under-researched. What evidence there is suggests that grief following bereavement takes the same form and follows the same course as it does at younger ages; it is normally characterized by initial numbness, followed by pangs of pining, restlessness, and anxiety, superimposed upon a background of more chronic dejection, difficulty with concentration, memory impairment, disturbed sleep and appetite, and social withdrawal (Parkes 1985). In most people, this grief reaction ameliorates with time, but in some individuals it is prolonged, inhibited, delayed, or followed by psychiatric disorder, usually some form of depression or anxiety state (Parkes 1965; Blazer 1982). Bereavement may also lead to the reappearance in old age of maladaptive coping strategies from earlier in life, such as alcohol abuse or disordered eating. It is not known if psychiatric disorder following bereavement is more or less common in the elderly than at younger ages although it has been argued that the timeliness of some losses in late life may reduce their impact (Neugarten 1979; Zisook *et al.* 1987; Murrell *et al.* 1988). Other factors thought to increase the likelihood of atypical grief and psychiatric morbidity following bereavement include post psychiatric history, circumstances of the death, ambivalent feelings towards the deceased, and lack of support by family and friends; there is little evidence concerning the relative importance of these in the elderly (Fasey 1990), although Dimond *et al.* (1987) found that the severity of depression shortly after bereavement was the best predictor of depression at two-year follow-up. The broader meaning of the bereavement for the elderly person is also important. In old age, widowhood may precipitate a number of other important changes in social and financial status, living arrangements, and social support, and these may also increase vulnerability to psychiatric disorder.

Retirement

In developed societies, retirement is a life event associated in many peoples' minds with the beginning of their 'old age'. However, its impact is incompletely understood; retirement is ranked low as a stressor by most elderly people, yet studies have shown an increase in psychiatric symptoms such as depression, anxiety, and somatization in a minority, for example, men who retire either early or late. What is the nature of the association between retirement and this psychological impairment? In both men and women, dissatisfaction with retirement is associated with lower education and income, reduced social contacts post-retirement, and poor physical health. In men, retirement stress is also associated with higher lifetime rates of reported stressful events (Blau *et al.* 1982; Matthews and Brown 1987). The nature of the retirement event is also important; early retirement tends to be associated with lower post-retirement income and less happiness, and unexpected or involuntary retirement is associated with higher levels of retirement stress in men (Patmore *et al.* 1984). There also appears to be an inverse relationship between prior work stress and mental health in retirement (Wheaton 1990). Bosse *et al.* (1992) make a distinction between the initial post-retirement period, when individuals are in transition, and the subsequent ongoing state of retirement, and provide some evidence that different social and personality factors are associated with perceived stress in these two periods. They also found that both transition stress and state stress were associated with higher rates of unrelated adverse life events and daily hassles, which suggests either that it is the presence of these other adverse circumstances that makes retirement stressful, or alternatively that some people are simply more vulnerable to the impact of events and difficulties in general.

Institutionalization

Admission into long-term institutional care in residential and nursing homes and hospitals is a unique and important life event experienced by a minority of elderly people. It is associated principally with loss– of independence, privacy, familiar social bonds– and for many elderly people it is seen as the beginning of the end of their lives. Most studies of people in institutional care focus on established residents, and show that all too often the quality of life in these settings is poor, with a substantial proportion of the residential population being significantly depressed (e.g. Mann *et al.* 1984). However, it is not possible to distinguish in these studies between the effect of the institutional environment and regime, and that of the transitional process. Longitudinal investigations of elderly people being admitted into institutional care have shown that various aspects of this process, such as selection bias, environmental discontinuity, and pre-admission effects, make an important contribution to residents' subsequent well-being (Tobin and Liebermann 1976). Selection bias refers to the fact that elderly people admitted to residential care are a vulnerable group, in that they are older and more physically and mentally frail than the elderly population living at home. Vulnerability to depression and other neurotic disorders may also be a factor determining whether or not an individual is admitted into residential care, particularly if they are socially isolated and it is thought that the experience of group living will be therapeutic. Environmental discontinuity, or the degree of difference between the home and the institution, is a measure of the loss that will be associated with moving from one to the other, and therefore of the stress associated with the transition. The pre-admission factors affecting outcome have to do with the manner in which the decision to admit into residential care is made, and the degree of choice and control that the elderly individual has in the process. Despite the fact that there has usually been a steady accumulation of problems, all too often the decision to admit into residential care is made following a crisis, such as a fall, and when the infrastructure of informal care collapses or is withdrawn. In these circumstances it is very difficult for the individual to exert any choice, even of the home they would like to be sent to (Willcocks *et al.* 1987). Murphy (1982) found that enforced change of residence was more frequent in depressed cases than controls.

Victimization and the fear of crime

The fear of crime is an important social issue because of the serious adverse impact it can have upon both individuals and the fabric of community life as a whole (Maxfield 1984). Studies repeatedly show that the elderly are particularly fearful of crime, despite the fact that they are the least victimized group in society. This paradox has received considerable attention from criminologists and policy-makers (Fattah and Sacco 1989), and their findings provide a valuable insight into the nature of the relationship between age and fearfulness in general. First and foremost, it is important to note that fear as defined by the criminologist is rather different from fear as understood by the psychiatrist. With few exceptions, crime surveys measure only the affective component of fear, and it is not possible to translate their categories into psychiatric diagnoses. Another important limitation of the concept of fear of crime as used in these surveys is that it is defined exclusively in terms of personal safety. Consequently, the reported association between age and fear of crime is primarily a reflection of the concern that elderly people feel about this issue; questions that tap worries about other crimes, such as burglary, do not reveal unduly high levels of concern in elderly people (Maxfield 1984). Another methodological problem is that victimization rates as reported in the crime statistics may significantly underestimate the true level of victimization of the elderly, since some crimes specifically directed against this age group, notably petty fraud, may not be reported by the victim. It is also the case that, while the global rates of reported victimization are low for the elderly, this is not true for all categories of crime. For certain offences, such as personal robbery involving contact with the thief, the levels of victimization do not fall significantly with age. Since elderly people are specifically concerned with the threat of physical attack, this may account for the the degree of fear of crime they express when this is defined in terms of feelings of personal safety.

The most plausible explanation for the apparently excessive fear of crime reported by the elderly is that this fear is associated less with the objective risk of victimization, and more with their perceived vulnerability. Elderly people have what Warr (1984) has termed a 'differential sensitivity to risk', that is, their high levels of fear of crime, as measured by crime surveys, reflect an evaluation of the severity of the consequences of victimization, whatever the likelihood of it occurring. If the result of an encounter with a mugger or a burglar is that you may well be killed or permanently disabled, then it makes sense to be careful about personal safety. When seen in this light, the concerns of elderly people look less like irrational fear and more like proper caution. A similar rationale probably underlies the higher levels of reported fear of crime by women of all ages, which prompts the speculation that it is young males who are in fact the most irrational group with respect to crime, since they alone believe themselves to be invulnerable to its consequences.

The process of risk evaluation by elderly people is determined by several factors, of which physical vulnerability, availability of social support, and integration within the local community appear to be particularly important (Hindelang *et al.* 1978; Yin 1982; Ginsberg 1984). It is factors such as these, rather than age alone, that should be taken into account when making judgements about the reasonableness or otherwise of the fears expressed by elderly people. In some individuals the evaluation of risk may be biased by their previous experience of victimization, or by depressive and anxious cognitions (Brillon 1987), resulting in irrational fears and behaviours, some of which may become very disabling (Feinberg 1981). Little is known about the rates of fear of crime associated with psychiatric disorders in the elderly, but the risk evaluation model suggests that they will be unreasonably high in individuals who are anxious and depressed.

Personal trauma and natural disaster

It has long been known that exposure to extreme trauma can cause significant psychological disturbance. Many of the symptoms of stress reactions and adjustment disorders also occur in other disorders, but their clear relationship to acute or ongoing trauma, together with certain specific features, has led to their being classed as separate clinical entities in DSM-III-R and ICD-10 (*International Classification of Diseases*, tenth revision). The paradigm stress reaction is post-traumatic stress disorder (PTSD), defined as a delayed and/or protracted response to a catastrophic event or situation, and characterized by intrusive memories, images, and dreams of the trauma which occur against a persistent background of anhedonia, emotional detachment, autonomic hyperarousal, depression, fear, avoidance, and occasional episodes of panic and aggression.

Little is known about the long-term effects of severe traumatic experiences, although PTSD can persist for many years, and ICD-10 recognizes a separate category (F62.0) of enduring personality change following catastrophic stress which may or may not be preceded by PTSD. The onset of PTSD can be also be very delayed, and may be precipitated by events occuring many years after the original trauma; Scaturo and Hayman (1992) suggest that retirement and leisure following the psychological distractions of work may be important in this respect. Many of the present elderly population were exposed to severe trauma both as military personnel and as civilians during the Second World War, and there is evidence to suggest that what would nowadays be diagnosed as PTSD was both common and persistent after these experiences. In one study of United States personnel who had been prisoners of war during the Second World War, 67 per cent had suffered from PTSD at the time, and only 27 per cent had fully recovered (Kluznik *et al.* 1986). Another study by Rosen *et al.* (1989) of Second World War combat veterans admitted to hospital with a psychiatric diagnosis other than PTSD found that 54 per cent met DSM-III criteria for past PTSD, and furthermore that 27 per cent met criteria for current PTSD in addition to their primary diagnosis. These studies suggest that traumatic wartime experiences continue to have a profound and enduring impact on a significant minority of elderly people, particularly those known to psychiatric services. Therefore, this aspect of elderly peoples' lives should be examined routinely in all psychogeriatric assessments, as long-standing PTSD may well have an effect on their course and outcome. The effect of chronic PTSD on the outcome of other psychiatric disorders, such as depression and anxiety, in old age needs to be researched.

As Goldberg and Huxley (1992) have pointed out, natural disasters are valuable experiments for students of social psychiatry, since they are severely stressful independent, non-normative life events affecting an entire population at one time. Studies of populations following such disasters have found a substantial increase in psychological symptoms in the weeks following the event, but that this disturbance subsides without treatment in all but a few individuals who are usually those who were particularly severely affected, having lost both homes and families (McFarlane 1987). In an interesting prospective study of the response of the elderly inhabitants of a poor rural region of the United States to two devastating floods, Phifer and Norris (1989) found that loss of property was associated with increased levels of anxiety and depression, but that this response was limited in all except those exposed to the worst catastrophe. Persistent psychological symptoms were associated more with loss to the community as a whole than with individual losses. The authors of this study point out that any psychological disturbance, persistent or not, was relatively mild, and that few of their subjects met the criteria for a diagnosis of PTSD. The resilience of many people in the face of such extreme experiences serves to remind us that personal vulnerability is a very important factor determining whether or not individuals develop psychiatric disorder.

EARLY EXPERIENCE

The work of Brown and Harris (1978) identifying early maternal loss as a vulnerability factor for depression in adulthood in young women has received considerable attention. Few studies have examined the developmental anteced-ents of other neurotic disorders in any detail, but there is some evidence from clinical and community studies which indicates that early parental loss is also a significant factor in these conditions. Faravelli *et al.* (1985) compared young adult patients with DSM-III agoraphobia and panic attacks with non-psychiatric controls, and found statistically significant associations between agoraphobia and early parental loss by death or divorce. Significant associations between agoraphobia with panic attacks and maternal death and parental separation have also been reported in a general adult community sample surveyed as part of the ECA study (Tweed *et al.* 1989). These researchers found no association between other anxiety disorders and early parental loss, or any specific associations with maternal or paternal loss, but these may have been obscured by the method used, which involved a simple comparison of screen-positive and screen-negative survey subjects with neither exclusion of borderline cases nor follow-up verification of case status. A re-analysis of data from the 1965 Queensbrook Survey in the United States, using DSM-III diagnostic categories, found a significant association between parental loss in childhood and generalized anxiety in adulthood among men; older men with disrupted childhoods were also at greater risk of depression (Zahner and Murphy 1989). There was no association between early parental loss and subsequent risk of psychiatric disorder in women in this sample. Few studies have examined this issue in a specifically elderly population. Murphy (1982) did not find that early parental loss was associated with depression in her sample; conversely, in a case–control study of a community sample of elderly people with phobic disorders, Lindesay (1991) found that phobias were associated with the loss of a parent, particularly the father, before the age of 18 years.

Bowlby's attachment theory has provided the conceptual foundation for the empirical study of the impact of parental death and separation (Bowlby 1977). This theory is:

. . . a way of conceptualizing the propensity of human beings to make strong affectional bonds to particular others and of explaining the many forms of emotional distress and personality disturbance, including anxiety, anger, depression and emotional detachment, to which unwilling separation and loss give rise.

This presupposes that it is the 'disruption of . . . affectional bonds' that leads to 'distress and personality disturbance' in the child, and so to the vulnerability to adverse life events which has been shown to be a significant factor in the aetiology of depression and anxiety later in life (Brown and Harris 1978; Finlay-Jones and Brown 1981). In fact, the evidence from studies of younger adults suggests that it is other experiences associated with parental loss and separation, such as parental conflict preceding separation or subsequent inadequate care (Parker 1983; Perris 1983; Brier *et al.* 1988) that are more important determinants of vulnerability to subsequent psychiatric disorder. For example, Tennant *et al.* (1982) found that marital discord and parental physical illness between the ages of five and fifteen years were predictive of psychopathology in adulthood, particularly depression. By contrast, Lindesay (1991) found that, while phobias in the elderly were associated with early parental death, parental divorce and separation was not an independent risk factor. This may be a reflection of generational differences, since death was a much commoner cause of early parental loss when today's elderly were young than it is now, when children are much more likely to experience parental divorce or separation.

Vulnerability to depression was found by Brown and Harris (1978) to be specifically associated with early maternal loss in young women. The evidence concerning the association between other disorders and the loss of one or other parent is relatively meagre. In an early case–record study (Webster 1953) the fathers of female agoraphobics were reported as being more often absent from the parental home than the fathers of other patient groups. Similarly, in the study of anxious individuals carried out by Finlay-Jones (1989) there was a suggestion that the vulnerability associated with parental divorce was associated with the father's departure. By contrast, in their comparison of community adults with and without DSM-III anxiety disorders, Tweed *et al.* (1989) found no specific associations with early loss of father or mother. In the elderly, Lindesay (1991) found a specific association between phobic disorders and early paternal death, but since there was also an excess of paternal over maternal deaths in the control group, this association may have been the result of a general factor, such as the First World War. increasing the likelihood of exposure of this age group to paternal death. Sex of the subject was not a significant effect modifier in relation to loss of either parent in this study.

SOCIAL RELATIONSHIPS

As part of the general social trend towards smaller and simpler households in developed societies, the proportion of elderly people living alone in the UK has risen substantially since the Second World War; for women aged 75 years and older, living alone is now the modal category of household composition. While living alone does not necessarily imply a lack of support by family and friends, and is not associated *per se* with psychiatric disorder in epidemiological surveys, this trend is usually taken to mean that increasing numbers of elderly people are at risk of social isolation and psychiatric disorder. To what extent is this in fact the case? Most studies have found that elderly people have extensive social networks and good support. In a recent review of the literature on social bonds in late life, Jerrome (1991) has emphasized their increasing complexity in a world where the birth rate is falling, people live longer, and divorce in all adult generations is increasing; rather than belonging to some past golden age, the transgenerational family is a modern and growing phenomenon, and we have yet to fully understand how it currently supports and sustains its older members. While the well-studied relationships with spouses and children are clearly of great importance, there is evidence that for many elderly people the most important bonds are with others such as siblings, friends, or even pets. The effect of these relationships upon individual well-being also merits study, particularly their therapeutic and protective effects, if any.

Studies of both clinical and general populations usually show the expected relationship between depression and neurotic disorder and reduced levels of social support. For example, in an elderly community sample resident in Hobart, Tasmania, Henderson *et al.* (1986) found that depression was associated with reduced levels of social interaction, although the subjects did not complain of this. In cross-sectional studies it is not possible to say with any certainty which comes first: does the disorder lead to social withdrawal, or does lack of social support increase vulnerability to disorder? One follow-up study of depression in an elderly community sample (Blazer 1983) found that depression was associated with *increased* levels of social support 13 months later, suggesting that the disorder may have resulted in improvements in social networks. In contrast, Oxman *et al.* (1992) found that reduced social support at three-year follow up was associated with increased depression.

It is the quality as much as the quantity of social relationships that is important in sustaining individuals' well-being, and the absence of a current confiding relationship has been found in some studies to be associated with psychiatric disorder, particularly depression, in the elderly (Lowenthal and Haven 1968; Murphy 1982; Blazer 1983; Kennedy *et al.* 1989), although in others this relationship is relatively weak (Henderson *et al.* 1986), perhaps due to methodological differences. There is more to the lack of a confidant than simply poor social support; intimacy as measured by the LEDS is a function of the capacity as well as the opportunity to form and maintain personal relationships, and it is argued by Murphy (1986) that the association between the absence of a confiding relationship and late-life depression is in fact due to a long-standing incapacity for intimacy that increases vulnerability to destabilizing events in old age.

In contrast to depression, there does not appear to be an association between anxiety and intimacy as measured by the LEDS, either in younger individuals (Finlay-Jones 1989) or in the elderly. Lindesay (1991) found no association between phobic disorder in the elderly and either the presence or absence of a current intimate confiding relationship. Among the more severe cases, however, there was a non-significant gradient relating phobic disorder and higher rates of intimate relationships. Cases in this study were also more likely to have living children than were controls, so it may be that the presence of close relationships acts to maintain phobic avoidance in elderly people. However, these were established cases, so it is also possible that their current capacity or opportunity for intimate relationships may have altered as a result of the phobic disorder. In a community study of elderly women in New Zealand, Walton *et al.* (1990) found that phobic subjects were less likely to have families of their own.

CONCLUSIONS

To date, most research into the psychosocial aspects of mental illness has concentrated on factors such as adverse life events that are associated with onset of disorder. However, it is clear that these events are a relatively minor component in the aetiology of illness episodes, and in future much more attention needs to be directed towards the underlying vulnerability. Why do certain people fall ill, and what are the critical affective, cognitive, and behavioural components of their vulnerability to adverse events? Future research should also focus on protective factors, and those which promote recovery. A better understanding of the social aspects of vulnerability to and recovery from mental illness will not only be of practical clinical value, but will also help to improve the currently low-profile and marginal status of the social sciences within psychiatric research.

REFERENCES

Baltes, P. B., and Baltes, M. M. (1990). Psychological perspectives on successful aging: the model of selective optimization with compensation. In *Successful aging: perspectives from the behavioural sciences* (ed. P. B. Baltes and M. M. Baltes), pp. 1–34. Cambridge University Press, Cambridge.

Blau, Z. S., Oser, G. T., and Stephens, R. C. (1982). Patterns of adaptation in retirement: a comparative analysis. In *Coping with medical issues: aging* (ed. A. Kolker and P. I. Ahmed), pp. 119–138. Elsevier Biomedical, New York.

Blazer, D. G. (1982). Late life bereavement and depressive neurosis. In *Depression in late life* (ed. D. G. Blazer). C. V. Mosby and Co., New York.

Blazer, D. G. (1983). Impact of late-life depression on the social network. *American Journal of Psychiatry*, **140**, 162–6.

Blazer, D. G., and Williams, C. D. (1980). The epidemiology of dysphoria and depression in an elderly population. *American Journal of Psychiatry*, **137**, 439–44.

Blazer, D. G., George, L. K., Landermann, R., Pennybacker, M., Melville, M. L., Woodbury, M., *et. al.* (1985). Psychiatric disorders: a rural/urban comparison. *Archives of General Psychiatry*, **42**, 651–6.

Blazer, D. G., George, L. K., and Hughes, D. (1991). The epidemiology of anxiety disorders: an age comparison. In *Anxiety in the elderly* (ed. C. Salzman and B. Lebowitz), pp. 17–30. Springer, New York.

Bosse, R., Levenson, M. R., Spiro, A., Aldwin, C. M., and Mroczek, D. K. (1992). For whom is retirement stressful? Findings from the Normative Aging Study. In *Facts and research in gerontology 1992* (ed. B. Vellas and J. L. Albarède), pp. 223–237. Springer, New York.

Bowlby, J. (1977). The making and breaking of affectional bonds. I: Aetiology and psychopathology in the light of attachment theory. *British Journal of Psychiatry*, **130**, 201–10.

Brier, A., Kelsoe, J. R., Kirwin, P. D., Beller, S. A., Wolkowitz, O. M., and Pickar, D. (1988). Early parental loss and the development of adult psychopathology. *Archives of General Psychiatry*, **45**, 987–93.

Brillon, Y. (1987). *Victimization and fear of crime among the elderly*. Butterworth, Toronto.

Brown, G. W. (1993). Life events and psychiatric disorder: replications and limitations. *Psychosomatic Medicine*, **55**, 248–59.

Brown, G. W., and Harris, T. O. (1978). *Social origins of depression*. Tavistock, London.

Brown, G. W., and Harris, T. O. (ed.) (1989) *Life events and illness*. Unwin Hyman, London.

Brown, G. W., Bifulco, A., and Harris, T. O. (1987). Life events, vulnerability and onset of depression: some refinements. *British Journal of Psychiatry*, **150**, 30–42.

Brown, G. W., Lemyre, L., and Bifulco, A. (1992). Social factors and recovery from anxiety and depressive disorders: a test of the specificity hypothesis. *British Journal of Psychiatry*, **161**, 44–54.

Champion, L. (1990). The relationship between social vulnerability and the occurence of severely threatening life events. *Psychological Medicine*, **20**, 157–61.

Coleman, P. G., Ivani-Chilian, C., and Robinson, M. (1993). Self-esteem and its sources: stability and change in later life. *Ageing and Society*, **13**, 171–92.

Dimond, M., Lund, D. A., and Caserta, M. S. (1987). The role of social support in the first two years of bereavment in an elderly sample. *Gerontologist*, **27**, 599–604.

Faravelli, C., Webb, T., Ambonetti, A., Fonessu, F., and Sessarego, A. (1985). Prevalence of traumatic early life events in 31 agoraphobic patients with panic attacks. *American Journal of Psychiatry*, **142**, 1493–4.

Fasey, C. N. (1990). Grief in old age: a review of the literature. *International Journal of Geriatric Psychiatry*, **5**, 67–75.

Fattah, E. A., and Sacco, V. F. (1989). *Crime and victimization in the elderly*. Springer-Verlag, New York.

Feinberg, N. (1981). The emotional and behavioural consequences of violent crime on elderly victims. *Victimology*, **6**, 355–7.

Fillenbaum, G. G., George, L. K., and Palmore, E. B. (1985). Determinants and consequences of retirement among men of different races and economic levels. *Journal of Gerontology*, **40**, 85–94.

Finlay-Jones, R. (1989). Anxiety. In *Life events and illness* (ed. G. W. Brown and T. O. Harris), pp. 95–112. Unwin Hyman, London.

Finlay-Jones, R., and Brown, G. W. (1981). Types of stressful life event and the onset of anxiety and depressive disorders. *Psychological Medicine*, **11**, 803–16.

Ginsberg, Y. (1984). Fear of crime amongst elderly Jews in Boston and London. *International Journal of Ageing and Human Development*, **20**, 257–68.

Goldberg, D., and Huxley, P. (1992). *Common mental disorders: a bio-social model*. Routledge, London.

Grundy, E. (1989). Living arrangements and social support in later life. In *Human aging and late life*: *multidisciplinary perspectives* (ed. A. M. Warnes), pp. 96–106. Edward Arnold, London.

Harris, T. O. (1988). Psychosocial vulnerability to depression. In *Handbook of social psychiatry* (ed. S. Henderson and G. Burrows). Elsevier, Amsterdam.

Henderson, A. S., Byrne, D. G., and Duncan-Jones, P. (1981). *Neurosis and the social environment*. Academic Press, Sydney.

Henderson, A. S., Grayson, D. A., Scott, R., Witsen, J., Rickwood, D., and Kay, D. W. K. (1986). Social support, dementia and depression among elderly living in the Hobart community. *Psychological Medicine*, **16**, 379–90.

Himmelfarb, S., and Murrell, S. A. (1984). The prevalence and corelates of anxiety symptoms in older adults. *Journal of Psychology*, **116**, 159–67.

Hindelang, M. J., Gottfredson, M. R., and Garofolo, J. (1978). *Victims of personal crime: an empirical foundation for a theory of personal victimisation*. Balinger, Cambridge, Massachusetts.

Jerrome, D. (1991). Social bonds in later life. *Reviews in Clinical Gerontology*, **1**, 297–306.

Kennedy, G. J., Kelman, H. R., and Thomas, C. (1989). Hierarchy of characteristics associated with depressive symptoms in an urban elderly sample. *American Journal of Psychiatry*, **146**, 220–22.

Kennedy, G. J., Kelman, H. R., and Thomas, C. (1990). The emergence of depressive symptoms in late life. The importance of declining health and increasing disability. *Journal of Community Health*, **15**, 93–104.

Khansari, D., Murgo, A., and Faith, R. (1990). Effects of stress on the immune system. *Immunology Today*, **11**, 170–4.

Kluznik, J. C., Speed, N., Van Valkenberger, C., and McGraw, R. (1986). Forty-year follow-up of United States prisoners of war. *American Journal of Psychiatry*, **143**, 1443–5.

Lin, N., and Ensel, W. M. (1984). Depression-mobility and its social etiology: the role of life events and social support. *Journal of Health and Social Behaviour*, **25**, 176–88.

Lindesay, J. (1991). Phobic disorders in the elderly. *British Journal of Psychiatry*, **159**, 531–41.

Lowenthal, M. F., and Haven, C. (1968). Interaction and adaptation intimacy as a critical variable. *American Sociological Review*, **33**, 20–30.

McFarlane, A. (1987). Life events and psychiatric disorder: the role of natural disaster. *British Journal of Psychiatry*, **151**, 362–7.

Matthews, A. M., and Brown, K. H. (1987). Retirement as a critical life event. *Research into Aging*, **9**, 548–71.

Mann, A. H., Graham, N., and Ashby, D. (1984). Psychiatric illness in residential homes for the elderly: a survey in one London borough. *Age and Ageing*, **13**, 257–65.

Maxfield, M. G. (1984). *Fear of crime in England and Wales*. HMSO, London.

Mertens, F., and Wimmers, M. (1987). Life-style of older people: improvement or threat to their health. *Ageing and Society*, **7**, 329–43.

Murphy, E. (1982). Social origins of depression in old age. *British Journal of Psychiatry*, **141**, 135–42.

Murphy, E. (1986). Social factors in late life depression. In *Affective Disorders in the Elderly* (ed. E. Murphy), pp. 79–96. Churchill Livingstone, London.

Murrell, S. A., Norris, F. H., and Goote, C. (1988). Life events in older adults. In: *Life Events and Psychological Functioning* (ed. L. H. Cohen). Sage, Newbury Park.

Neugarten, B. (1979). Time, age and the life cycle. *American Journal of Psychiatry*, **136**, 887–94.

Office of Population Censuses and Surveys (1986). *General Household Survey 1984*. HMSO, London.

Oxman, T. E., Berkman, L. F., Kasl, S., Freeman, D. H., and Barratt, J. (1992). Social support and depressive symptoms in the elderly. *American Journal of Epidemiology*, **135**, 356–68.

Parker, G. (1983). 'Parental affectionless control' as an antecedent to adult depression. *Archives of General Psychiatry*, **134**, 138–47.

Parkes, C. M. (1965). Bereavement and mental illness. Part 2: A classification of bereavement reactions. *Journal of Medical Psychology*, **38**, 13–26.

Parkes, C. M. (1985). Bereavement. *British Journal of Psychiatry*, **146**, 11–17.

Patmore, E. B., Fillenbaum, G. G., and George, L. K. (1984). Consequences of retirement. *Journal of Gerontology*, **39**, 109–16.

Perris, H. (1983). Deprivation in childhood and life events in depression. *Archiv für Psychiatrie und Nervenkrankenheit*, **23**, 489–98.

Phifer, J. E., and Norris, F. H. (1989). Psychological symptoms in older adults following natural disaster: nature, timing, duration and course. *Journal of Gerontology*, **44**, 207–17.

Prudo, R., Brown, G. W., Harris, T. O., and Dowland, J. (1981). Psychiatric disorder in a rural and in an urban population: 2. Sensitivity to loss. *Psychological Medicine*, **11**, 601–16.

Rosen, J., Fields, R. B., Hand, A. M., Falsettie, G., and Van Kammen, D P.

(1989). Concurrent posttraumatic stress disorder in psychogeriatric patients. *Journal of Geriatric Psychiatry and Neurology*, **2**, 65–9.

Scaturo, D. J., and Hayman, P. M. (1992). The impact of combat trauma across the family life cycle: clinical considerations. *Journal of Trauma and Stress*, **5**, 273–88.

Seiden, R. H. (1981). Mellowing with age: factors influencing the nonwhite suicide rate. *International Journal of Aging and Human Development*, **13**, 265–84.

Tennant, C., Bebbington, P., and Hurry, J. (1982). Social experiences in childhood and adult psychiatric morbidity: a multiple regression analysis. *Psychological Medicine*, **12**, 321–7.

Tobin, S. S., and Liebermann, M. A. (1976). *Last home for the aged*. Jossey-Bass, San Francisco.

Tweed, J. L., Schoenbach, V. J., George, L. K., and Blazer, D. G. (1989). The effects of childhood parental death and divorce on six-month history of anxiety disorders. *British Journal of Psychiatry*, **154**, 823–8.

Walton, V. A., Romans-Clarkson, S. E., Mullen, P. E., and Herbison, G. P. (1990). The mental health of elderly women in the community. *International Journal of Geriatric Psychiatry*, **5**, 257–63.

Warr, M. (1984). Fear of victimization: why are women and elderly more afraid? *Social Science Quarterly*, **65**, 681–702.

Webster, A. S. (1953). The development of phobias in married women. *Psychological Monographs*, **67**, No. 367.

Weissman, M. M., Bruce, M. L., Leaf, P. J., Florio, L. P., and Holzer, C. (1991). Affective disorders. In *Psychiatric disorders in America* (ed. L. N. Robins and D. A. Regier), pp. 53–80. Free Press, New York.

Wheaton, B. (1983). Stress, personal coping resources and psychiatric symptoms: an investigation of interactive models. *Journal of Health and Social Behaviour*, **24**, 208–30.

Wheaton, B. (1990). Life transitions, role histories and mental health. *American Sociology Review*, **55**, 209–33.

Willcocks, D., Peace, S., and Kelleher, L. (1987). *Private lives in public places*. Tavistock, London.

Yin, P. (1982). Fear of crime as a problem for the elderly. *Social Problems*, **30**, 240–5.

Zahner, G. E. P., and Murphy, J. M. (1989). Loss in childhood: anxiety in adulthood. *Comprehensive Psychiatry*, **30**, 553–63.

Zisook, S., Shuchter, S. R., and Lyons, L. E. (1987) Predictors of psychological reactions during the early stages of widowhood. *Psychiatric Clinics of North America*, **10**, 355–68.

5

Biological factors
MICHAEL P. PHILPOT

INTRODUCTION

Research into biological factors involved in late-life neurosis is in its infancy. Much of this chapter is based, therefore, on studies conducted in young subjects and ends with a few speculations as to how the suggested models of neurosis might be modulated by age. It is possible to glean some information about neurosis from studies of late-life depression in which the symptom profile or the neurotic subtype have been identified. Unfortunately, early studies have tended to concentrate on patients with endogenous depression or those admitted to hospital, and it is only now being recognized that these patients might represent atypical and unrepresentative cases: in other words, psychobiological research has not so far been particularly epidemiologically sound. There have also been problems with study design, with cross-sectional studies being favoured over longitudinal studies, and the identification of 'old age' as a state defined by social factors (that is, retirement) rather than biological ones. These and other problems are discussed more fully elsewhere (Macdonald 1991; Philpot 1994).

A major complication for the researcher concerns the classification of the neuroses (q.v. Introduction). Holmes (1993) has reiterated the problem of the 'splitters' and the 'lumpers'. As will become apparent in this review, evidence from psychopharmacological studies tends to support the 'splitters' while that from clinical genetic studies supports the 'lumpers'. Given the tendency for all manner of data to become more variable with increasing age, it is likely that the lumpers will win the day in this respect, as elderly patients seem to fit less well into the neat categories of the international classification systems. Indeed, attempts to isolate biological factors for specific neurotic disorders have been frustrated by the problem of co-morbidity, even in young patients.

With regard to age-specific factors, it is still fashionable to ask whether there are biological features specific to neurosis in the elderly, and if so, whether they are related to brain ageing *per se* or simply secondary manifestations of other pathology associated with being old. Given the general preoccupation with research into affective disorders it is impossible to avoid discussion of depression, although, as mentioned above, it is often difficult to know whether specific subtypes of the disorder are being studied.

Psychobiologists indulge in at least two scientific activities: the attempted discovery of the physical aetiology of mental disorders (or factors increasing vulnerability to them), and the identification of state or trait markers that might assist in making a diagnosis or identifying subjects at risk. This chapter will concentrate on the former and will omit many worthy topics, including peripheral markers studied in blood, urine, and cerebrospinal fluid.

GENETICS

Clinical studies have identified a definite genetic contribution to the aetiology of depression but, to date, the search for the genes responsible has not been successful. Two approaches have been taken to the study of the genetics of neurosis: first, to determine the heritability of personality factors which might contribute to neuroticism, such as shyness, timidity, and fear; and second, to determine the heritability of clinically defined states.

Neuroticism

In infancy and childhood, monozygotic (MZ) twins are more alike than dizygotic (DZ) twins with respect to characteristics of fearfulness and inhibition (Goldsmith and Gottesman 1981). Questionnaire measures of neuroticism are also more similar in MZ twins, particularly those reared apart (Bouchard *et al.* 1990). Mackinnon *et al.* (1990) found that genetic factors and shared environment significantly accounted for the variability of these scores among twin pairs. However, variations in mood and anxiety were not related to these factors but were triggered by adverse life events. Genetic factors play a strong part in the heritability of other neurotic traits, physiological measures of arousal, and galvanic skin response (reviewed by Marks 1986). Other self-reported fears and simple phobias also aggregate in families (Fyer *et al.* 1990).

Anxiety disorders

The prevalence of anxiety disorder in first-degree relatives of anxious probands is higher among female relatives and is, overall, two or three times that of the general population (Marks 1986). Concordance rates for anxiety disorder are predictably higher in MZ twins than DZ twins (56 per cent versus 40 per cent), but this difference may only be a factor in men (Torgersen 1983). Although co-morbidity is common, Torgersen (1990) has presented twin data that suggest that pure anxiety disorders, particularly patients with panic disorder, may be genetically distinct from pure depression or mixed states.

The first-degree relatives of panic disorder probands also have an increased lifetime risk of panic disorder: 25 per cent versus 2 per cent in the general population in one study (Crowe 1990). Again, there was considerable co-morbidity with 61 per cent of first-degree relatives displaying some symptomatology.

Depression

In a classic twin study, Shapiro (1970) failed to find evidence for genetic factors in neurotic depression. However, Englund and Klein (1990) re-analysed this data using diagnostic criteria rather than hospitalization to define concordance and found that MZ twins did in fact show greater concordance than DZ twins. Torgersen (1986) found that neurotic depression clustered in families largely because of the shared environment rather than because of any additive genetic factor. In support of this, McGuffin and Katz (1989) reported that the tendency to experience threatening life events as well as depression itself was inherited, and concluded that life-event-related depression (not synonymous with neurotic depression) occurred in hazard-prone individuals rather than stress-susceptible ones.

Obsessive–compulsive disorder (OCD)

OCD is highly heritable, being present in 40–50 per cent of parents, 19–39 per cent of siblings and 16 per cent of children of OCD probands (reviewed by Marks 1986). Black *et al.* (1992) found that anxiety disorders and obsessional traits and symptoms—but not OCD itself—were more common in families of OCD probands than in control families. This supports the idea that an anxiety diathesis is inherited which is not always expressed as OCD.

General neurotic syndrome

Andrews *et al.* (1990) studied the inheritance of six neurotic disorders and demonstrated that while there was a significant genetic contribution to neurotic vulnerability, this did not extend to specific disorders. Kendler *et al.* (1992) also found that depression and generalized anxiety in female twins were influenced by the same genetic factors, and that environmental influences largely determined which illness the women presented with. Winokur and Coryell (1992) reported that probands with 'depression spectrum disease' (that is, probands with family histories of alcoholism) had more first-degree relatives with anxiety and somatization disorders than pure depression. They also tended to have a more neurotic form of depression.

Effects of ageing

A number of studies have shown that the genetic influence diminishes with age in affective disorders. The earliest relevant study (Hopkinson 1964) was performed on in-patients with depression and showed that relatives of probands aged over 50 years had two-and-a-half times less risk of depression than young probands. Rice *et al.* (1984) also found that genetic influence fell with the age of the proband. While not contradicting these findings, Maier *et al.* (1991) found that relatives of probands with late-onset depression still had an increased rate of depression over relatives of a control sample. However, an adoption study by Gatz *et al.* (1992) found that heritability of depression was greater in twins of 60 years and over, especially for individual symptoms such as psychomotor retardation.

There have been suggestions that different coping styles may modulate the expression of 'neurosis' genes, and that these may themselves be genetically determined (McGuffin and Katz 1989; Kendler *et al.* 1991). Is it possible that the apparent reduction in genetic influence with age results from the increased expression of a gene for coping, or from the environmental benefits of experience?

NEURORADIOLOGY

As has been stated above, many of the studies cited in this chapter have focused on affective disorders, particularly in in-patient samples. Their relevance to the study of neurosis may, then, be only peripheral. Technical details of imaging methods will not be given here, but the interested reader is referred to the reviews by Beats (1991), Baldwin (1993), and Joyce (1991).

Brain structure

Volumetric analysis
Early studies using semi-subjective visual ratings of computerized tomography (CT) scan appearance have largely been superseded by more sophisticated methods of quantitative analysis, no doubt in an attempt to capture subtle changes in structure undetected by the eye. Most studies have sought to determine the mean differences between experimental and control groups using quantitative measures (e.g. Andreasen *et al.* 1990). A quite different approach has been to identify patients in the experimental group with abnormal scans and then compare them to those with normal scans (e.g. Jacoby and Levy 1980). The two approaches have produced somewhat conflicting results.

Jacoby and Levy (1980) found no differences in the mean ventricular-brain ratio (VBR) of depressed in-patients and age-matched controls. However, 9 of 41 patients had scans reported as showing enlarged ventricles. These patients had significantly lower anxiety scores and higher Newcastle scale scores, implying that the more neurotically depressed patients had more normal scans. Those with enlarged ventricles were older and had a higher mortality at 2-year follow-up but no comment is made about the destiny of the others (Jacoby *et al.* 1981, 1983). Bird *et al.* (1985) re-scanned just over half the control group used in these studies after an average of 2 years and found that the new cases of depressive illness (including those with bereavement reactions) had higher initial mean VBRs.

Some studies have shown that younger patients also have significantly raised

VBRs in comparison to age-matched controls (Targum *et al.* 1983; Dolan *et al.* 1985), but many others have failed to confirm this in cognitively normal depressed patients of middle and old age (Scott *et al.* 1983; Schlegel and Kretschmer 1987*a*; Andreasen *et al.* 1990; Pearlson *et al.* 1989; Abas *et al.* 1990; Beats *et al.* 1991). The last three reports cited involve elderly patients exclusively, but none comments on the clinical features of the patients, although the sample investigated by Abas *et al.* (1990) all had endogenous depression. Alexopoulos *et al.* (1992) compared late-onset with early-onset elderly depressed cases. VBR and severity of cognitive impairment were increased in the late-onset patients, suggesting that they may have been in the early stages of dementia. There was no comment on clinical subtypes of depression, but ventricular size correlated positively with symptom severity. Beats *et al.* (1991) found increased third-ventricle size which correlated positively with age as well as duration of depressive symptoms, and negatively with the frequency of episodes and age of onset.

A number of studies have used magnetic resonance imaging (MRI) to measure ventricular size and cerebral atrophy. Rabins *et al.* (1991), using a visual scoring method, found greater cortical and subcortical atrophy and enlargement of the lateral and third ventricles in elderly depressed patients, whereas Coffey *et al.* (1993), using a quantitative method, found differences only in the frontal lobes, which were smaller in elderly depressed patients. The patients in the latter study had been referred for electroconvulsive therapy and it is unlikely that many of them suffered from mild or neurotic depression. Reduction in the size of the putamen (Husain *et al.* 1991) and thickening of the anterior and posterior quadrants of the corpus callosum similar to that found in schizophrenia (Wu *et al.* 1993) have also been demonstrated.

Lastly, in a search for the determinants of ventricular enlargement in middle-aged patients with chronic affective and neurotic disorders, Johnstone *et al.* (1986) found a higher-than-expected rate of hypothyroidism in those with large ventricles. In view of the well-known association between thyroid status and mood (Szabadi 1991), this finding is worth further exploration.

Regional brain density

Jacoby *et al.* (1983) found that regional brain density was reduced in the left temporal region and right thalamus, but these findings were largely attributable to those patients with enlarged ventricles, again implying that the more neurotic patients had normal scans. Pearlson *et al.* (1991) showed that brain density in the white matter of the centrum semiovale was reduced in the cognitively normal as well as the cognitively impaired depressed. The centrum-semiovale slice is more apical than those usually chosen for study and may be more sensitive to age-related changes. However, Beats *et al.* (1991) found no differences in white-matter or grey-matter density in the frontal and parietal regions, but there was increased brain density in both caudate nuclei and reduced density in the right thalamus. These findings confirm those of studies in younger patients (Schlegel and Kretschmer 1987*b*).

Focal changes in white and grey matter

MRI has distinct advantages over CT in terms of its resolution and ability to differentiate grey from white matter. On the other hand, MR scanners are less readily available and the procedure is lengthy and can lead to some discomfort for the patient. Interest has centred on subtle changes such as patchy white-matter hyperintensities. There has been some confusion caused by the synonymous use of terms to identify these abnormalities, but Baldwin (1993) has clarified the issue and lists periventricular hyperintensities (PVH) and subcortical white-matter and grey-matter lesions (SCWML and SCGML) as being of chief importance. Briefly, there is agreement that elderly depressed patients have a higher frequency of white-matter and grey-matter lesions in subcortical areas (Coffey *et al.* 1990; Rabins *et al.* 1991), but that PVH has been increased in some studies but not others (Baldwin 1993). Studies referring to 'white-matter hyperintensities' have in general found a greater prevalence or severity of lesions in depressed elderly subjects (Zubenko *et al.* 1990; Lesser *et al.* 1991), and that these lesions are possibly more prevalent in late-onset cases (Krishnan *et al.* 1988; Churchill *et al.* 1991; Figiel *et al.* 1991). This may simply be related to the observation that with age these lesions increase in prevalence in normal subjects (George *et al.* 1986; Jernigan *et al.* 1991; Awad *et al.* 1986*a*).

There is some controversy as to the pathological nature of the white-matter hyperintensities. État criblé—a state in which the perivascular parenchyma shrinks and fills with fluid giving a sieve-like appearance—has been found to correspond to the MRI lesions (Awad *et al.* 1986*b*), but tiny infarcts and areas of demyelination have also been found (Baffman *et al.* 1988).

The questions relating to structural imaging which remain unanswered to date are: do the abnormalities discovered predate the onset of psychiatric disorder and act as a risk factor; do they arise as a result of the disorder or its treatment; or are they related to a common factor such as cardiovascular disease and/or hypertension (Awad *et al.* 1986*a*; Coffey *et al.* 1990; Lesser *et al.* 1991; Howard *et al.* 1993)?

Functional imaging

Cerebral blood flow

Absolute rates of global and regional cerebral blood flow (rCBF) may be measured using inhalation techniques, such as the xenon-133 (involving single photon emission tomography: SPET) or oxygen-15 (involving positron emission tomography: PET). Relative rCBF may be measured using lipophilic tracers labelled with technetium-99m (e.g. hexamethylpropylene-amine oxime: HMPAO). Under normal circumstances rCBF is closely tied to local metabolic requirements. Theoretically, this linkage may be dysfunctional in elderly subjects, but no studies specifically testing this hypothesis have yet been carried out.

Studies of depressive illness again prevail but unfortunately there is little consistency in the literature. In young and middle-aged patients, global cerebral blood flow in unipolar depression has been reported as unchanged (Gur *et al.* 1984; Silfverskiold and Risberg 1989; Berman *et al.* 1993; Bench *et al.* 1993), increased (Rosenberg *et al.* 1988), and decreased (Schlegel *et al.* 1989; Sackeim *et al.* 1990). Focal reductions in rCBF have been identified in the frontal (Schlegel *et al.* 1989; Sackeim *et al.* 1990; Bench *et al.* 1992; Austin *et al.* 1992), central (Sackeim *et al.* 1990; Kanaya and Yonekawa 1990), parietal (Schlegel *et al.* 1990; 1989; Sackeim *et al.* 1990; Austin *et al.* 1992), temporal lobes (Schlegel *et al.* 1989; Sackeim *et al.* 1990; Kanaya and Yonekawa 1990; Austin *et al.* 1992), and basal ganglia (Austin *et al.* 1992). In addition, increased rCBF has been demonstrated in the right temporal lobe (Amsterdam and Mozley 1992), left posterior cingulate gyrus (Bench *et al.* 1993), and cerebellum (Bench *et al.* 1992). Studies have variously demonstrated a predominance of left-hemisphere abnormalities (Kanaya and Yonekawa 1990; Bench *et al.* 1992), right-hemisphere abnormalities (Schlegel *et al.* 1989; Amsterdam and Mozley 1992), or no hemispheric asymmetry (Sackeim *et al.* 1990; Austin *et al.* 1992). Deficits in rCBF have been found to correlate with depression severity in a number of studies (Kanaya and Yonekawa. 1990; Sackeim *et al.* 1990; Austin *et al.* 1992) but not in all (e.g Schlegel *et al.* 1989).

Austin *et al.* (1992) demonstrated a strong positive relationship between scores on the Newcastle scale and rCBF in the cingulate and frontal areas, and Schlegel *et al.* (1989), using a different rating scale, found no positive effect of endogenicity although patients with reactive symptoms had lower rCBF. Bench *et al.* (1993) sought associations between rCBF and clinical factors derived from a standardized interview schedule. The factor incorporating anxiety, agitation, somatization, and insomnia correlated positively with rCBF in the right posterior cingulate gyrus and the bilateral inferior parietal lobules.

To date three studies, all using HMPAO-SPET, have included only elderly patients. Upadhyaya *et al.* (1990) found no significant differences in relative rCBF using HMPAO when comparing 18 elderly depressed patients with 12 age-matched controls, although an average measure of global cerebral blood flow was lower in depressed patients. On visual inspection, areas of impaired perfusion were found in 30–40 per cent of depressed patients and only 10–15 per cent of controls. Half of the patients were cases of depressive neurosis, but there is no comment on the effect of subtype save the observation that occipital rCBF correlated negatively with the Newcastle score. There was no significant correlation between rCBF and depression severity *per se*. Our study (Philpot *et al.* 1993) compared 10 elderly depressed patients with 9 age-matched controls in a split-dose paradigm measuring rCBF during a resting state and during a verbal fluency task. At rest, reduced flow was found in the left parietal and temporal regions and the basal ganglia of the depressed patients. There were no correlations between rCBF and either severity of depression or degree of endogenicity, but rCBF did correlate negatively with anxiety and somatic symptoms and positively with psychotic symptoms. During activation, the relative rCBF in the patients increased, particularly in the frontal regions, such that differences between the depressed group and the controls were abolished. In the largest study to date, 20 elderly depressed patients were compared to 30 normal subjects and 20 patients with Alzheimer's disease (Curran *et al.* 1993). Differences between the depressed patients and controls were only found for men; reductions were discovered in tracer uptake in the right anterior cingulate, both temporal and frontal cortices, and the caudate and thalamic nuclei. Cognitive impairment in some male patients may have led to this pattern of results. Unfortunately, no mention was made of the relationship between rCBF and clinical subtype or Newcastle score, even though this was used. There were no differences between early-onset and late-onset cases but good outcome was possibly related to higher rCBF in the subcortical areas, the right parietal and posterior cingulate cortex.

Reports of rCBF in anxiety disorders are only just emerging. O'Carroll *et al.* (1993) analysed rCBF in ten phobic patients during a relaxation tape and during a taped description of exposure to the feared stimulus. rCBF fell in occipital and posterior temporal regions during the provocation of anxiety. The authors argued that the changes may reflect activation of inhibitory gamma-aminobutyric acid (GABA) receptors which are concentrated in these regions. The results of this study are broadly similar to those from Zohar *et al.* (1989), who found reduced flow in compulsive hand-washers, although Mountz *et al.* (1989) found that reductions in global and regional rCBF disappeared when corrected for associated hypocapnia and hyperventilation. Increased medial frontal rCBF in association with reduced caudate nucleus rCBF has been demonstrated in obsessive–compulsive disorder (Machlin *et al.* 1991; Rubin *et al.* 1992*b*) and depersonalization (Hollander *et al.* 1992) These findings must be set against those of two recent studies (McGuire *et al.* 1994; Rauch *et al.* 1994) which reported changes occurring in rCBF during activation. Patients were scanned at rest and during exposure to anxiety-provoking situations which induced obsessional thoughts. Both studies found that rCBF increased in the right caudate nucleus and right orbitofrontal cortex. McGuire *et al.* (1994) found that additional changes in the right globus pallidus and right thalamus were associated with the urge to perform compulsive movements, while increases in the left hippocampus and left posterior cingulate cortex were associated with anxiety.

Regional cerebral metabolism

Positron emission tomography can be used to study cerebral metabolism *in vivo*, as well as neuroreceptor number and function. Reductions in left frontal metabolism have been demonstrated in a number of studies of unipolar depression (Phelps *et al.* 1984; Baxter *et al.* 1989). These reductions correlated with the severity of depression. Reductions in basal-ganglia and temporal lobe metabolism (Cohen *et al.* 1989) have also been shown. Wu *et al.* (1993) found reduced callosal metabolic activity in depressed patients with a thickened corpus callosum. Results from depressed patients with obsessive–compulsive disorder (Baxter *et al.* 1989) and Parkinson's disease (Mayberg *et al.* 1990) suggest that the left frontal abnormalities are related to low mood *per se*.

Wu *et al.* (1991) have studied fluorine-18-labelled glucose metabolism in patients with generalized anxiety disorder. At rest, absolute metabolic rates were lower in basal ganglia and white matter, but relative rates were increased in the left occipital lobe, right posterior temporal lobe, and precentral frontal gyrus. Activation during an anxiety-provoking vigilance task showed an increase in relative basal-ganglia metabolism, and benzodiazepine administration reduced metabolic rate in cortical, basal ganglia, and limbic areas. Patients given placebo showed correlations between the change in anxiety scores and changes in metabolism in these areas.

Baxter *et al.* (1992) demonstrated abnormalities in caudate-nucleus metabolism in obsessive–compulsive disorder and argued, by analogy with invertebrate physiology, that OCD involves dysfunction in the central serotonergic system. Cortical abnormalities similar to those found in depression have also been reported (Swedo *et al.* 1989).

Summary

The studies reviewed above provide a bewildering array of regional abnormalities, many of which involve regions of the frontal lobes. This is comforting, as these areas are supposed to be involved in the integration of higher brain function. There appear to be differences between affective and anxiety disorders in terms of abnormalities of functional scanning. As imaging methods achieve greater powers of resolution, it is to be hoped that more specific abnormalities or networks of dysfunction will be identified. Unfortunately, the current picture is one of inconsistency and lack of specificity.

NEUROENDOCRINOLOGY

Hypothalamic–pituitary–adrenal (HPA) axis

From modest beginnings in the 1970s, the dexamethasone suppression test (DST) developed from a simple putative diagnostic indicator of melancholia (Carroll 1982) to a means of assessing the integrity of a complex neuro-humoral system which might hold the key to the link between the body's reaction to stressful events and functional and structural brain changes. This is an example of the almost mythical status that neuroendocrine challenge tests have acquired. The relationship between stress, depression, and high basal levels of serum cortisol has long been observed (Cushing 1932), but the DST emerged at a critical moment in the history of psychobiology as a possible objective sign of mental distress. Unfortunately, after more than 20 years of experimentation, it is clear that an abnormal DST response is far from specific to any one psychiatric disorder, and is influenced by diverse factors such as age, cognitive state, and the ability to absorb dexamethasone (Gastpar *et al.* 1992). In elderly patients, McKeith (1984) found that the DST differentiated well between endogenous and non-endogenous depression, but unfortunately abnormal responses were also common in patients with depression and dementia (Katona and Aldridge 1985; Abou-Saleh *et al.* 1987).

The HPA axis may be stimulated artificially by corticotrophin-releasing factor (CRF), which acts directly on the anterior pituitary. In depression, CRF produces a blunted adrenocorticotrophic hormone (ACTH) response in combination with a normal or exaggerated cortisol response (Holsboer 1992). As a result, it has been suggested that raised CRF is the basis for the hypersecretion of cortisol. This is borne out by the increased CRF levels found in the CSF of depressed patients (Nemeroff *et al.* 1988). Von Bardeleben and Holsboer (1991) administered the CRF test to a group of depressed patients after pre-treatment on the previous day with dexamethasone: in normal subjects cortisol response to CRF was inhibited and was not affected by the subjects' age, but in depressed subjects cortisol rose sharply and the magnitude of this effect correlated positively with age and severity of depression. This seemed to indicate that impairment of brain corticosteroid receptors in depression could be accentuated by the ageing process.

The HPA axis is under the control of the noradrenergic system from the brainstem via the ventral noradrenaline bundle (Checkley 1992). It is thought that this pathway is only active under stressful conditions, but other neurotransmitter systems also affect the axis.

Administration of high levels of corticosterone has been found to damage pyramidal neurones in the rat brain (Woolley *et al.* 1990) and primate hippocampus (Sapolsky *et al.* 1990), and adrenalectomy results in a loss of cells from the dentate gyrus. Thus, McEwen *et al.* (1992) have argued that the hippocampus, which contains the highest concentration of type-I corticosteroid receptors, is particularly vulnerable to damage by chronically high levels of circulating cortisol as might be found in depression or chronic stress. In an excellent review of this increasingly complex area, Checkley (1992) placed more emphasis on the role of type-II corticosteroid receptors and argued that antagonists at these sites, such as metyrapone, might offer vulnerable individuals protection against the vicissitudes of adverse life events.

Other neuroendocrine challenges

The thyroid-stimulating hormone (TSH) response to thyrotrophin-releasing hormone (TRH) is usually blunted in depression (Szabadi 1991) and in normal elderly subjects (Targum *et al.* 1992). Maes *et al.* (1989*b*) found that the response was relatively normal in women with minor depression, but Molchan *et al.* (1991) found reduced responses in elderly depressed patients.

Growth-hormone response to clonidine (an α_2 adrenoreceptor agonist) has been reported as blunted in generalized anxiety disorder (Abelson *et al.* 1991), panic disorder (Abelson *et al.* 1992), and depression (Checkley *et al.* 1981). This may indicate a non-specific dysfunction, possibly post-synaptic receptor subsensitivity. On the other hand, it is normal in obsessive–compulsive disorder (Lee *et al.* 1990) and the balance of evidence suggests that dysfunction of the serotonergic system predominates in this condition (Insel 1992).

Melatonin secretion from the pineal gland is under beta-adrenergic control and reaches a peak during the early hours of the morning. Melatonin production falls off with age (Thomas and Miles 1989; Rubin *et al.* 1992*a*) and the peak secretion has been found by some to be reduced in endogenous depression (Thompson *et al.* 1988) but not others (Rubin *et al.* 1992*a*).

NEUROIMMUNOLOGY

It is generally supposed that stress and depression affect the immune system (Fox 1985). However, this view has been challenged on the basis that deaths among particular patient groups and bereaved persons are more often the result of cardiovascular disease than disorders of the immune system (Stein *et al.* 1991). In general, studies of immune function in patients with depression have reached conflicting and inconclusive results (Stein *et al.* 1991). Those few that have focused on older subjects have been more suggestive of a relationship. Schleifer *et al.* (1983) demonstrated significant impairment of lymphocyte function in vitro in a study of men before and after the death of their wives. Similar abnormalities were found in patients suffering from major depressive disorder (Schleifer *et al.* 1984) but were later found to be limited to depressed patients over the age of 60 years (Schleifer *et al.* 1989). Aldwin *et al.* (1991) also reported that older depressed men who had experienced recent adverse life events were more likely to have abnormalities of thymosin-alpha-1 (TA-1), which is required for the differentiation and development of T-cells. Hypercortisolaemia may produce these changes in white-cell function (Lowy *et al.* 1984), and it has been found that this effect may be exaggerated in older patients with melancholia (Maes *et al.* 1989*a*). Spurrell and Creed (1993) have recently demonstrated that while reduced lymphocyte function was associated with high depression scores in bereaved subjects it was associated with low scores in those anticipating bereavement. The inverted U-shaped curve describing the relationship between the two variables in this study may explain some of the inconsistencies found in previous work mentioned above, but it may also reflect the differences between anticipatory stress and reaction to completed events. The observations identifying reduced immunity in mental disorders refer to *in vitro* challenge tests of white-cell function. Their significance for the living human is, surprisingly, still debated (Stein *et al.* 1991).

NEUROBIOLOGICAL MODELS OF NEUROTIC DISORDERS

Model or theory generation is a way of making sense of any collection of data. However, as a general rule the more broad and encompassing such models are, the less they actually explain. The ideal model should generate hypotheses which can be tested and re-tested.

Anxiety and panic disorders

Neuroanatomy

Gray (1982) has hypothesized that the hippocampus, septum, amygdala, and frontal cortex all play a crucial part in the modulation of anxiety. The septo-hippocampal region is linked to the noradrenergic nuclei in the locus coeruleus and the serotonergic centre in the raphe nuclei. The locus coeruleus receives innervation from the peripheral autonomic organs via the solitary nucleus and the medullary chemosensitive area. Essentially, the frontal cortex assesses the danger and the amygdala–septal–hippocampal system generates the fearful emotions. Kalin (1993) has suggested that innervation from the latter areas stimulates the hypothalamus to release CRF, which links into the HPA axis. The system has a feedback loop, since the hippocampus is rich in corticosteroid receptors (see p. 81). Experiments in rhesus monkeys have shown that selective response to fearful stimuli develops at about the time that the formation of synapses in the prefrontal cortex and amygdala reaches a peak (Kalin 1993). The same happens in humans between seven and twelve months, when children begin to show a marked fear of strangers. Perhaps the reverse process occurs as a result of ageing or dementia, leading to increasingly inappropriate fear responses, anxiety and/or panic. George and Ballenger (1992) postulate that the right parahippocampal region acts as an important component of Gray's circuit, and cite evidence to show that lesions or stimulation of any point in the pathway can induce panic attacks.

Neurochemistry

The discovery that panic attacks can be induced in susceptible individuals by chemical means has led to the present focus of research in this disorder. The ability to generate panic symptoms under laboratory conditons has obvious attractions, since physiological and chemical changes occurring during the course of an attack may be investigated under controlled circumstances. Numerous methods of panic induction have been described, and are reviewed by Nutt and Lawson (1992). Most popular is the use of sodium lactate infusions; although the mechanism of action is unknown, bilateral increase in temporal and superior collicular rCBF has been observed on PET (Reiman *et al.* 1989). The possible harmful effects of inducing such attacks probably account for the paucity of studies involving elderly subjects.

Three neurotransmitter systems have been implicated in the pathogenesis of panic: the benzodiazepine, noradrenaline, and serotonin systems. It has been thought that an endogenous ligand that blocks or stimulates the benzodiazepine receptor might be responsible for panic symptoms (Nutt and Lawson 1992). This would have to be released on an intermittent basis, and candidate substances include diazepam-binding inhibitor (DBI), tribulin and desmethyl-diazepam.

Abnormalities of the benzodiazepine receptor have also been hypothesized (Nutt 1990). Chronic benzodiazepine administration produces a shift in receptor function such that the effects of agonists and antagonists become paradoxical; such an alteration could be inherited. Dysfunction of the benzodiazepine / GABA receptor complex has also been considered. Like corticosteroid receptors, benzodiazepine / GABA receptors are concentrated in the hippocampus and the limbic system.

The noradrenaline hypothesis is based on the discovery of raised levels of noradrenaline and its metabolites in the cerebrospinal fluid and peripheral circulation of anxious and panic-disordered patients (Charney *et al.* 1992). In addition, direct stimulation of the locus coeruleus in animals can produce panic-like features (Redmond 1986). Noradrenergic agonists such as yohimbine stimulate the locus coeruleus and can produce anxiety in normal human subjects (Charney *et al.* 1992). Conversely, clonidine, an α_2 agonist, inhibits the locus coeruleus and reduces anxiety (Charney *et al.* 1992) as well as blocking the effects of lactate-induced panic (Coplan *et al.* 1992). Nutt and Lawson (1992) conclude that evidence in this area points to subsensitivity of the post-synaptic α_2 adrenoreceptors.

The serotonin theory derives from the discovery that the 5-hydroxy-tryptamine (5-HT) agonist *m*-chloro-phenyl-piperazine (mCPP) produces anxiety in both panic-disordered patients and normal subjects (Charney *et al.* 1987). Interestingly, this substance has also been tested in patients with Alzheimer's disease and normal elderly controls, and minimal anxiety was observed (Lawlor *et al.* 1989). It is possible that the body becomes less responsive to challenge tests with increasing age. Selective serotonergic re-uptake inhibitors also produce anxiety in the initial stages of use (Cowen 1991). It is thought that 5-HT receptors are initially hypersensitive and then become subsensitive during chronic administration. Buspirone, which has agonist effects on 5-HT_{1A} receptors and reduces anxiety in generalized anxiety disorder, may exacerbate the symptoms of panic disorder, particularly in higher doses (Nutt and Lawson 1992).

Neurotic depression

Despite early studies that reported changes in brainstem serotonergic and noradrenergic activity which might predispose elderly persons to depression (Robinson *et al.* 1972), there has been no confirmation of this finding (Cheetham *et al.* 1991). Frontal-lobe 5-hydroxy-indole-acetic acid (5-HIAA) levels are reduced in elderly depressed patients dying from natural causes (Ferrier and Perry, 1992) but reductions are greater and more consistent in suicide victims (Cheetham *et al.* 1991). Although serotonin receptor binding sites fall in number with age (Sparks 1989), frontal 5-HT_2 receptors may be raised in elderly depressed patients (McKeith *et al.* 1987; Yates *et al.* 1990). Leake *et al.* (1991) suggested that this was due to down-regulation of pre-synaptic receptor sites.

Unfortunately *post mortem* studies such as those cited above concentrate on those with severe depression, often ex-inhabitants of long-stay wards, so that it is unclear what relevance these findings have for neurotic depression. A more detailed account of neurochemical and brain-receptor changes found in major depressive disorder may be found elsewhere (Delgado *et al.* 1992; Ferrier and Perry, 1992).

Goldberg and Huxley (1992) have attempted to integrate the endocrine, immune, and central nervous systems, particularly the limbic-system control of the HPA axis, into a model linking the physical impact of stressful life events and the experience of depression and/or anxiety. Although they abandon the traditional categorical view of mental disorders, their model does have the advantage that it sets up testable hypotheses.

Obsessive–compulsive disorder (OCD)

Certain features of OCD may be seen in brain diseases such as Huntington's chorea, Sydenham's chorea, and lesions of the globus pallidus. All the obsessionally slow OCD patients studied by Hymas *et al.* (1991) had soft neurological signs and demonstrated some features of Parkinson's disease. Limbic leucotomy, involving lesions in the cingulate gyrus and the lower medial quadrant of the orbitofrontal cortex, is used to treat persistent OCD (Freeman 1993) and Gilles de la Tourette syndrome (Sawle *et al.* 1993). Insel (1992) has hypothesised that a functional circuit involving the orbitofrontal cortex, the basal ganglia, the substantia nigra, and the ventrolateral pallidum may be dysfunctional in OCD. In common with other disorders described here, the serotonergic system has been the recent focus for attention (Murphy *et al.* 1989). Indeed, Benkert *et al.* (1993) have suggested abandoning the usual classification of clinical disorders and propose instead a 'serotonin dysfunction syndrome' which embraces the neuroses. This idea is the result of the observed lack of specificity of all the neurotransmitter abnormalities described above, and merely reflects the current practice of attempting to treat every disorder with the same type of drug.

Functional psychiatric disorders following stroke

The onset of depression following cerebrovascular accident is a much-investigated field. Work in this area was stimulated by the Johns Hopkins group (Robinson *et al.* 1983), who found a high prevalence of depressive disorder following stroke. The severity of depression did not correlate with the degree of disability but with nearness of the lesion to the left frontal pole and its size (Robinson *et al.* 1984). Evidence to support the view that depression might be a direct effect of the lesion came from animal studies in which experimental lesions made in corresponding areas of the rat brain produced depressive behaviour (Starkstein and Robinson 1989).

Initial attempts to replicate this finding were unsuccessful (Sinyor *et al.* 1986; Wade *et al.* 1987; Ebrahim *et al.* 1987; House *et al.* 1990), and it was suggested that emotional lability or emotionalism, rather than depression, had been observed (House *et al.* 1989). However, Eastwood *et al.* (1989) and, more recently, Hermann *et al.* (1993) have found supportive evidence for the importance of lesion location, and Sharpe *et al.* (1990) found that severity of depression about two years after the stroke correlated with the size of left-hemisphere lesions. Hermann *et al.* (1993) found that depression scores were higher in patients with non-fluent aphasias, but this only applied to patients tested within three months of their stroke.

The original hypothesis, which referred to cortical lesions, has now been extended as a result of the study of subcortical regions. Starkstein *et al.* (1987) found that lesions of the left basal ganglia were also associated with depression. Furthermore, depressed and non-depressed stroke patients matched for size and location of the cortical lesions were found to be different with regard to the size of the lateral and third ventricles, suggesting that subcortical atrophy might be a necessary associated condition for the development of depression (Starkstein *et al.* 1988). Hermann *et al.* (1993) also found that aphasic patients with major depression had lesions of the basal ganglia and internal capsule as well as the left frontal lobe.

Attention has now turned to post-stroke anxiety disorders. Sharpe *et al.* (1990) found that anxiety scores were correlated with the size of left-hemisphere lesions, but not to their location. Starkstein *et al.* (1990) compared post-stroke patients with major depression and anxiety, anxiety alone, major depression alone, and no psychiatric disorder. The mixed anxiety/depression group had a higher frequency of cortical lesions and the depression-alone group a higher number of subcortical lesions. Lastly, Castillo *et al.* (1993) reported that patients with right-hemisphere lesions were more likely to have pure anxiety states and those with left-hemisphere lesions more likely to have depressive illness (with or without anxiety). These results indicate that while anxiety disorders may well arise from a different pattern of lesions than affective disorders, there is, once more, inconsistency in the detail regarding location.

CONCLUSIONS

As was stated earlier, there has been little research into the biological aspects of neurosis in elderly people, as studies have primarily targeted the seriously depressed or cognitively impaired. Work carried out on younger patients suggests that there are genetic and physiological differences between the affective disorders and the neuroses, and this in itself should stimulate psychogeriatric research in this area. Within the neuroses, it is apparent that obsessive–compulsive disorder may be biologically distinct from other anxiety disorders, although having some genetic factors in common with them. The relative rarity of the condition in late life is also of interest.

Our knowledge of ageing factors in general predicts that the body's response to destabilizing events or physical changes will be dysfunctional, but this may have positive as well as negative aspects. For example, there may be advantages in not perceiving threat, or in responding less swiftly to it. Similarly, the body's homeostatic feedback mechanisms may be sluggish or diminished as a result of reduced receptor sensitivity. On the other hand, the ability to accommodate physical stress reactions, such as increased heart rate, blood pressure, or serum-cortisol level may be reduced and, in the long term, these conditions may be more damaging. What are needed, as the first if imperfect steps, are comparative studies of old and young patients, proceeding to longitudinal studies as advocated by Spurrell and Creed (1993).

Returning to the questions posed in the introduction, it is not yet known whether there are any specific markers of late-life neurosis. However, it is becoming clearer that certain brain lesions increase vulnerability to and precipitate neurotic disorders. As to whether brain ageing *per se* is a risk factor, this can only be determined when there are adequate independent markers of biological age.

REFERENCES

Abas, M. A., Sahakian, B. J., and Levy, R. (1990). Neuropsychological deficits and CT scan changes in elderly depressives. *Psychological Medicine*, **20**, 507–20.

Abelson, J. L., Glitz, D., Cameron, O. G., Lee, M. A., Bronzo, M., and Curtis, G. C. (1991). Blunted growth hormone response to clonidine in patients with generalized anxiety disorder. *Archives of General Psychiatry*, **48**, 57–62.

Abelson, J. L., Glitz, D., Cameron, O. G., Lee, M. A., Bronzo, M., and Curtis, G. C. (1992). Endocrine, cardiovascular and behavioural responses to clonidine in patients with panic disorder. *Biological Psychiatry* **32**, 18–25.

Abou-Saleh, M. T., Spalding, E. M., Kellett, J. M., and Coppen, A. (1987). Dexamethasone suppression test in dementia. *International Journal of Geriatric Psychiatry*, **2**, 59–65.

Aldwin, C. M., Spiro, A., Clark, G., and Hall, N. (1991). Thymic peptides, stress and depressive symptoms in older men: a comparison of different statistical techniques for small samples. *Brain, Behaviour and Immunity*, **5**, 206–18.

Alexopoulos, G. S., Young, R. C., and Shindeldecker, R. D. (1992). Brain computed tomography findings in geriatric depression and primary degenerative dementia. *Biological Psychiatry*, **31**, 591–9.

Amsterdam, J. D., and Mozley, P. D. (1992). Temporal lobe asymmetry with iofetamine (IMP) SPECT imaging in patients with major depression. *Journal of Affective Disorders*, **24**, 43–53.

Andreasen, N. C., Swayze, V., Flaum, M., Alliger, R., and Cohen G. (1990). Ventricular abnormalities in affective disorder: clinical and demographic correlates. *American Journal of Psychiatry*, **147**, 893–900.

Andrews, G., Stewart, G., Allen R., and Henderson, A. S. (1990). The genetics of six neurotic disorders: a twin study. *Journal of Affective Disorders*, **19**, 23–9.

Austin, M.-P., Dougall, N., Ross, M., Murray, C., O'Carroll, R. E., Moffoot, A., et al. (1992). Single photon emission tomography with ⁹⁹mTc-exametazime in major depression and the pattern of brain activity underlying the psychotic/neurotic continuum. *Journal of Affective Disorders*, **26**, 31–44.

Awad, I. A., Speltzer, R. F., Hodak, J. A., Awad, C. A., and Carey, R. (1986a).

Incidental subcortical lesions identified on magnetic resonance imaging in the elderly. I: Correlation with age and cerebrovascular risk factors. *Stroke*, **17**, 1084–9.

Awad, I. A., Johnson, P. C., and Speltzer, R. F. (1986*b*). Incidental subcortical lesions identified on magnetic resonance imaging in the elderly. II: Postmortem correlations. *Stroke*, **17**, 1090–7.

Baffman, B. H., Zimmerman, R. A., Trojanowski, J. Q., Gonatas, N. K., Hickley, W. F., and Schlaepfer, W. W. (1988). Brain MR: pathologic correlation with gross and histopathology. 2. Hyperintense white-matter foci in the elderly. *American Journal of Neuroroentgenology*, **9**, 629–36.

Baldwin, R. C. (1993). Late life depression and structural brain changes: a review of recent magnetic resonance imaging research. *International Journal of Geriatric Psychiatry*, **8**, 115–23.

Baxter, L., Schwartz, J., Phelps, M., Mazziotta, J., Guze, B., Selin, C., *et al.* (1989). Reduction of prefrontal cortex glucose metabolism common to three types of depression. *Archives of General Psychiatry*, **46**, 243–50.

Baxter, L., Schwartz, J., Bergman, K. S., Phelps, M., Guze, B., and Gerner, R. (1992). Caudate glucose metabolic rate changes with both drug and behaviour therapy for obsessive–compulsive disorder. *Archives of General Psychiatry*, **49**, 681–9.

Beats, B., (1991). Structural imaging in affective disorder. *International Journal of Geriatric Psychiatry*, **6**, 419–23.

Beats, B., Levy, R., and Förstl, H. (1991). Ventricular enlargement and caudate hyperdensity in elderly depressives. *Biological Psychiatry*, **30**, 452–8.

Bench, C. J., Friston, K. J., Brown, R. G., Scott, L. C., Frackowiak, R. S. J., and Dolan, R. J. (1992). The anatomy of melancholia—focal abnormalities of cerebral blood flow in major depression. *Psychological Medicine*, **22**, 607–15.

Bench, C. J., Friston, K. J., Brown, R. G., Frackowiak, R. S. J., and Dolan, R. J. (1993). Regional cerebral blood flow in depression, measured by position emission tomography: the relationship with clinical dimensions. *Psychological Medicine*, **23**, 579–90.

Benkert, O., Wetzel, H., and Szegedi, A. (1993). Serotonin dysfunction syndromes: a functional common denominator for classification of depression, anxiety, obsessive–compulsive disorder. *International Clinical Psychopharmacology*, **8**, Supp. 1, 3–14.

Berman, K. F., Doran, A. R., Pickar, D., and Weinberger, D. R. (1993). Is the mechanism of prefrontal hypofunction in depression the same as in schizophrenia? Regional cerebral blood flow during cognitive activation. *British Journal of Psychiatry*, **162**, 183–92.

Bird, J. M., Levy, R., and Jacoby, R. J. (1985). Computed tomography in the elderly. Changes over time in a normal population. *British Journal of Psychiatry*, **147**, 80–5.

Black, D. W., Noyes, R., Goldstein, R. B., and Blum, N. (1992). A family study of obsessive–compulsive disorder. *Archives of General Psychiatry*, **49**, 362–8.

Bouchard, T. J., Lykken, D. T., McGue, M., Segal, N. L., and Tellegen, A. (1990). The Minnesota study of twins reared apart. *Science*, **250**, 223–8.

Carroll, B. J. (1982). The dexamethasone suppression test for melancholia. *British Journal of Psychiatry*, **140**, 292–304.

Castillo, C. S., Starkstein, S. E., Federoff, J. P., Price, T. R., and Robinson, R. G. (1993). Generalised anxiety disorder after stroke. *Journal of Nervous and Mental Diseases*, **181**, 102–8.

Charney, D. S., Woods, S. W., Goodman, W. K., and Heninger, G. R. (1987).

Neurobiological mechanisms of panic anxiety: biochemical and behavioural correlates of yohimbine-induced panic attacks. *American Journal of Psychiatry*, **144**, 1030–6.

Charney, D. S., Woods, S. W., Krystal, J. H., Nagy, L. M., and Heninger, G. R. (1992). Noradrenergic neuronal dysregulation in panic disorder: the effects of intravenous yohimbine and clonidine in panic disorder patients. *Acta Psychiatrica Scandanavica*, **86**, 273–82.

Checkley, S. (1992). Neuroendocrine mechanisms and the precipitation of depression by life events. *British Journal of Psychiatry*, **160**, Supp. 15, 7–17.

Checkley, S. A., Slade, A. P., and Shur, E. (1981). Growth hormone and other responses to clonidine in patients with endogenous depression. *British Journal of Psychiatry*, **138**, 51–5.

Cheetham, S. C., Katona, C. L. E., and Horton, R. W. (1991). Post-mortem studies of neurotransmitter biochemistry in depression and suicide. In *Biological aspects of affective disorders* (ed. R. Horton and C. Katona), pp. 191–222. Academic Press, London.

Churchill, C. M., Priolo, C. V., Nemeroff, C. B., Krishnan, K. R. R., and Breitner, J. C. S. (1991). Occult subcortical magnetic resonance findings in elderly depressives *International Journal of Geriatric Psychiatry*, **6**, 213–16.

Coffey, C. E., Figiel, G. S., Djang, W. T., and Weiner, R. D. (1990). Subcortical hyperintensity on magnetic resonance imaging: a comparison of normal and depressed elderly subjects. *American Journal of Psychiatry*, **147**, 187–9.

Coffey, C. E., Wilkinson, W. E., Weiner, R. D., Parashos, J. A., Djang, W. T., Webb, M. C., *et al.* (1993). Quantitative cerebral anatomy in depression. A controlled magnetic resonance imaging study. *Archives of General Psychiatry*, **50**, 7–16.

Cohen, R., Semple, W., Gross, M., Nordahl, T., King, A. C., Pickar, D., and Post, R. (1989). Evidence for common alterations in cerebral glucose metabolism in major affective disorders and schizophrenia. *Neuropsychopharmacology*, **2**, 241–54.

Coplan, S. P., Davies, S. O., Martinez, R., and Klein, D. F. (1992). Noradrenergic function in panic disorder. Effects of intravenous clonidine pretreatment on lactate induced panic. *Biological Psychiatry*, **31**, 135–46.

Cowen, P. J. (1991). Serotonin receptor subtypes: implications for psychopharmacology. *British Journal of Psychiatry*, **159**, Supp. 12, 7–14.

Crowe, R. R. (1990). Panic disorder: genetic considerations. *Journal of Psychiatry Research*, **24**, 129–34.

Curran, S. M., Murray, C. M., Van Beck, M., Dougall, N., O'Carroll, R. E., Austin, M. P., *et al.* (1993). A single photon emission computerised tomography study of regional brain function in elderly patients with major depression and with Alzheimer-type dementia. *British Journal of Psychiatry*, **163**, 155–65.

Cushing, H. (1932). The basophil adenomas of the pituitary body and their clinical manifestations (pituitary basophilism). *Bulletin of the Johns Hopkins Hospital*, **50**, 137–95.

Delgado, P. L., Price, L. H., Heninger, G. R., and Charney, D. S. (1992). Neurochemistry. In *The handbook of affective disorders* (ed. E. S. Paykel), pp. 267–88. Churchill Livingstone, Edinburgh.

Dolan, R. J., Calloway, S. P., and Mann, A. H. (1985). Cerebral ventricular size in depressed patients. *Psychological Medicine*, **15**, 873–8.

Eastwood, M. R., Rifat, S. L., Nobbs, H., and Ruderman, J. (1989). Mood disorders following cerebrovascular accident. *British Journal of Psychiatry*, **154**, 195–200.

Ebrahim, S., and Nouri, F. (1987). Affective disorder after stroke. *British Journal of Psychiatry*, **151**, 52–6.

Englund, S. A., and Klein, D. N. (1990). The genetics of neurotic-reactive depression: a reanalysis of Shapiro's (1970) twin study using diagnostic criteria. *Journal of Affective Disorders*, **18**, 247–52.

Ferrier, I. N., and Perry, E. K. (1992). Post-mortem studies in affective disorder. *Psychological Medicine*, **22**, 835–8.

Figiel, G. S., Krishnan, K. R. R., Doraiswamy, P. M., Rao, V. P., Nemeroff, C. B., and Boyko, O. B. (1991). Subcortical hyperintensities on brain magnetic resonance imaging: a comparison between late age onset and early onset elderly depressed subjects. *Neurobiology of Aging*, **12**, 245–7.

Fox, R. A. (1985). Immunology of aging. In *Textbook of geriatrics and gerontology* (3rd edn) (ed. J. C. Brocklehurst), pp. 82–104. Churchill Livingstone, Edinburgh.

Freeman, C. P. (1993). ECT and other physical therapies. In *Companion to psychiatric studies* (5th edn) (ed. R. E. Kendell and A. K. Zealley), pp. 847–68. Churchill Livingstone, Edinburgh.

Fyer, A. J., Mannuzza, S., Gallops, M. S., Martin, L. Y., Aaronson, C., Gorman, C., et al. (1990). Familial transmission of simple phobias and fears. *Archives of General Psychiatry*, **47**, 252–6.

Gastpar, M., Gilsdorf, U., Abou-Saleh, M. T., and Ngo-Khac, T. (1992). Clinical correlates of response to DST. The dexamethasone suppression test in depression: a World Health Organization collaborative study. *Journal of Affective Disorders*, **26**, 17–24.

Gatz, M., Pedersen, N. L., Plomin, R., Nesselroade, J. R., and McClearn, G. E. (1992). Importance of shared genes and shared environments for symptoms of depression in older adults. *Journal of Abnormal Psychology*, **101**, 701–8.

George, A. E., de Leon, M. J., Kalnin, A., Rosner, L., Goodgold, A., and Chase, N. (1986). Leukoencephalopathy in normal and pathologic aging. 2: MRI of brain lucencies. *American Journal of Neuroroentgenology*, **7**, 567–70.

George, M. S., and Ballenger, J. C. (1992). The neuroanatomy of panic disorder: the emerging role of the right parahippocampal region. *Journal of Anxiety Disorders*, **6**, 181–8.

Goldberg, D., and Huxley, P. (1992). *Common mental disorders. A biosocial model*, pp. 133–47. Routledge, London.

Goldsmith, H. H., and Gottesman, I. I. (1981). Origins of variation in behavioural style; a longitudinal study of temperament in young twins. *Child Development*, **52**, 91–103.

Gray, J. (1982). *The neuropsychology of anxiety*. Oxford University Press, Oxford.

Gur, R. E., Skolnik, B. E., Gur, R. C., Caroff, S., Rieger, W., Obrist, W. D., et al. (1984). Brain function in psychiatric disorders. II. Regional cerebral blood flow in medicated unipolar depressives. *Archives of General Psychiatry*, **41**, 695–9.

Hermann, M., Bartels, C., and Wallesch, C.-W. (1993). Depression in acute and chronic aphasia: symptoms, pathoanatomical–clinical correlations and functional implications. *Journal of Neurology, Neurosurgery and Psychiatry*, **56**, 672–8.

Hollander, E., Carrasco, J. L., Mullen, L. S., Trungold, S., DeCaria, C. M., and Towey, J. (1992). Left hemisphere activation in depersonalization disorder: a case report. *Biological Psychiatry*, **31**, 1157–62.

Holmes, J. (1993). Neuroses and personality disorders. Editorial overview. *Current Opinion in Psychiatry*, **6**, 177–8.

Holsboer, F. (1992). The hypothalamic–pituitary–adrenocortical system. In *The handbook of affective disorders* (ed. E. S. Paykel), pp. 267–88. Churchill Livingstone, Edinburgh.

Hopkinson, G. (1964). A genetic study of affective illness in patients over 50. *British Journal of Psychiatry*, **110**, 244–54.

House, A., Dennis, M., Molyneux, A., Warlow, C., and Hawton, K. (1989). Emotionalism after stroke. *British Medical Journal*, **298**, 991–4.

House, A., Dennis, M., Warlow, C., Hawton, K., and Molyneux, A. (1990). Mood disorders after stroke and their relation to lesion location—a CT scan study. *Brain*, **113**, 1113–29.

Howard, R. J., Beats, B., Förstl, H., Graves, P., Bingham, J., and Levy, R. (1993). White matter changes in late onset depression: a magnetic resonance imaging study. *International Journal of Geriatric Psychiatry*, **8**, 183–5.

Husain, M. M., McDonald, W. M., Doraiswamy, P. M., Figiel, G. S., Na, C., Escalona, P. R., et al. (1991). A magnetic resonance imaging study of putamen nuclei in major depression. *Psychiatry Research*, **40**, 95–9.

Hymas, N. F., Lees, A. J., Bolton, D., Epps, K., and Head, D. (1991). The neurology of obsessional slowness. *Brain*, **114**, 2203–33.

Insel, T. R. (1992). Neurobiology of obsessive compulsive disorder: a review. *International Clinical Psychopharmacology*, **7**, Supp. 1, 31–33.

Jacoby, R. J., and Levy, R. (1980). Computed tomography in the elderly. 3. Affective disorder. *British Journal of Psychiatry*, **136**, 270–5.

Jacoby, R. J., Levy, R., and Bird, J. M. (1981) Computed tomography and the outcome of affective disorder: a follow-up study of elderly patients. *British Journal of Psychiatry*, **139**, 288–92.

Jacoby, R. J., Dolan, R. J., Levy, R., and Baldy, R. (1983). Quantitative computed tomography in elderly depressed patients. *British Journal of Psychiatry*, **143**, 124–7.

Jernigan, T. L., Archibald, S. L., Berhow, M. T., Sowell, E. R., Foster, D. S., and Hesselink, J. R. (1991). Cerebral structure on MRI. Part I: Localisation of age-related changes. *Biological Psychiatry*, **29**, 55–67.

Johnstone, E. C., Owens, D. G. C., Crow, T. J., Colter, N., Lawton, C. A., Jagoe, R., et al. (1986). Hypothyroidism as a correlate of lateral ventricular enlargement in manic–depressive and neurotic illness. *British Journal of Psychiatry*, **148**, 317–22.

Joyce, E. M. (1991). Cerebral blood flow and metabolism in affective disorders. *International Journal of Geriatric Psychiatry*, **6**, 423–30.

Kalin, N. H. (1993). The neurobiology of fear. *Scientific American*, **268**, 54–60.

Kanaya, T., and Yonekawa, M. (1990). Regional cerebral blood flow in depression. *Japanese Journal of Psychiatry and Neurology*, **44**, 571–6.

Katona, C. L. E., and Aldridge, C. R. (1985). The dexamethasone suppression test and depressive signs in dementia. *Journal of Affective Disorders*, **8**, 83–9.

Kendler, K. S., Kessler, R. C., Heath, A. C., Neale, M. C., and Eaves, L. J. (1991). Coping: a genetic epidemiological investigation. *Psychological Medicine*, **21**, 337–46.

Kendler, K. S., Neale, M. C., Kessler, R. C., Heath, A. C., and Eaves, L. J. (1992). Major depression and generalized anxiety disorder. Same genes, (partly) different environments? *Archives of General Psychiatry*, **49**, 716–22.

Krishnan, K. R. R., Goli, V., Ellinwood, E. H., France, R. D., Blazer, D. G., and Nemeroff, C. B. (1988). Leukoencephalopathy in patients diagnosed as major depressive. *Biological Psychiatry*, **23**, 519–22.

Lawlor, B. A., Sunderland T., Mellow, A. M., Newhouse, P. A., and Murphy, D. L. (1989). A preliminary study of the effects of intravenous *m*-chloro-phenyl-piperazine, a serotonin agonist in elderly subjects. *Biological Psychiatry*, **25**, 679–86.

Leake, A., Fairburn, A. F., McKeith, I. G., and Ferrier, I. N. (1991). Studies on the serotonin uptake binding site in major depressive disorder and control post-mortem brain: neurochemical and clinical correlates. *Psychiatry Research*, **39**, 155–65.

Lee, M. A., Cameron, O. G., Gurguis, G. N., Glitz, D., Smith C. B., Hariharan, M., *et al.* (1990). Alpha-2 adrenoreceptor status in obsessive–compulsive disorder. *Biological Psychiatry*, **27**, 1083–93.

Lesser, I. M., Miller, B. L., Boone, K. B., Hill-Gutierrez, E., Mehringer, C. M., Wong, K., *et al.* (1991). Brain injury and cognitive function in late-onset psychotic depression. *Journal of Neuropsychiatry and Clinical Neuroscience*, **3**, 33–40.

Lowy, M. T., Reder, A. T., Antel, J. P., and Meltzer, H. Y. (1984). Glucocorticoid resistance in depression. The DST and lymphocyte sensitivity to dexamethasone. *American Journal of Psychiatry*, **141**, 1365–8.

Macdonald, A. J. D. (1991). Old age depression and organic brain damage. In *Recent advances in psychogeriatrics 2*, (ed. T. Arie), pp. 45–58. Churchill Livingstone, Edinburgh.

Machlin, S. R., Harris, G. J., Pearlson, G. D., Hoehn-Saric, R., Jeffrey, P., and Camargo, E. E. (1991). Elevated medial–frontal cerebral blood flow in obsessive–compulsive patients: a SPECT study. *American Journal of Psychiatry*, **148**, 1240–2.

Mackinnon, A. J., Henderson, A. S., and Andrews, G. (1990). Genetic and environmental determinants of the lability of trait neuroticism and the symptoms of anxiety and depression. *Psychological Medicine*, **20**, 581–90.

Maes, M., Bosmans, E., Suy, E., Minner, B., and Raus, J. (1989*a*). Impaired lymphocyte stimulation by mitogens in severely depressed patients. A complex interface with HPA-axis hypersecretion, noradrenergic activity and the ageing process. *British Journal of Psychiatry*, **155**, 793–8.

Maes, M., Vandewoude, M., Maues, L., Schotte, C., and Cosyns, P. (1989*b*). A revised interpretation of the TRH test result in female depressed patients. Part 1: TSH responses. Effects of severity of illness, thyroid hormones, monoamines, age, sex hormonal, corticosteroid and nutritional state. *Journal of Affective Disorders*, **16**, 203–13.

Maier, W., Lichtermann, D., Minges, J., Heun, R., Hallmayer, J., and Klinger, T. (1991). Unipolar depression in the aged: determinants of familial aggregation. *Journal of Affective Disorders*, **23**, 53–61.

Marks, I. M. (1986). Genetics of fear and anxiety disorders. *British Journal of Psychiatry*, **149**, 406–18.

Mayberg, H. S., Starkstein, S. E., Sadzot, B., Preziosi, T., Andrezejewski, P. L., Dannals, R. F., *et al.* (1990). Selective hypometabolism in the inferior frontal lobe in depressed patients with Parkinson's disease. *Annals of Neurology*, **28**, 57–64.

McEwen, B. S., Gould, E. A., and Sakai, R. R. (1992). The vulnerability of the hippocampus to protective and destructive effects of glucocorticoids in relation to stress. *British Journal of Psychiatry*, **160**, Supp. 15, 18–24.

McGuffin, P., and Katz, R. (1989). The genetics of depression: current approaches. *British Journal of Psychiatry*, **155**, Supp. 6, 18–26.

McGuire, P. K., Bench, C. J., Frith, C. D., Marks, I. M., Frakowiak, R. S. J., and Dolan, R. J. (1994). Functional anatomy of obsessive-compulsive phenomena. *British Journal of Psychiatry*, **164**, 459–68.

McKeith, I. G. (1984). The clinical use of the DST in a psychogeriatric population. *British Journal of Psychiatry*, **145**, 389–94.

McKeith, I. G., Marshall, E. F., Ferrier, I. N., Armstrong, M. M., Kennedy, W. N., Perry, R. H., *et al.* (1987). 5-HT receptor binding in post-mortem brain from patients with affective disorder. *Journal of Affective Disorders*, **13**, 67–74.

Molchan, S. E., Lawlor, B. A., Hill, J. L., Mellow, A. M., Davis, C. L., Martinez, R., *et al.* (1991). The TRH stimulation test in Alzheimer's disease and major depression: relationship to clinical and CSF measures. *Biological Psychiatry*, **30**, 567–76.

Mountz, J. M., Modell, J. G., Wilson, M. W., Curtis, G. C., Lee, M. A., Schmaltz, S., *et al.* (1989). Positron emission tomographic evaluation of cerebral blood flow during state anxiety in simple phobia. *Archives of General Psychiatry*, **46**, 501–4.

Murphy, D. L., Zohar, J., Benkelfat, C., Pato, M. T., Piggott, T. A., and Insel, T. R., (1989). Obsessive–compulsive disorder as a 5-HT subsystem-related behavioural disorder. *British Journal of Psychiatry*, **155**, Supp. 8, 15–24.

Nemeroff, C. B. (1988). The role of corticotrophin-releasing factor in the pathogenesis of major depression. *Pharmacopsychiatry*, **21**, 76–82.

Nemeroff, C. B., Knight, D. L., Krishnan, R. R., Slotkin, T. A., Bissette, G., Melville, M. L., *et al.* (1988). Marked reduction in the number of platelet-tritiated imipramine binding sites in geriatric depression. *Archives of General Psychiatry*, **45**, 919–23.

Nutt, D. (1990). The neurochemistry of anxiety. *Progress in neuropsychopharmacology and biological psychiatry*, **14**, 737–52.

Nutt, D., and Lawson, C. (1992). Panic attacks. A neurochemical overview of models and mechanisms. *British Journal of Psychiatry*, **160**, 165–78.

O'Carroll, R. E., Moffoot, A. P. R., Van Beck, M., Dougall, N., Murray, C., Ebmeier, K. P., *et al.* (1993). The effect of anxiety induction on the regional uptake of ^{99m}Tc-exametazime in simple phobia as shown by single photon emission tomography (SPET). *Journal of Affective Disorders*, **28**, 203–10.

Pearlson. G. D., Rabins, P. V., Kim, W. S., Speedie, L. J., Moberg, P. J., Burns, A., *et al.* (1989). Structural brain CT changes and cognitive deficits in elderly depressives with and without reversible dementia ('pseudodementia'). *Psychological Medicine*, **19**, 573–84.

Pearlson, G. D., Rabins, P. V., and Burns, A. (1991). Centrum semiovale white matter CT changes associated with normal ageing, Alzheimer's disease and late life depression with and without reversible dementia. *Psychological Medicine*, **21**, 321–8.

Phelps. M. E., Mazziotta, M., Baxter, L., and Gerner, R. (1984). Positron emission tomographic study of affective disorders. Problems and strategies. *Annals of Neurology*, **15**, Supp. 1, 149–156.

Philpot, M. P. (1994). The biology of functional psychiatric disorders. In *Functional psychiatric disorders of the elderly* (ed. E. Chiu and D. Ames), pp. 355–76. Cambridge University Press, Cambridge.

Philpot, M. P., Banerjee, S., Needham-Bennett, H., Costa, D. C., and Ell, P. J. (1993). ^{99m}Tc-HMPAO single photon emission tomography in late life depression: a pilot study of regional cerebral blood flow at rest and during a verbal fluency task. *Journal of Affective Disorders*, **28**, 233–40.

Rabins, P. V., Pearlson, G. D., Aylward, E., Kumar, A. J., and Dowell, K. (1991). Cortical magnetic resonance imaging changes in elderly inpatients with major depression. *American Journal of Psychiatry*, **148**, 617–20.

Rauch, S. L., Jenike, M. A., Alpert, N. M., Baer, L., Breiter, H. C., Sarage, C. R., *et al.* (1994) Regional cerebral blood flow measured during symptom provocation in obsessive-compulsive disorder using oxygen 15-labelled carbon dioxide and positron emission tomography. *Archives of General Psychiatry*, **51**, 62–70.

Redmond, D. E. (1986). The possible role of locus coeruleus noradrenergic activity in anxiety-panic. *Clinical Neuropharmacology*, **9**, Supp. 4, 40–2.

Reiman, E. M., Raichle, M. E., Robins, E., Muntin, M. A., Fusselman, M. J., Fox, P. T., *et al.* (1989). Neuroanatomical correlates of a lactate-induced anxiety attack. *Archives of General Psychiatry*, **46**, 493–500.

Rice, J., Reich, T., Andreasen, N. C., Lavori, P. W., Endicott, J., Clayton, P. J., *et al.* (1984). Sex-related differences in depression. Familial evidence. *Journal of Affective Disorders*, **71**, 199–210.

Robinson, D. S., Davies, J. M., Nies, A., Colburn, R. W., Davis, J. N., Bourne, H. R., *et al.* (1972). Ageing, monoamines and monoamine oxidase levels. *Lancet*, **i**, 290–1.

Robinson, R. G., Starr, L. B., Kubos, K. L., and Price, T. R. (1983). A two-year longitudinal study of post-stroke mood disorders: findings during initial evaluation. *Stroke*, **14**, 736–41.

Robinson, R. G., Kubos, K. L., Starr, L. B., Rao, K., and Price, T. R. (1984). Mood disorders in stroke patients—importance of location of lesion. *Brain*, **107**, 81–93.

Rosenberg, R., Vorstrup, S., Anderson A., and Bolwing, T. (1988). Effects of ECT on cerebral blood flow in melancholia assessed with SPECT. *Convulsive Therapy*, **4**, 62–73.

Rubin, R. T., Heist, E. K., McGeoy, S. S., Hanada, K., and Lesser, I. M. (1992*a*). Neuroendocrine aspects of primary endogenous depression. XI. Serum melatonin measures in patients and matched control subjects. *Archives of General Psychiatry*, **49**, 558–67.

Rubin, R. T., Villanueva-Meyer, J., Anath, J., Trajmar, P. G., and Mena, I. (1992*b*). Regional xenon[133] cerebral blood flow and cerebral technetium[99m] HMPAO uptake in unmedicated patients with obsessive–compulsive disorder and matched control subjects: determination by high-resolution single-photon emission computed tomography. *Archives of General Psychiatry*, **49**, 695–702.

Sackeim, H. A., Prohovnik, I., Moeller, J. R., Brown, R. P., Apter, S., Prudic, J., *et al.* (1990). Regional cerebral blood flow in mood disorders: I. Comparison of major depressives and normal controls at rest. *Archives of General Psychiatry*, **47**, 60–70.

Sapolsky, R. M., Hideo, U., Rebert, C. S., and Finch, C. E. (1990). Hippocampal damage associated with prolonged glucocorticoid exposure in primates. *Journal of Neuroscience*, **10**, 2897–902.

Sawle, G. V., Lees, A. J., Hymas, N. F., Brooks, D. J., and Frackowiak, R. S. J. (1993). The metabolic effects of limbic leucotomy in Gilles de la Tourette syndrome. *Journal of Neurology, Neurosurgery and Psychiatry*, **56**, 1016–19.

Schlegel, S., and Kretschmer, K. (1987*a*). Computed tomography in affective disorders. Part I: Ventricular and sulcal measurements. *Biological Psychiatry*, **22**, 4–14.

Schlegel, S., and Kretschmer, K. (1987*b*). Computed tomography in affective disorders. Part II: Brain density. *Biological Psychiatry*, **22**, 15–23.

Schlegel, S., Aldenhoff, J. B., Eissner, D., Lindner, P., and Nickel, O. (1989). Regional cerebral blood flow in depression: association with psychopathology. *Journal of Affective Disorders*, **17**, 211–18.

Schleifer, S. J., Keller, S. E., Camerino, M., Thorton, J. C., and Stein, M. (1983). Suppression of lymphocyte stimulation following bereavement. *Journal of the American Medical Association*, **250**, 374–7.

Schleifer, S. J., Keller, S. E., Meyerson, A. T., Raskin, M. J., Davis, K. L., and Stein,

M. (1984). Lymphocyte function in major depressive disorder. *Archives of General Psychiatry*, **41**, 484–6.

Schleifer, S. J., Keller, S. E., Bond, R. N., Cohen, J., and Stein, M. (1989). Major depressive disorder and immunity. Role of age, sex, severity and hospitalisation. *Archives of General Psychiatry*, **46**, 81–7.

Scott, M. L., Golden, C. J., Ruedrich, S. L., and Bishop, R. J. (1983). Ventricular enlargement in major depression. *Psychiatry Research*, **8**, 91–3.

Shapiro, R. W. (1970). A twin study of non-endogenous depression. *Acta Jutlandica*, **42**, 2.

Sharpe, M., Hawton, K., House, A., Molyneux, A., Sandercock, P., Bamford, J., *et al.* (1990). Mood disorders in long-term survivors of stroke: associations with brain lesion location and volume. *Psychological Medicine*, **20**, 815–28.

Silfverskiold, P., and Risberg, J. (1989). Regional cerebral blood flow in depression and mania. *Archives of General Psychiatry*, **46**, 253–9.

Sinyor, D., Amato, P., Kaloupek, D. G., Becker, R., Goldenberg, M., and Coopersmith, H. (1986). Post-stroke depression: relationship to functional impairment, coping strategies and rehabilitation outcome. *Stroke*, **17**, 1102–7.

Sparks, L. D. (1989). Ageing and Alzheimer's disease. Altered cortical serotonergic binding. *Archives of Neurology*, **46**, 138–40.

Spurrell, M. T., and Creed, F. H. (1993). Lymphocyte response in depressed patients and subjects anticipating bereavement. *British Journal of Psychiatry*, **162**, 60–4.

Starkstein, S. E., and Robinson, R. G. (1989). Affective disorders and cerebral vascular disease. *British Journal of Psychiatry*, **154**, 170–82.

Starkstein, S. E., Robinson, R. G., and Price, T. R. (1987). Comparison of cortical and subcortical lesions in the production of post-stroke mood disorders. *Brain*, **110**, 1045–59.

Starkstein, S. E., Robinson, R. G., and Price, T. R. (1988). Comparison of patients with and without poststroke major depression matched for size and location of lesion. *Archives of General Psychiatry*, **45**, 247–52.

Starkstein, S. E., Cohen, B. S., Federoff, P., Parikh, R. M., Price, T. R., and Robinson, R. G. (1990). Relationship between anxiety disorders and depressive disorders in patients with cerebrovascular injury. *Archives of General Psychiatry*, **47**, 246–51.

Stein, M., Miller, A. H., and Trestman, R. L. (1991). Depression, the immune system and health and illness. Findings in search of a meaning. *Archives of General Psychiatry*, **48**, 257–63.

Swedo, S. E., Schapiro, M. B., Grady, C. L., Cheslow, D. L., Leonard, H. L., Kumar, A., *et al.* (1989). Cerebral glucose metabolism in childhood-onset obsessive–compulsive disorder. *Archives of General Psychiatry*, **46**, 518–23.

Szabadi, E. (1991). Thyroid dysfunction and affective illness. *British Medical Journal*, **302**, 923–4.

Targum, S. D., Rosen, L. N., Delisi, L. E., Weinberger, D. R., and Citrin, C. M. (1983). Cerebral ventricular size in major depressive disorder: association with delusional symptoms. *Biological Psychiatry*, **18**, 329–36.

Targum, S. D., Marshall, L. E., and Fishman, P. (1992). Variability of TRH test response in depressed and normal elderly subjects. *Biological Psychiatry*, **31**, 787–93.

Thomas, D. R., and Miles, A. (1989). Melatonin secretion and age. *Biological Psychiatry*, **25**, 365–7.

Thompson, C., Franey, C., Arendt, J., and Checkley, S. A. (1988). A comparison of melatonin secretion in depressed patients and normal subjects. *British Journal of Psychiatry*, **152**, 260–5.

Torgersen, S. (1983). Genetics of neurosis: the effects of sampling variation upon the twin concordance ratio. *British Journal of Psychiatry*, **142**, 126–32.

Torgersen, S. (1986). Genetic factors in moderately severe and mild affective disorders. *Archives of General Psychiatry*, **43**, 222–6.

Torgersen, S. (1990). Comorbidity of major depression and anxiety disorders in twin pairs. *American Journal of Psychiatry*, **147**, 1199–202.

Upadhyaya, A. K., Abou-Saleh, M. T., Wilson, K., Grime, S. J., and Critchley, M. (1990). A study of depression in old age using single-photon emission computerised tomography. *British Journal of Psychiatry*, **157**, Supp. 9, 76–81.

Von Bardeleben, U., and Holsboer, F. (1991). Effects of age on the cortisol response to human corticotrophin-releasing hormone in depressed patients pretreated with dexamethasone. *Biological Psychiatry*, **29**, 1042–50.

Wade, D. T., Leigh-Smith, J. E., and Hewer, R. A. (1987). Depressed mood after stroke: a community study of its frequency. *British Journal of Psychiatry*, **151**, 200–5.

Winokur, G., and Coryell, W. (1992). Familial subtypes of unipolar depression: a prospective study of familial pure depressive disease compared to depression spectrum disease. *Biological Psychiatry*, **32**, 1012–18.

Woolley, C., Gould, C., and McEwen, B. S. (1990). Exposure to excess glucocorticoids alters dendritic morphology of adult hippocampal pyramidal neurons. *Brain Research*, **531**, 225–31.

Wu, J. C., Buchsbaum, M. S., Hershey, T. G., Hazlett, E., Sicotte, N., and Johnson, J. C. (1991). PET in generalised anxiety disorder. *Biological Psychiatry*, **29**, 1181–199.

Wu, J. C., Buchsbaum, M. S., Johnson, J. C., Hershey, T. G., Wagner, E. A., Teng, C., *et al.* (1993). Magnetic resonance and positron emission tomography imaging of the corpus callosum: size, shape and metabolic rate in unipolar depression. *Journal of Affective Disorders*, **28**, 15–25.

Yates, M., Leake, A., Candy, J. M., Fairburn, A. F., McKeith, I. G., and Ferrier, I. N. (1990). 5-HT$_2$ receptor changes in major depression. *Biological Psychiatry*, **27**, 489–96.

Zohar, J., Insel, T. R., Berman, K. F., Foa, E. B., Hill, J. L., and Weinberger, D. R. (1989). Anxiety and cerebral blood flow during behavioural challenge. *Archives of General Psychiatry*, **46**, 505–10.

Zubenko, G. S., Sullivan, P., Nelson, J. P., Belle, S. H., Huff, J., and Wolf, G. L. (1990). Brain imaging abnormalities in mental disorders of late life. *Archives of Neurology*, **47**, 1107–11.

6

Psychological treatments I: Behavioural and cognitive approaches
R. T. WOODS

INTRODUCTION

Cognitive behaviour therapy (CBT), in a variety of manifestations, has become established as a major treatment approach for the range of neurotic disorders in adults. Arguably, for a number of conditions—such as phobias, obsessive–compulsive disorders (OCD), and panic—it is the treatment strategy of choice. Given the possible harmful effects of some of the pharmacological alternatives, it is perhaps surprising that CBT has not been used more widely with older adults presenting with similar difficulties. The major reason for this comparative neglect is almost certainly the ageism of service providers, who have focused their efforts on younger adults. Furthermore, the current generation of older people lacks familiarity with psychological treatment and continues with an expectation of receiving medication for psychological difficulties, and little has been done to modify these assumptions. The tendency to view phobic anxiety, for which the earliest effective behavioural treatments were developed, as a symptom of depression in older people has also not been helpful in this respect.

CBT brings together the behavioural and cognitive approaches, which probably were never really applied in isolation. Behaviour therapy has its roots in learning-theory concepts of conditioning, avoidance, and reinforcement; cognitive therapy addresses the role of thought processes in the development and maintenance of this learning, drawing attention to the importance of the person's attributions, catastrophic thinking, assumptions—about themselves, the world, and the future—and of the ways in which the person's thoughts can distort their perceptions. Together they offer a developing repertoire of techniques but—more importantly—a powerful means of conceptualizing the person's difficulties, leading to an individual treatment plan. The emphasis in this chapter is on the adaptations and special considerations that might be required with older people in the application of CBT. Readers requiring fuller details of the CBT approach are referred to texts such as Williams (1992) and Hawton *et al.* (1989).

The impact of physical health and sensory loss in this age group is perhaps the major reason for adaptations being required. CBT has an emphasis on tasks, homework, and increased activity; the person's health clearly will place constraints on what they can manage, and on the pace of the therapy. Sensory difficulties will require careful attention to individualizing written information, supplying audio-tapes, and ensuring that this does not become a barrier. Like physical disability, sensory loss may place limits on what goals can be achieved, or entail the identification of alternative strategies for reaching the desired ends. Therapists sometimes have difficulty in establishing whether there is a physical cause for the person's symptoms. Close collaboration with a physician experienced with the less specific presentations of physical illness in older people is invaluable. However, even when all the tests are negative, experience suggests that the patient may still be right, and a confrontational approach is seldom helpful.

Cumulative losses must also be recognized. For some older people it becomes difficult to distinguish what is a normal reaction to loss, an experience of low morale as opposed to depression. When there are limited opportunities for new activities and meaningful relationships, and when the compensatory strategies that are recommended seem woefully inadequate, the CBT therapist may experience hopelessness also. Thus an elderly widow, who has no children living near and is too frail to go out alone may be taken to a day-centre once a week because she is 'lonely'. There she is sat between a lady who is deaf and another who is pleasantly confused; her isolation is not helped; her loneliness in any case reflects a lack of deep, intimate contact, not superficial chat. The hope for the CBT therapist is that, while difficult life circumstances are associated with depression, alone they are not sufficient to cause it. A number of older people have such difficulties and are not depressed; they differ from their depressed contemporaries in not having negative cognitions (Lam *et al.* 1987), suggesting that it may be the attributions regarding the adversity that are the key to depression, and which are therefore the interest of CBT. There are no easy answers to such adversity, but there is ample scope for more creative responses than older people with depression so often currently receive.

It has been suggested that the normal cognitive changes with ageing may present problems for cognitive therapy, which requires abstract thinking (Church 1983). It should be noted that there is wide diversity in rates of change of cognitive function in late life, with most decline in those with health problems of various kinds (Holland and Rabbitt 1991). What is needed is an individualized approach, checking at each stage that the person has understood what is expected— having them repeat back instructions, and taking away details of home-work tasks in writing if remembering them seems a problem. Some patients do respond better to a more active, behavioural approach; others are able to focus more on automatic thoughts and their association with mood or anxiety. Flexibil-ity is thus needed, with a wide range of abilities and styles being encountered.

ASSESSMENT

The core of assessment for CBT is a thorough, careful description of the presenting problem: its nature, frequency, history, and previous attempts at change, in the context of the patient's personal, medical, and social history. In some cases, of course, the problem initially presented is not that which eventually becomes the focus of therapy, and the history-taking process involves clarifying issues for both therapist and patient.

The next stage is to look in even more detail at the problem behaviour. This may involve a behavioural test, for the therapist to see the difficulty in action, or detailed record keeping, examining the *antecedents* of each occurrence, the *behaviour* that actually occurred, and the resulting *consequences* (the ABC model). In an in-patient setting, where a patient is showing behavioural disturbances arising from anxiety or depression, care staff would be asked similarly to chart the problem in this format. The person may be set a homework task of identifying and writing down thoughts associated with the occurrence of the behaviour, or to keep a diary charting their mood in relation to their activity and thoughts. For a problem such as panic attacks, the aim will be to obtain a baseline estimate for the frequency of attacks, as well as to begin to gather data for a formulation of the factors leading to and maintaining the attacks. In a case of depression, the aim at this stage may be to chart variations in mood, to begin to draw links between thoughts, activity, and mood, and to identify environmental factors that might be contributing.

Standardized assessment procedures have been used more routinely in depression than anxiety. The Beck Depression Inventory (BDI—reproduced in Williams (1992)) is the standard self-report measure of depressed mood used in CBT with younger patients, and is often used to monitor progress in therapy and as an outcome measure. Reliability and some normative data for older people are provided by Gallagher *et al.* (1982). Its response format, involving choice of one of four options for each item, can be difficult for some, and concern is often expressed about items in such scales tapping somatic symptoms that may not be good indicators of depression in older people (e.g. poor sleep, tiredness). Alternative self-report scales have been devised, most notably the Geriatric Depression Scale (GDS—Yesavage *et al.* (1983)), with each item simply answered 'yes' or 'no', and the 12-item SELFCARE (D) scale (Bird *et al.* 1987). Scales have also been devised to tap other areas of interest to the cognitive therapist, such as the Automatic Thought Questionnaire, the Dysfunctional Attitude Scale, and the Hopelessness Scale (see Williams 1992). These scales were used by Lam *et al.* (1987), who provide data on elderly depressed and non-depressed subjects, but these will probably be of more use in a research than a clinical context with older people.

PHOBIC AND OBSESSIVE–COMPULSIVE DISORDERS

There are surprisingly few reports of psychological therapy for older people experiencing phobias, given the effectiveness of these approaches and the proportion of older people (perhaps 10 per cent (Lindesay *et al.* 1989)) experiencing them. Most are single-case reports, e.g. fear of going out (Woods and Britton 1985) or fear of dogs (Thyer 1981), and larger studies tend to involve elderly people in institutions with fears of aspects of institutional life such as using lifts (Hussian 1981) or being raised on a hoist and lowered into a whirlpool bath (Downs *et al.* 1988). Experience would suggest that graded exposure can be a helpful procedure, especially when combined with the person learning skills to monitor and control their anxiety level, using relaxation and breathing procedures, distraction, or positive coping self-talk. Graded exposure involves working up a hierarchy of gradually more feared situations, coping with and mastering each before moving on to the next; a patient with a fear of going out would simply stand at the door, then go a few feet, then a little further. Each step is under the person's control; homework tasks to consolidate progress made in sessions would be an important treatment component. Few therapists would attempt flooding with an elderly patient; this involves exposing the person directly to the feared stimulus, and remaining in the feared situation until the anxiety subsides, and there is a concern that the high levels of arousal that might be generated could be counter-productive. However, there is a dearth of research addressing such technical issues with older populations. It should be noted that the behavioural focus of these approaches does not detract from the importance of cognitive processes; a recent patient, treated for a fear of falling after recovery from a hip-replacement operation, was maintaining her anxiety by thinking, 'I'm going to fall, I'm going to fall,' whenever a piece of furniture or other safe object was out of reach. During the process of graded exposure she learned to distract herself from this thought, and, as her range of walking successfully increased, was able to dispense with it.

Obsessive–compulsive disorder (OCD) is relatively rarely encountered in older people. Effective treatment procedures have been developed with younger patients; response prevention, for example, would be worth attempting with an elderly person with compulsive behaviour. Obsessional ruminations—such as thinking about blaspheming or killing babies—are difficult to treat, but some success has been achieved with repeatedly exposing the person to the rumination. The rationale here is that it is removing the thought that reduces anxiety and so maintains the rumination, which becomes linked with anxiety relief. Habituating to the rumination may break the paradoxically rewarding sequence of mental events.

PANIC AND GENERALIZED ANXIETY

The best documented account to date of CBT with elderly patients suffering from generalized anxiety and panic is provided by King and Barrowclough (1991), who report a series of ten cases with a mean age of 73 years (range 66–78). All ten patients had a diagnosis including panic (five) or generalized anxiety disorder (two) or both (three). Seven also were judged to have depression, two of these also showing hypochondriasis. Six showed evidence of agoraphobia. Three had significant medical conditions. Seven of the patients had previously been treated with benzodiazepines or antidepressants with no effect. All lived in the community. They were seen for an average of eight sessions.

The crux of the CBT view of panic is the notion of a 'catastrophic cognition'. This occurs when the person believes they are experiencing a life-threatening illness or disastrous event, such as a heart attack, inability to breathe, a collapse, a loss of control, or death. Often this occurs in the context of hyperventilation, which produces a number of physical sensations that are open to such misinterpretations: dizziness, tremor, chest pain, and nausea. In essence, the treatment involves helping the patient re-interpret the symptoms experienced as non-threatening, so that the catastrophic cognition can be challenged and its power diminished. In the King and Barrowclough study (1991), the procedures adopted to achieve this included identification of thoughts and behaviour (including avoidance) leading to anxiety, both during sessions and through homework tasks; reattributions were encouraged using cognitive restructuring procedures, involving self-monitoring and behavioural experiments, and techniques such as controlled breathing to reduce the effects of hyperventilation.

The outcome for these ten patients was encouraging. All but one showed a decrease in symptoms following intervention, and these improvements were generally maintained at follow-up 3 to 6 months post-treatment, with eight patients showing no symptoms at all at that stage. A number of patients showed improvement post-treatment on standardized measures (the Beck Anxiety and Depression Inventories); five of the seven patients who were initially depressed moved into the non-depressed range post-treatment, supporting the utility of this approach even where depression is also present. This approach also has much to commend it where hypochondriasis is the major presenting problem; while such patients will, of course, resist any suggestion that 'it's all in the mind', many are able to accept that anxiety-reduction procedures may be helpful in coping with any symptom, pain or discomfort that is being experienced—as indeed health psychology has demonstrated in a variety of health problems.

Holden (1988) describes in more detail approaches to helping patients reduce hyperventilation. These include the provocation test, which is used routinely with younger patients; here the person is encouraged to hyperventilate under controlled conditions with the aim of helping them experience the link between their symptoms and their breathing. Holden warns that this should be used cautiously with older patients, and recommends the use of controlled breathing procedures.

Ost (1992) reports a case of 'choking phobia', where a 68-year-old woman could not swallow fluids for fear that she would get water into her windpipe and accordingly (her catastrophic misconception) suffocate and die. An exposure and modelling approach was attempted first, with only limited effects. Only when the catastrophic cognition was targeted, through educational input and behavioural experiments, was there a dramatic change in the patient's fluid consumption, maintained at one year follow-up.

In relation to general anxiety, Arena *et al.* (1988) have demonstrated the effectiveness of relaxation therapy for long-standing tension headache in older people, aged 62 to 80 years. Therapy consisted of seven sessions of progressive muscle relaxation training; over half the subjects taking medication were able to reduce the amount used.

Finally, Shapiro (1989) has described an interesting technique of 'eye movement desensitization' in the treatment of post-traumatic stress disorder in a 63-year-old woman. This involves eliciting from patients a series of rhythmic saccadic eye movements while they visualize the traumatic scene and rehearse the negative cognitions associated with it. The technique has yet to be fully and formally evaluated, but in individual cases it is reported to result in very rapid and lasting reduction in anxiety, flashbacks, and intrusive thoughts associated with memory of the trauma. The mechanism underlying this remarkable strategy is not known.

COGNITIVE BEHAVIOUR THERAPY FOR DEPRESSION

The most systematic work in this area has been reported by Gallagher and Thompson and their colleagues. Their treatment approach is well described in Thompson *et al.* (1986). The link between mood and thought is the focus of the approach. In a collaborative relationship with the therapist, the patient is encouraged to become aware of automatic thoughts—negative cognitions that feed into the depressed mood, such as 'I'm useless; I can't do anything right.' A number of thought patterns may be identified that systematically distort the person's view of themselves, the world, and their future; these may include over-generalizing from one instance to all situations, attending specifically to the negative aspects of a situation, and ignoring positive aspects and misattributing events to reflect badly upon themselves. So for example, a patient goes out for the first time again to the local shop; a neighbour passes in the street, and, in a hurry, does not acknowledge the patient who reports back: 'It was a complete disaster; my neighbour ignored me because I'm such an awful person; no one ever takes any notice of me.' Bringing these thoughts into awareness allows them to be evaluated and in some cases tested out. The person's assumptions, or schemata, which underlie these thought patterns need also to be identified, and reappraised in relation to their current utility.

The behavioural approach used by this group involves assisting the person to become more active and involved in activities they find enjoyable, on the basis that depression is associated with reduced levels of reinforcement. In clinical practice such activation would be part of the overall CBT package, with the associated cognitions providing rich material for discussion. However, in a series of outcome studies with elderly depressed out-patients, cognitive, behavioural, and brief psychotherapy approaches have been compared with a waiting-list control group (Thompson *et al.* 1987). The key finding is that all three treatment modalities performed equally well, with identical outcomes at up to 2 years follow-up. Therapy consisted of 16–20 individual sessions, over a 4 month period. Over half the 91 patients involved became non-depressed post-treatment and, in all, 70 per cent showed substantial improvement. At 2 years follow-up 70 per cent were not at all depressed (Gallagher-Thompson *et al.* 1990).

The absence of differences in outcome may indicate that despite the apparent differences in style, approach, and technique, they are working in similar ways. Gallagher-Thompson *et al.* (1990) suggest that the common theme is in encouraging patients to take greater control over emotions and activities, perhaps leading to a greater sense of self-efficacy, and Whitehead (1991) similarly points to the importance of perceived control for psychological well-being. However, there are suggestions that there may be individual differences in the amount of control that is desired, and this is clearly an area where further work is required (Reich and Zautra 1990). To date, a comparison of psychological therapies and antidepressant medication has not been reported in the elderly; it would also be of interest to have information on whether their combined use has any beneficial effect compared with their use separately.

Identifying patients who will respond more or less well to a particular therapy is of some importance. In the Thompson *et al.* (1987) study, those showing a good response initially were those with the best outcome at follow-up. Non-responders received a variety of therapies, including medication, in the intervening period, with little overall effect. Patients with coexisting personality disorder have been reported to have poorer outcomes (Thompson *et al.* 1988; Leung and Orrell 1993); there is certainly scope for developing with older people strategies for treating such difficulties. Although the presence of endogenous symptoms initially is associated with poorer outcome (Gallagher and Thompson 1983), one-third of the endogenous-depression group in this study did recover from their depression following treatment, and many others showed notable improvements.

BEREAVEMENT AND LOSS

Some care needs to be taken to avoid the assumption that bereavement is always a problem requiring *treatment*, rather than a natural process of adjustment. Many would agree that interventions should be reserved for those going through an abnormal or difficult grief reaction, but there are problems in identification of such cases, in view of the large variability in normal grief reactions (defined as those that resolve without intervention). Passage of time is not a wholly reliable guide, although many clinicians have rules of thumb that need to be used cautiously; after six months or a year, say, some easing of grief might be expected. Diagnosis of a psychiatric condition may be problematic, as normal bereavement reactions have many features in common with depression, such as dysphoria, tearfulness and difficulty sleeping, and may also include hallucinatory experiences, perhaps seeing the dead person in the familiar places of the home. Even the continuing avoidance of talking about the loss, of entering the process of grief work, which many would see as a sign of impending difficulty, has been suggested to be part of normal variation, and for some a healthy way of coping (Stroebe and Stroebe 1991).

Assessment for intervention needs therefore to take into account a number of factors, including the amount of time that has elapsed, what change there has been already, the person's habitual style of coping with problems, and the impact on the person's basic survival functioning. In addition are those risk factors for difficult grief reactions identified by Parkes (1980): a particularly traumatic or unexpected death, lack of social/family supporters in whom the person can confide, an ambivalent relationship with the person who has died and multiple losses. In the context of older people specifically, these may be elaborated to include relationships where the couple were completely enmeshed ('We lived for each other, did everything together; we never needed anyone else'); where the death was untimely, such as the loss of their adult child or even grandchild; or where the death followed a long period of debilitating illness in the person, for whom they acted as a care-giver. In contrast with younger people, older people generally do not benefit from the anticipatory grieving such a situation allows, perhaps in view of the stresses of the care-giving role, and perhaps because the death is seen as 'timely' in an older person whether or not it is specifically anticipated.

Kavanagh (1990) outlines possible interventions in a CBT framework. Where avoidance is seen as a key part of the difficulty, when all reminders of the dead person are avoided, but the person does not wish to maintain this as a strategy, gradual exposure to bereavement-related cues in a safe, supported environment is recommended. With one patient this process of guided mourning began with looking at photographs of the couple together, supporting her as she cried, and eventually visiting the cemetery, as she learned that she could express her emotions without being completely overwhelmed.

A second strategy involves beginning to take up roles and activities once again; this is especially difficult for someone who did everything with his/her spouse and feels incompetent alone. Where roles within a relationship have been fairly rigid, learning of new skills may be needed in order to develop an independent lifestyle, whether it be learning to cook or to manage finances. The role of the therapist is to help the patient develop strategies for problem-solving, identifying goals for change and ways of breaking down each goal into manageable tasks—beginning with steps the person feels able to tackle immediately. Some steps may involve negotiation with other family members, who may have become involved in the aftermath of the bereavement, but who may need to gradually withdraw their input alongside the person's increased activity, to ensure that unnecessary dependency is not reinforced.

The third aspect of therapy is assisting the person to identify sources of social support, in part to compensate for that which has been lost, in part recognizing the protective effects it may have. Again this needs to be seen in the context of the family; their immediate response may have been such that the person feels no need of additional social contact and support, but the family may have intended this level of input to be purely temporary. Building up new contacts, developing friendships, joining new groups are not easy tasks for an elderly person on their own, and again a problem-solving approach may help in tackling this.

Kavanagh's fourth suggested strategy involves the use of cognitive therapy techniques for evaluating with the person excessively negative cognitions. Amongst these may be thoughts involving guilt and self-blame: 'If only I had . . .' The person is invited to examine these thoughts and the evidence for them; sometimes it is helpful to ask the person how the person who has died would answer these thoughts; this can assist the process of the person letting go of these troubling cognitions. Sometimes, the person may be ignoring those positive aspects that do remain; becoming aware of these again may be helpful in achieving a more balanced view of what has been lost.

Bereavement is of course not the only form of loss, and many older people must also cope with losses of physical health and function. Where these losses are associated with depression and anxiety, acknowledging the extent of what has been lost is a necessary first step before the person can begin to move on to develop compensatory strategies, finding ways around the problem or identifying alternative ways of achieving enjoyment and pleasure. Denial of the loss may well not be a sustainable strategy in this context, and emotional processing of what has to be borne is then unavoidable. The ease with which some older people seem to be able to make adjustments should not obscure the real difficulties involved in changing lifelong patterns. For example, a person who develops a difficulty with mobility may be reluctant to be seen using a walking-aid, and so stops going out; they might be encouraged to evaluate whether other people's reactions are more important than their own pleasure, and to check out whether their perception of those reactions is in fact accurate.

For some patients, the extent of the health problems or disabilities is such that finding alternative ways of responding is a great challenge. In such instances, treatment has to start from a recognition of the depth of the person's loss, and then in collaboration with the person, seek to identify the coping resources and strengths the person has brought with them to this phase of life. One effective way of doing this might be through the process of structured evaluative life review, where the therapist assists the person in re-evaluating the experiences of the person over their life span (Haight and Dias 1992). Drawing up a life chart and/or a genogram is often helpful in this process. This approach should be differentiated from 'reminiscence therapy', which may involve the recounting of past memories in a more random fashion, with less emphasis on appraising the meaning of the experience in the context of the person's whole life.

RELATIONSHIP PROBLEMS

Even when the person is being seen individually, maintaining a view of the person in his/her social network is vital in identifying resources that can assist the person's progress, as well as those relationships that are perhaps contributing to the maintenance of the difficulties. The initial assessment should include consideration of the key relationships in the person's life, but the full picture may not emerge until later in the course of therapy— perhaps on a home visit. If the patient is living with a partner it is often worthwhile to see the other person, with the patient's permission, fairly soon to obtain a broader view of the difficulties the patient is experiencing. Where the couple have a generally positive communication system, the partner may become involved in therapy, encouraging the person in identifying and carrying out homework tasks, and ensuring that the person has opportunities to exercise control in areas of day-to-day life where this has been relinquished though anxiety or depression.

Where the relationship is more strained, and appears to be contributing to the patient's difficulties, it may be appropriate to seek to work directly on the relationship issues. The timing of this work will need to be considered carefully; for example, if the patient is receiving in-patient care for severe depression, the relationship work may best be tackled when the person has begun to recover and plans for the return home are being considered. With a less severely depressed out-patient, work on relationships may be an immediate priority. It is essential to gain the relative's co-operation with attending and participating in sessions; a non-judgemental approach and a willingness to listen to the relative's perspective will be helpful here. Relatives may readily feel blamed if suggestions are made immediately that they should behave differently or respond in a new way to the anxious or depressed person. The problems may well have had a considerable, unwanted impact on their lives also, and this should be acknowledged.

Behavioural couple therapy has as a key component the aim of improving communication; simple, but effective, procedures such as asking each person to allow the other to speak uninterrupted, and listening to each other's point of view are a useful starting point. Each is encouraged to take responsibility for their own feelings for example, 'You make me so angry when . . .' becomes 'I feel so angry when you . . .' Positive aspects of the relationship and of each person are elicited alongside mutual complaints. Agreeing a contract based on mutual exchanges is another strategy: 'If you come shopping with me, I won't complain when you go to Bingo.' This may be particularly useful when there seems to be a pattern of turn-taking in terms of who presents as unwell; for instance, when, as one recovers from depression, the other becomes more dependent. Recognizing that both partners have strong unmet—and probably uncommunicated—needs leads the way to finding more appropriate ways of these being met.

Identifying the negative interaction patterns that rapidly spiral into a blazing row, as each person hits home, almost automatically after years of practice, at the other's vulnerable areas, can assist motivated couples to break out of the vicious circle before emotions run high. For some couples the negative interaction runs so deep, and so much damage has been inflicted and received over the years, that commitment to change is minimal on both sides. Clear communication can at least clarify the situation, and the couple may be able to agree strategies for spending time apart and developing separate interests/lives that are mutually acceptable.

In many instances more than one relative will be involved, and it may be helpful to convene a family meeting, inviting all members of the family who wish to come and take part. Again the primary aim is to establish effective communication, and to encourage each person to listen to the views of other family members, with a further aim of mobilizing the resources of the family to generate strategies for tackling the current difficulties. An ethos is established where the answers do not lie within the one family member who is identified as the patient, but where tackling broader family issues might be helpful to all concerned. Systemic family therapy is beginning to be used more widely where the identified patient is an older person (Benbow *et al.* 1990), and may well have a great deal to offer to situations where individual CBT cannot begin to address the long-standing family tensions contributing to the maintenance of the psychological disorder. Whether or not a formal family therapy approach is utilized, issues of power, control, safety, and security—so important in depression and anxiety—can be addressed in the context of family meetings. For example, the person who has become depressed may be reacting to a loss of power and control in the family circle; they may feel that they are considered to have lost status, with the family now revolving around their children's generation. Alternatively, an individual's symptoms of anxiety may be exerting control over other family members, for example by preventing them going away. Talking about these issues may enable more appropriate ways of meeting these powerful needs to be evolved. Working in this way is demanding, and it is recommended that at least two therapists are present; where the patient's anxiety or depression is severe, or the person has difficulty in communicating, it is useful for one therapist who knows the person well to sit with the person and ensure their voice is heard.

GROUP TREATMENTS

There are a number of reports of the use of CBT in a group setting. Some have tackled problems of anxiety (e.g. Garrison 1978; Woods 1982) but more often the groups have focused on depression. Yost *et al.* (1986) have produced a useful, detailed treatment manual for such groups. Working in groups may have advantages in terms of savings in therapists' time and in bringing to bear the powerful motivating force of peer support. However, as Steuer and Hammen (1983) relate, there are some drawbacks to the group approach. These include heterogeneity of group members, making it more difficult to build on shared experiences and common understanding, which are essential for group cohesion and for members to be able to learn from each other's experiences. Individual differences may arise in a large variety of ways: age, health, background, education, ability to grasp certain aspects of the therapeutic approach, hearing problems, social networks, severity of depression, and so on. Bringing together a homogenous group of anxious or depressed older people is not an easy task; in a recent group, for example, one member, who had never married, clearly felt quite isolated when all the other members spoke of the loss of their spouses. A member whose depression is more severe may find confirmation of unworthiness in their inability to match the progress of their less depressed peers. More positively, Steuer and Hammen (1983) note that social pressure from group members was particularly helpful in tackling some group members' reluctance to try new strategies, or to modify long-standing patterns of response. They received strong encouragement from their peers to at least make an attempt and not to hold too firmly to the idea that they were too old to change.

Outcome studies comparing the effectiveness of group and individual CBT for depression in older people would be useful. The evidence, to date, appears to be that studies which have used a group format (e.g. Steuer *et al.* 1984; Beutler *et al.* 1987) have had lower success rates, in terms of the proportion of patients moving into the non-depressed range post-treatment, than studies using individual therapy. However, there are many potential differences between studies in terms of patient population, outcome measures, duration of treatment, and so on, so this can only be an extremely tentative conclusion. Indeed, a recent uncontrolled study of group CBT (Leung and Orrell 1993) reports an identical response rate (70 per cent) to that reported by Thompson *et al.* (1987) for individual therapy. Whether in a clinical context the benefits might outweigh a small reduction in effectiveness also requires evaluation. What is clear is that group CBT is not an easy option, and issues of selection, preparation of potential group members and work on developing cohesion throughout the group must be carefully addressed. It is surprising that there has not been more interest in anxiety-management groups, where there can be a more active task-centred focus, with exercises such as relaxation training, controlled breathing, and goal setting, for graded exposure carried out on a group basis. Although not specifically a CBT group, there is much to be said for relapse-prevention groups, such as those described by Ong *et al.* (1987) and Culhane and Dobson (1991), for those who have made some recovery from depression. Such groups can meet a need for a place of security, safety, and attachment, whilst enhancing the person's own sense of control and worth by giving a setting where the person is able to give support to others as well as receiving it.

STRATEGIC ADAPTATIONS

What are the features that distinguish the application of CBT to older adults from its use with younger adults with neurotic disorders? Generally there are more similarities than differences, but there are several issues that—allowing for individual differences—do need to be considered, particularly with the older age group.

First, the goals of treatment may need to be more limited. This may arise from constraints imposed by the person's physical health or disabilities; for example, Woods and Britton (1985) describe the successful treatment of an agoraphobic patient, where the goals were simply to reach the local shops and social centre; Hussian (1981) reports a treatment programme helping four elderly residents in an institutional setting overcome anxiety about using the lift. Relatively small goals may none the less have an important impact on the person's life, particularly if they open up the way for the person to regain involvement in activities they enjoy. The person's whole lifestyle may have developed around these problems, which may have become an integral part of their self-concept, and so quite difficult to relinquish. This should not be taken to imply that treatment should not be attempted with individuals with long-standing problems, but rather that the goals should initially be set realistically low, to enable the person to achieve something worthwhile to them, but not to raise false hopes of a 'cure', which when dashed would add further to the person's negative self-image.

Secondly, a number of issues are raised for therapists working with this client group. Amongst these are a change in emphasis in the therapeutic relationship, where the therapist will virtually always be younger (often considerably so) than the patient. The patient may view the therapist along similar lines to their own children or grandchildren; conversely, the therapist may be affected by issues that relate to their relationship with their own parents or grandparents. Knight (1986) discusses these issues, which are as relevant to the practice of CBT as they are to more dynamic psychotherapies, and which therapists need to be aware of in reflecting on their casework. More generally, the therapist brings into the treatment session their own perceptions of ageing, which may themselves include cognitive distortions, such as unrealistically negative expectations of the person's potential for learning and for change, and making unjustified generalizations about all old people from specific instances (such as one's own relatives). The advice usually given to therapists is to ensure they have contact with the whole range of older people, including those who are functioning well, enjoying life, and coping well with difficulties. However, it must be recognized that for some patients the real-life hardships are so great that difficulty does arise in distinguishing between helplessness and hopelessness arising from depression and a valid self-appraisal of a life now constricted by, for example, severe ill health, or loss of all the important relationships in their life. Therapists must be aware of their own need for support in entering into the suffering and pain of older people in such circumstances.

It has been suggested that older patients may be more likely to require treatment socialization (Emery 1981). This is on the basis that they are less likely to be psychologically minded, less used to what psychological therapy might involve, and more inclined to seek external solutions rather than the more active approach of CBT, with its emphasis on the patient's own input both during and between sessions. The experience of many therapists in this area concurs with that expressed by Steuer and Hammen (1983) that there is great individual variation in psychological sophistication, and age is probably a less important variable in this respect than education and social background. With any age-group it is good practice to offer the person sufficient orientation to the treatment approach to enable them to have realistic expectations; this must be judged on an individual basis. For those who seem to have more difficulty with the cognitive aspects such as identifying automatic negative thoughts, there remains the option of adopting a more active behavioural approach at first.

Finally, therapists are often encouraged to be more active with older patients (e.g. Sparacino 1978), even intervening directly in their lives. How much practical help should be given? There is a real danger of taking over, and of disempowering the patient further, colluding with phobic avoidance, and feeding into the depressive dynamic of helplessness. However, at times, a little practical help can enable the person by opening a door that had appeared to them to be blocked. This must be the basis of the judgement to be made —will my intervention remove an obstacle that is beyond the patient's ability to tackle, or am I taking power out of the person's hands? Is there a way of assisting the patient obtain the help needed from another source, which could be a resource in future, outside of the therapy context? On a home visit the therapist may readily change a light bulb for the patient whose immobility prevents them climbing the step-ladder, but this indicates a need to work on developing a social network to call on next time.

FUTURE DIRECTIONS

There are several areas where CBT has not been sufficiently implemented: first, in behavioural management of disturbed behaviours in severe depression, in in-patient and family contexts, where the work of Church (1986) stands out as a plea for a multimodal approach. It is too easy to write off such behaviour as 'manipulative' or 'attention seeking' without beginning to examine the reasons why the natural process of seeking to meet one's own needs (i.e. manipulating the environment) should produce unacceptable demands in the context of some people with depression, or why the particular way in which the depressed person seeks attention is deemed inappropriate. Gilbert (1993) has written about defence and safety systems in relation to depression. Being demanding may be a manifestation of seeking safety cues, searching for reassurance and protection. The non-reactive demobilization of depression is seen as a defensive state, which may be associated with either issues of separation and rejection or of power and subordination. Recognizing some of the basic mechanisms that may underlie some of the behavioural difficulties encountered in such patients may lead the way to the new treatment options that are required.

Secondly, further work is needed with the 'hard to treat' group who fail to respond to any kind of therapy. This group probably includes a number with difficult personalities, where CBT is now being applied to younger patients. Clinically some of these patients seem to have experienced damage early on in life; there has been little attention as yet to post-traumatic stress disorder in older people, despite the trauma so many have lived through in times of war and hardship. The possibility of childhood abuse, including sexual abuse, having had long-term effects should be considered; clinically, recent publicity regarding sexual abuse of children has led to several patients talking of their own experience, for the first time in some instances. One patient, for example, reported frequent intrusive flashback memories of the experience, nearly 70 years after its occurrence.

Thirdly, there is scope for developing cognitive theories of depression in late life, and in particular the role of autobiographical memory (Morris and Morris 1991); it is well known that depressed people are more likely to recall negative events; there is also evidence that recall in depression will produce a less specific, more general memory (Williams 1992). The interaction of such changes with age-related changes would be well worth evaluating, and, as Morris and Morris (1991) suggest, could lead to additional therapeutic techniques involving the cueing of specific, positive memories.

REFERENCES

Arena, J. G., Hightower, N. E., and Chong, G. C. (1988). Relaxation therapy for tension headache in the elderly: a prospective study. *Psychology and Ageing*, **3**, 96–8.

Benbow, S., Egan, D., Marriott, A., Tregay, K., Walsh, S., Wells, J., and Wood, J. (1990). Using the family life cycle with later life families. *Journal of Family Therapy*, **12**, 321–40.

Beutler, L. E., Scogin, F., Kirkish, P., Schretlen, D., Corbishley, A., Hamblin, D., *et al.* (1987). Group cognitive therapy and alprazolam in the treatment of depression in older adults. *Journal of Consulting and Clinical Psychology*, **55**, 550–6.

Bird, A. S., Macdonald, A. J. D., Mann, A. H., and Philpot, M. P. (1987). Preliminary experience with the SELFCARE (D): a self-rating depression questionnaire for use in elderly, non-institutionalised subjects. *International Journal of Geriatric Psychiatry*, **2**, 31–8.

Church, M. (1983). Psychological therapy with elderly people. *Bulletin of the British Psychological Society*, **36**, 110–2.

Church, M. (1986). Issues in psychological therapy with elderly people. In *Psychological therapies for the elderly* (ed. I. G. Hanley and M. Gilhooly), pp. 1–21. Croom Helm, London.

Culhane, M., and Dobson, H. (1991). Groupwork with elderly women. *International Journal of Geriatric Psychiatry*, **6**, 415–18.

Downs, A. F. D., Rosenthal, T. L., and Lichstein, K. L. (1988). Modelling therapies reduce avoidance of bath-time by the institutionalised elderly. *Behaviour Therapy*, **19**, 359–68.

Emery, G. (1981). Cognitive therapy with the elderly. In *New directions in cognitive therapy* (ed. G. Emery, S. D. Hollon, and R. C. Bedrosian). Guilford, New York.

Gallagher, D. E., and Thompson, L. W. (1983). Effectiveness of psychotherapy for both endogenous and non-endogenous depression in older adult out-patients. *Journal of Gerontology*, **38**, 707–12.

Gallagher, D. E., Nies, G., and Thompson, L. W. (1982). Reliability of the Beck Depression Inventory with older adults. *Journal of Consulting and Clinical Psychology*, **50**, 152–3.

Gallagher-Thompson, D., Hanley-Peterson, P., and Thompson, L. W. (1990). Maintenance of gains versus relapse following brief psychotherapy for depression. *Journal of Consulting and Clinical Psychology*, **58**, 371–4.

Garrison, J. E. (1978). Stress management training for the elderly: A psychoeducational approach. *Journal of the American Geriatrics Society*, **26**, 397–403.

Gilbert, P. (1993). Defence and safety: their function in social behaviour and psychopathology. *British Journal of Clinical Psychology*, **32**, 131–53.

Haight, B. K., and Dias, J. K. (1992). Examining key variables in selected reminiscing modalities. *International Psychogeriatrics*, **4**, (Supp. 2) 279–90.

Hawton, K., Salkovskis, P. M., Kirk, J., and Clark, D. M. (1989). *Cognitive behaviour therapy for psychiatric problems: a practical guide*. Oxford University Press, Oxford.

Holden, U. P. (1988). Hyperventilation. In *Neuropsychology and ageing: definitions, explanations and practical approaches* (ed. U. P. Holden), pp. 177–92. Croom Helm, London.

Holland, C. A., and Rabbitt, P. (1991). The course and causes of cognitive change with advancing age. *Reviews in Clinical Gerontology*, **1**, 81–96.

Hussian, R. A. (1981). *Geriatric psychology: a behavioural perspective*. Van Nostrand Reinhold, New York.

Kavanagh, D. J. (1990). Towards a cognitive–behavioural intervention for adult grief reactions. *British Journal of Psychiatry*, **157**, 373–83.

King, P., and Barrowclough, C. (1991). A clinical pilot study of cognitive–behavioural therapy for anxiety disorders in the elderly. *Behavioural Psychotherapy*, **19**, 337–45.

Knight, B. (1986). *Psychotherapy with older adults*. Sage, Beverly Hills.

Lam, D. H., Brewin, C. R., Woods, R. T., and Bebbington, P. E. (1987). Cognition and social adversity in the depressed elderly. *Journal of Abnormal Psychology*, **96**, 23–6.

Leung, S. N. M., and Orrell, M. W. (1993). A brief cognitive behavioural therapy group for the elderly: who benefits? *International Journal of Geriatric Psychiatry*, **8**, 593–8.

Lindesay, J., Briggs, K., and Murphy, E. (1989). The Guys / Age Concern survey: prevalence rates of cognitive impairment, depression and anxiety in an urban elderly community. *British Journal of Psychiatry*, **155**, 317–29.

Morris, R. G., and Morris, L. W. (1991). Cognitive and behavioural approaches with the depressed elderly. *International Journal of Geriatric Psychiatry*, **6**, 407–13.

Ong, Y., Martineau, F., Lloyd, C., and Robbins, I. (1987). A support group for the depressed elderly. *International Journal of Geriatric Psychiatry*, **2**, 119–23.

Ost, L. (1992). Cognitive therapy in a case of choking phobia. *Behavioural Psychotherapy*, **20**, 79–84.

Parkes, C. M. (1980). Bereavement counselling. *British Medical Journal*, **281**, 3–6.

Reich, J. W., and Zautra, A. J. (1990). Dispositional control beliefs and the consequences of a control-enhancing intervention. *Journal of Gerontology*, **45**, 46–51.

Shapiro, F. (1989). Eye movement desensitization: a new treatment for post-traumatic stress disorder. *Journal of Behavioural Therapy and Experimental Psychiatry*, **20**, 211–17.

Sparacino, J. (1978). Individual psychotherapy with the aged: a selective review. *International Journal of Ageing and Human Development*, **9**, 197–217.

Steuer, J. L., and Hammen, C. L. (1983). Cognitive–behavioural group therapy for the depressed elderly; issues and adaptations. *Cognitive Therapy and Research*, **7**, 285–96.

Steuer, J. L., Mintz, J., Hammen, C. L., Hill, M. A., Jarvik, L. F., McCarley, T., *et al.* (1984). Cognitive–behavioural and psychodynamic group psychotherapy in treatment of geriatric depression. *Journal of Consulting and Clinical Psychology*, **52**, 180–92.

Stroebe, M., and Stroebe, W. (1991). Does 'grief-work' work? *Journal of Consulting and Clinical Psychology*, **59**, 479–82.

Thompson, L. W., Davies, R., Gallagher, D. E., and Krantz, S. E. (1986). Cognitive therapy with older adults. In *Clinical gerontology: a guide to assessment and intervention* (ed. T. L. Brink), pp. 245–79. Haworth, New York.

Thompson, L. W., Gallagher, D. E., and Breckenridge, J. S. (1987). Comparative effectiveness of psychotherapies for depressed elderly. *Journal of Consulting and Clinical Psychology*, **55**, 385–90.

Thompson, L. W., Gallagher, D. E., and Czirr, R. (1988). Personality disorder and outcome in the treatment of late-life depression. *Journal of Geriatric Psychiatry*, **21**, 133–46.

Thyer, B. A. (1981). Prolonged in-vivo exposure therapy with a 70 year old woman. *Journal of Behaviour Therapy and Experimental Psychiatry*, **12**, 69–71.

Whitehead, A. (1991). Twenty years a-growing: some current issues in behavioural psychotherapy with elderly people. *Behavioural Psychotherapy*, **19**, 92–9.

Williams, J. M. G. (1992). *The psychological treatment of depression: a guide to the theory and practice of cognitive behaviour therapy* (2nd edn). Routledge, London.

Woods, R. T. (1982). The psychology of ageing: Assessment of deficits and their management. In: *The Psychiatry of Late Life* (eds R. Levy and F. Post), pp. 68–113. Blackwell, Oxford.

Woods, R. T., and Britton, P. G. (1985). *Clinical psychology with the elderly*. Croom Helm / Chapman Hall, London.

Yesavage, J. A., Brink, T. L., and Rose, T. L. (1983). Development and validation of a geriatric depression scale: a preliminary report. *Journal of Psychiatric Research*, **17**, 37–49.

Yost, E. B., Beutler, L. E., Corbishley, M. A., and Allender, J. R. (1986). *Group cognitive therapy: a treatment approach for depressed older adults*. Pergamon Press, Oxford.

7

Psychological treatments II: Psychodynamic approaches
BRIAN MARTINDALE

INTRODUCTION

Some knowledge of psychodynamics is of therapeutic value in most encounters between health professionals and elderly patients, whether they be diagnostic, supportive, management orientated, or formally psychotherapeutic. A receptive and empathic attitude on the part of the therapist helps considerably in gaining knowledge and understanding of the complex personal struggles that lie behind any fellow human being's request for professional help, and the usefulness of some psychodynamic expertise is well established in the clinical management of younger age groups by general practitioners and psychiatrists (Balint 1957; Balint and Norell 1975; Taylor 1987; Yorke *et al.* 1989). This chapter outlines the important psychodynamic factors that lie at the root of the developmental preoccupations and impasses that concern older people, and describes some of the psychodynamically based treatments that can be effective.

COMMON PREOCCUPATIONS AND DIFFICULTIES

Loss

King (1980) has summarized some of the principal preoccupations that emerged in her work with middle-aged and elderly people. Losses of various kinds are central to all of the themes that she adduces—not only actual loss, but also worries about possible future loss or losses can lead to psychopathology and suffering. Important actual or anticipated losses include:

(1) the fear of diminution or loss in sexual potency and the impact this would have on relationships;

(2) the threat of redundancy or displacement in work roles;

(3) anxieties arising in marital relationships after children have left home and

parents can no longer use them to mask problems arising in their relationship with each other;

(4) the awareness of the implications of their own ageing, in terms of illness and dependence;

(5) the inevitability of death, and the realization that important goals may not be achieved, and that important experiences and pleasures may not be experienced.

Difficulties in assimilating

In his analysis of the stages of life, Erikson (1959) has summarized the eighth and last as a crisis between integrity and despair. By 'integrity', Erikson means the ability to assimilate the value of one's life experience, 'to be, through having been', balancing despair from 'facing not being'. Hildebrand (1986) has also emphasized that there are developmental struggles specific to later life, beyond those specifically related to loss. By way of example, he quotes evidence from Gutmann *et al.* (1977) suggesting that men before the end of midlife tend to be active and controlling, and adopt a stance of mastery at the expense of their capacity for tenderness, sensuality, and dependence. These latter attributes are normally more able to be assimilated in later life, together with a lessening interest in producing and an increased concern with what is produced for them. He agrees with Gutmann that late-onset disturbance in both men and women may sometimes reflect an inability to assimilate certain traits, and not only be a result of loss.

Earlier trauma

Most psychodynamic therapists believe that traumatic experiences and developmental distortions at earlier stages in the life cycle usually have a profound influence on the capacity to manage difficulties later in life, particularly when these difficulties are significantly connected with earlier traumas or humiliations, and threaten powerful defences that have been constructed against the associated memories and painful affects. These defences, however, lead to difficulties in working through losses of various kinds and in the assimilation of certain characteristics, especially those connected with dependency.

Physical dependency and dying

Old age is associated with a return to preoccupation with physical needs, physical survival, and the quality of that survival. Thoughts of illness and physical dependency may revive from childhood deep anxieties connected with the reliability of the body, both one's own and, perhaps more importantly, that of others. The prospect of physical dependency in old age may threaten individuals with previously successful defences against dependency as well as those with dependent characters. This is one of the commonest reasons why symptomatic disturbances and breakdowns may happen for the first time in late life.

The preoccupation with physical dependency is often intimately linked with that of dying. Most elderly patients are intensely preoccupied with fantasies concerning the manner of their dying and the responses of their caretakers. Many symptoms of depression, anxiety, panic, and paranoia are linked more with these fears than with death itself. All the worst experiences in a patient's life or those of the people with whom they are most identified may be reawoken in this anticipation of a terrifying dying experience.

So far as death itself is concerned, listening to many elderly patients confirms Freud's view that the unconscious seems inaccessible to the idea of death as an absence (Freud 1915). Most people talk about death as an active state of continuing experience (pleasurable or painful) and not as a final ending of personal experience.

Late-life envy

Tolerating ageing involves accepting the loss of certain attributes, and eventually the separation by death from life and those who continue to live. Sometimes it is an older person's destructive envy that causes havoc by actively interfering with younger peoples' lives.

Case 1

Miss J was an 82-year-old woman who was repeatedly referred as an 'emergency' to the local psychogeriatric team. It was initially unclear what was precipitating these emergencies, in which Miss J would be very dramatically distraught. A young, attractive, and modest woman psychologist started to see her regularly to try and unravel the issues. Miss J was often very flattering of the psychologist, and made comments concerning the wonderful personal life that such an attractive young woman must have with her partner. However, the psychologist would also be left feeling angry and frustrated, as Miss J made only haphazard use of her appointment sessions, but would ring up the hospital late at night and irritate the junior doctors by making them feel helpless. Following supervision, the psychologist was able to talk with Miss J about how overwhelmed with envy was Miss J at what she thought was the psychologist's wonderful life compared with her own lonely one, and how out of control the expression of her envy was in her unconscious intentions to mess up the psychologist's appointments and disrupt the doctors' sleep at night. What was most important was the patient's fear that, if the extent of her envious destructive wishes towards the psychologist were to be revealed, she would be rejected. Following this frank discussion there were no further emergency calls and the patient was maintained on regular monthly out-patient visits.

Time

The psychology and psychopathology of the perception of time is not often given much consideration in thinking about developmental processes of the elderly. In the first half of life it is fairly normal to behave as if the realities that the passage of time presents will be conquerable. Most healthy young people seem to feel that in time they will be able to accomplish much of what they would like to do in life. To come to terms with the realities of one's mortality and therefore the finiteness of the time available, requires a letting go and modification of some of these aspirations. This requires a capacity to mourn the fact that many ambitions may not be achieved. Jacques (1965) suggests that it is this capacity to be able to mourn, i.e. to face feelings of loss of functions, relationships, and also of ideas and ambitions, that is a central key in determining personal creativity within the confines of finite time in later life.

Psychodynamics and organic brain disease

The fact that an elderly person has an organic cerebral disorder does not mean that psychodynamic factors and mental mechanisms are not relevant or useful in understanding their experiences and difficulties. Indeed, defence mechanisms may play an important part in early dementia in protecting the individual from the reality of what is happening to their mental functioning.

Case 2

Mrs F was an 80-year-old Jewish lady who could not avail herself of the facilities of a day hospital when she developed a dementing illness. Her premorbid character, which included both marked masochistic and paranoid traits, probably contributed significantly to her difficulty in being cared for; however, it is likely that her horrific Holocaust memories were also reawoken as she hurried out of the hospital asking why all the people were lined up.

MENTAL MECHANISMS AND DEFENCES IN LATER LIFE

The psychodynamic model of mental functioning concentrates specifically on the fate of unconscious phantasy, feelings, and drives, and their effects on the self and others. Its central tenets are the power of unconscious phantasy in determining conscious experiences, behaviour, and symptoms, and also the existence of unconscious defence mechanisms for dealing with unacceptable or unbearable feelings and thoughts, and the important role of these in adaptation and maladaptation. Symptoms are the result of a varying degree of breakdown in these defences, and compromises between defences and unconscious forces seeking expression.

In these respects, the mental mechanisms of elderly people are no different from those of the young. The explanatory theories of Klein on the paranoid–schizoid and depressive positions (Segal 1979), of Kohut on self psychology (Deitz 1991), of Winnicott on the stages of concern and primary maternal preoccupation (Winnicott 1958, 1963), and of Bion on containment and attacks on linking (Bion 1988), are immensely helpful and relevant to understanding the problems of the elderly and the variety of their reactions to their internal and external circumstances.

Primitive defence mechanisms

These are defences in which the primary aim is to disown or rid the mind of unbearable or unacknowledgeable qualities. Denial, projection, projective identification, omnipotence, idealization and denigration, splitting, and reaction formation are those most commonly described. In the Kleinian paranoid–schizoid position, the view of oneself and others is not integrated but split—there are no loved features or good qualities coexisting in the same person alongside the hated ones, and the survival of the self is constantly threatened by aggressive and other feared qualities such as neglect. In this state of mind, objective qualities in oneself and others are not easily distinguished by the subject from phantasies, so a person is dominated by phantasies of highly idealized or terrifyingly aggressive or uncaring objects, and their external world is felt to be fully inhabited by similar persons.

In people whose states of mind are dominated by these primitive defences, old age, and the possible dependency on others for physical and emotional needs are terrifying and threatening, and may be massively denied. These people are at great risk of driving away or avoiding potential family and professional carers because of the extent of their hatred, contempt, and lack of trust.

More mature defence mechanisms

The depressive position

In contrast to the primitive paranoid–schizoid position, individuals in the depressive position or 'stage of concern' (Winnicott 1963) do not feel so vulnerable. Psychological survival is more assured, and there is an increased awareness of the capacity of the individual to hurt those that they care about. In the depressive position, others are more real and integrated, a balance of loved and hated characteristics, and the individual tries to mitigate harmful impulses out of concern for others.

All individuals have the capacity to move back and forth between paranoid–schizoid and depressive position modes of functioning towards the key persons in their lives. Factors that determine these movements include repression, sublimation, self-esteem, and the amount of hatred aroused in the self and the capacity for its containment. This degree of hatred may itself depend upon the capacities of persons that the individual is dependent on to contain the subject's hatred, dependency, and envy in addition to their own. The capacity for containment of affect is an important determinant of the quality of a health service's provision for the elderly, since if a society can contain the affects aroused by the dependency and needs of its elders, then it is likely that provision for those needs will be more equitable and appropriate.

Examples of defence mechanisms

The following vignettes illustrate the operation of manic denial (Case 3) and projective identification (Case 4) in elderly patients:

Case 3

A 66-year-old single man, Mr B, presented to his general practitioner with panic attacks. Although he had had coronary artery grafts and replacement hips, he insisted on going on holidays only with younger persons and engaging frantically in activities that would have taxed the physical capacities of a 30-year-old. There was a clear idealization of youth. He committed suicide a few weeks later. From the interviews, it was apparent that he was unable to consciously contemplate the future because it might bring to the surface disturbing phantasies of the consequences for him of less treatable physical ailments in years to come. Unconsciously, he was adopting an omnipotent solution of being able to retain his youthful vigour and immortality. However, his panic attacks represented the breaking down of these manic/omnipotent denial defences.

Case 4

A 75-year-old man, Mr T, was in group therapy and would always talk in a very superior way as if he were the expert on, and had solutions for, whatever subject was being discussed. In contrast to this view that he offered of himself, he was full of contempt for the uselessness and incompetence of every other person in any position of authority. He felt that these people should all be ashamed of themselves for being so incompetent. However, he would repeatedly say that there was one part of his life that he was not prepared to discuss. This irritated some of the group members. On one occasion Mr T let slip the fact that before his first hospital admission he had led a tramp-like existence for a period. Following this, he flew into a rage and left the room saying that the group members and the therapist should be ashamed of themselves. Mr T was disowning and projecting into others unbearable thoughts of an incompetent, useless, and shameful aspect of himself and his past. He also projected into others the expectation that his weakness would be treated with the same degree of contempt that he had been expressing for the weakness of others.

IMPLICATIONS FOR ASSESSMENTS OF THE ELDERLY

Because many aspects of ageing revive anxieties that have their origins in the vital dependent relationships of early life, a detailed personal history, concentrating particularly on the relationship with both parents throughout childhood and adolescence, may be most helpful in gaining a full understanding of the patient's current vulnerabilities. It should however be kept in mind that this information may have been subject to distortion by the unconscious mechanisms described above. Identifying the predominant defence mechanisms and their strength may be as useful as the subjective history. Clues to these defences may be gleaned from the patterns of ways in which the person relates to past and contemporary key figures, including the interviewer; it is particularly helpful to know as much as possible about how important relationships have ended. An understanding of patients' defences is necessary if professionals are to avoid perpetuating malign cycles by acting out the negative roles that the paranoid–schizoid patients will project into them, or colluding with the idealizing tendencies of others. It is always necessary to carefully evaluate the capacity of the patient to hold on to a more balanced (depressive position) view of their care-givers, for example, in determining the frequency of appointments.

It sometimes transpires that the anxieties expressed by patients turn out to be partly based on identifications with what happened to parents or other key persons in the last period of their lives (introjective identification). It is therefore important to assess whom the elderly person is most identified with, or fears being identified with, and the nature of these identifications.

Case 5

A 72-year-old man, Mr B, had attended an out-patient clinic every two months for a number of years after a depressive illness following his wife's death. He had seen a series of junior doctors at the clinic, and the latest of these decided that Mr C could be discharged as he had been symptom-free for two years. Mr C was stunned but could not say why. Six weeks later he was readmitted in a severely depressed state. It became clear that the two-monthly visit to the clinic had been sufficient for Mr C to maintain a view of himself as being worthwhile and as someone who would not get forgotten if in difficulties. In his childhood, he had suffered a very lengthy difficult period of feeling abandoned and unwanted when he lost emotional contact with both his father, after his parents' marriage ended, and his mother, who was preoccupied with his younger siblings. He had recovered considerably when he went to boarding-school. Following the loss of his wife, Mr C had established a similar sustaining institutional attachment with the clinic.

Case 6

An 87-year-old woman, Mrs C, had shown a marked capacity for survival and independence in Britain after loosing all of her family and her husband in the Holocaust. There was a certain cost attached to her staunchly independent character, as she was regarded by those who knew her well as rather self-centred, and this played a part in her one surviving younger relative keeping some distance from her. Her depression was brought about by the unexpected potential loss of her flat to a 'selfish and greedy landlord' and the consequent possibility of having to move well away from the area in which she had built up her life over the last 45 years. She said that she had survived losing everything and everyone once in her life, but was sure that she would not be able to do it again. Although she did not lose her flat, she needed the occasional visit to both the medical and psychiatric departments of the hospital to give external symbolic confirmation that potential care-givers were well disposed towards her when her internal fears of encountering persons similar to her 'selfish' landlord returned.

The very telling of their history is a means through which the elderly patient begins to establish a psychotherapeutic relationship. Indeed, life review or reminiscence has been identified by several workers as an integral part of the psychotherapy of older people (Butler 1963; Pincus 1970).

FORMAL PSYCHODYNAMIC TREATMENTS

Psychodynamic therapies cannot be learned from reading a textbook. Those who are interested but inexperienced in these approaches should ensure that they are carefully supervised by an experienced and trained practitioner in psychoanalytic psychotherapy who is also familiar with problems of the elderly. There are many pitfalls for the enthusiastic novice and their patient, particularly when there is a gap of a generation or more between their ages (Martindale 1989). Here is just one example of the common problem of misplaced therapeutic zeal:

Case 7

A 74-year-old woman, Miss P, had had many contacts with the mental health profession during her life. These had been of some help, but she remained a vulnerable and fragile personality. After a five year period without professional help, the death of a friend and the illness of another led to a further referral to the mental health service for what her family doctor described as an anxiety state. A woman doctor saw Miss P and embarked on a therapeutic endeavour that seemed aimed at changing her fragile personality. Miss P's anxiety state became much worse and the doctor more frantic in her ministrations until eventually the doctor wisely sought consultation for herself about the case. Careful reassessment of the referral revealed that Miss P's previous family doctor had recently retired. This fact, combined with the recent experience of death and illness, led to Miss P becoming very anxious that there might not be suitable professional help available to her in the event of her needing further psychological support. Contact with her new general practitioner had not sufficiently allayed her anxieties, hence the referral to specialist services. Miss P became terrified that the hospital doctor was now trying to change her in a way with which experts had only had limited success in earlier times, and lived in fear that this new doctor, whom she otherwise liked, would reject her if she did not improve. All Miss P had wanted was to know that there was a kindly competent doctor available if she were in difficulties. The doctor recognized her omnipotent aims, and recognized that she should *do* far less and concentrate on listening more attentively to the symbolic significance of Miss P's worries, and demonstrate her availability. She offered fortnightly regular twenty-minute appointments, and there was a rapid improvement in Miss P which was sustained until the doctor rotated to another job. At this time the doctor needed a further consultation to deal with her own difficulty of letting go, based on an exacerbation of her omnipotence, believing that no other professional could help Miss P as much as she had done.

Brief individual psychodynamic psychotherapies

For many years, Hildebrand and his staff at the Tavistock Clinic in London have been offering elderly patients brief (usually 15 sessions) analytic psychotherapy based on transference interpretations (Hildebrand 1986). In the hands of these psychoanalytically trained and experienced practitioners, the outcomes of this treatment are good. Many of their patients are not severely troubled individuals likely to need the help of psychiatric services. However, they are clearly suffering greatly from difficulties in making the necessary developmental and adaptational shifts that stem from reaching particular points in their life cycle. These patients are followed up at yearly intervals, and it is important to bear in mind the psychological significance to patients of this follow-up, as this may well mean a temporary goodbye rather than a final one. The work of Malan (1976) on outcome in brief psychotherapy shows convincingly the therapeutic benefit of the skilled elicitation of hostile feelings towards the therapist about the ending of the therapeutic relationship.

Indications

Brief psychoanalytic psychotherapy is indicated for the following elderly patients:

(1) those with a considerable degree of ego strength;

(2) those with circumscribed problems related to some of the developmental issues of getting older;

(3) those who recognize that their problems are internal;

(4) those who are clearly motivated to be understood and make sense of their difficulties;

(5) those who are not unconsciously seeking excessive gratification of dependency needs from the therapeutic relationship;

(6) those who are in pathological mourning and unable to cope with unexpected emotion.

Supportive psychotherapy

Elderly people can receive a great deal of benefit from psychotherapy that is limited and supportive in its aims, involving more activity and giving on the part of the therapist than occurs in interpretive therapies (Pfeiffer 1971). The aims of supportive psychotherapy are: to assist patients in minimizing the consequences of their current problems for themselves and others; to assist patients to make the maximum use of their existing strengths; and to relieve, intervene or even take over, in a judicious manner, areas of responsibility that the patient cannot manage at that point in time. Unlike other dynamic therapies, supportive psychotherapy does not aim at improvements beyond symptomatic relief, or aspire to any degree of character change. However, the fact that the aims of supportive psychotherapy are usually limited does not in any way minimize the importance of its interventions either to the patient or to society as a whole. Supportive psychotherapy requires considerable skill and understanding of the psychodynamics and character structure of the patient and the therapist, and the dynamics that develop between the two. It would be wrong to suggest that these interventions should never be interpretative, as research shows that all psychodynamic therapies have a mixture of both supportive and interpretative elements (Luborsky *et al.* 1988; Wallerstein 1986; de Jonghe 1992).

The physical aspects of the supportive treatments need to be carefully considered in the elderly, and much important supportive therapy can and indeed should happen in patients' own homes. This of course may be necessary for immediate practical reasons and may also have great symbolic value for the patient, providing that the therapist is very careful not to arouse unrealistic expectations. Support must be offered in a way that both succeeds in preventing deterioration, but at the same time does not facilitate a more malignant regression by over-gratifying the patient or facilitating too much secondary gain. The main problems occurring in supportive therapies stem from the failure of staff to recognize the powerful, often idealized fantasies that they may be silently arousing in the patient. These may disturb the inexperienced professional, who may drop his patient when they emerge.

Much important supportive psychotherapy can occur between the members of groups. These groups can be both formal and informal, arranged by medical, social work, occupational, art, music, and drama therapy staff in community, day-centre, day-hospital, and ward settings. The staff have an important role in providing the reliable setting for these groups to occur, facilitating the supportive capacities of the members of the groups, and intervening when the difficulties of particular members overstretch the capacities of the group to respond.

Case 8

A young female social worker was seeing a seriously depressed, lonely man in his own home, and would have tea with him on a regular weekly visit. It transpired that this man had a penchant for young ladies and that his depression was connected with the recent sudden departure of a care assistant with whom he had a very strong fantasy relationship. The social worker was not trained to handle the transference phenomena that inevitably surfaced, and, although her own behaviour had been entirely professional up to that point, she now dropped the patient at that critical point out of her embarrassment when she realized that the elderly man had formed an erotic attachment to her.

In the planning of services, those offering support will often need a secure forum to share and support one another in the emotional strains that this can involve, preferably with the assistance of a fully trained facilitator.

Longer-term individual psychodynamic psychotherapy and psychoanalysis

A number of issues are important when considering the indications for longer-term psychoanalysis and depth-psychoanalytic psychotherapy with elderly patients. The first is to make a clear distinction between the problems of the patient and the patient's suitability for treatment from the availability of such treatments. Although this may seem obvious, in practice the two issues are frequently muddled. In the UK, intensive psychoanalytic psychotherapy is only available at a very few National Health Service (NHS) centres for a limited number of younger adults and children. In other Western European countries however (e.g. The Netherlands, Germany, Finland, France, and Sweden), intensive analytic psychotherapy is more widely available in the public sector and is not age restricted. The following remarks will therefore be confined to (a) non-intensive (weekly) open-ended psychoanalytic psychotherapy, which is somewhat more widely available and occasionally mentioned as being offered to the elderly in the NHS (Porter 1991), and (b) single case reports of elderly people treated by psychoanalysts in private practice.

If one had to summarize the essential aim of analytic psychotherapy and psychoanalysis, it would be to help individuals form a more satisfying and more realistic internal relationship with themselves and the world that they live in. This is accomplished by creating a private setting in which the individual and the therapist can slowly explore the unconscious factors that shape the individual's inner life, and how this inner world interacts and distorts external reality. The therapist will work particularly with the patient on their use of more primitive defence mechanisms, and try and help the patient find his way to conditions in which integration of disowned affects and aspects of self and object relations can be recovered. The analyst's verbalizations (interpretations) are informed especially from the way in which the patient communicates with, experiences, and uses the analyst. The analyst maintains a relatively opaque position (apart from interpretations and empathic interventions) in order to minimize his or her influence on what the patient brings, and is thereby able to see more clearly what are the patient's internal problems. The analyst and psychoanalytic psychotherapist should have had an intensive therapy or analysis themselves in order to minimize the tendency to impose understandings and solutions on the patient, and to be able to tolerate better whatever the patient may bring. Reference has already been made in this chapter to breakdowns in treatment being sometimes due to professionals being unable to handle the intensity of their patients' love, hatred, contempt, envy, guilt, erotic pressures, loss, or fear of dying. Although there are important qualitative differences, as a very broad generalization, less intensive psychoanalytic psychotherapies attempt to do on a much smaller scale what a psychoanalysis would try to achieve.

To illustrate a few points particularly relevant to therapy with this age group, the following is a more detailed account of one patient's once-a-week psychoanalytic psychotherapy over five years.

Case 9

Mr M was 69 years old when he was eventually referred for psychotherapy by a consultant psychiatrist. For several years, starting just before he retired, Mr M had been suffering from depression, severe anxiety states, sleep disturbance, and psychosomatic problems. He had been offered a wide variety of symptomatic treatments, pharmacological, psychological, supportive, social, and diversionary. These all helped a little but never in any enduring way, and he would readily relapse, especially at the end of any intervention.

He had always prided himself on being the breadwinner, enjoying his family's dependency on him, and had never previously received any psychological help until just before his retirement. There was little difficulty in seeing that retirement had been the precipitating factor, but until his analytic therapy there was no attempt to explore the significance of this with him in any sophisticated way. Even before he had seen the clinic, let alone the psychotherapist, Mr M had developed very powerful and disturbing fantasies about the significance of the referral. For Mr M, these fantasies felt very real and he had been in a very distressed state between the time of the referral and the appointment. He saw the referral as a sign that he was being got rid of—that he was a terrible burden to the previous doctor, who was sending him away just as an uncle had been sent away never to return home again when Mr M was a child. Without needing to elicit the past history at this point, the therapist listened very carefully to these current worries, sensing that they held the clues to Mr M's terrors of retirement. The therapist interpreted that Mr M's worry was made worse from fear that the psychotherapist would also soon find him too much of a burden and get rid of him. Although this interpretation did not diminish his fears, Mr M agreed that that fear had been disturbing him greatly and he felt some relief at both being understood and that the therapist was able to allow him to discuss without criticism or defensiveness his (Mr M's) private terrors. He was then able to tell more about these worries in a way that deepened the rapport. Mr M made it clear that the fear of being abandoned by his wife was never absent. He told of terrible fears that the family would be impoverished as a result of his retirement and that they would never forgive him. Mr M was aware in one part of his mind that his wife had shown no signs of abandoning him, in spite of the torment that she must suffered from the endless worrying that Mr M was unable to keep to himself. He also knew that in external reality there was no significant financial hardship.

Mr M was offered once-weekly analytic psychotherapy. Over the succeeding months a number of related trends became central to his communications. The therapy and the therapist became extremely important. Slowly, he became aware for the first time that his other symptoms were connected with worries about his possible abandonment. Mr M had cautious hopes for the first time that it might be possible to unravel some of what he now realised were fears coming from within him. He increasingly looked forward to his weekly sessions, and as they became more important the worries that he would be abandoned by the therapist increased.

At this point, Mr M started to try and be very helpful to the therapist. He would wait at the top of the stairs instead of the downstairs waiting room 'to save the younger therapist's legs'. He started to ask if the sessions could be briefer or less frequent. Mr M would put this in a way that was initially difficult not to agree with, but the therapist managed to wait long enough before making any particular response. It was soon apparent that this helpfulness was all in order to try and prevent the therapist abandoning him. For example, Mr M was quite certain that by coming weekly he was putting such a strain on the therapist that at any moment the latter would bring the treatment to an end as had happened several times in recent years. After a while, the therapist was able to understand and interpret that cutting down the sessions would be confirmation that the therapist was indeed getting so fed up with Mr M that he had to reduce the contact and that Mr M would then have external justification for his fears. Mr M laughed as he appreciated this, but his worries about the therapist persisted, functioning as he was in the paranoid–schizoid position in which he felt totally at the mercy of a very uncaring therapist who could readily and precipitately discard him.

In parallel with these developments, there was a gradual elaboration of Mr M's personal history, especially his adolescence in which there had been a crucial character development that had helped him considerably until his retirement. Mr M had been the middle of six children living in two cramped rooms. He recalls no particular personal affection from either parent and thinks he was rather timid and lacking in confidence as a child. Following his father's sudden death when he was twelve, the family were exceedingly poor. During the course of the therapy, Mr M came to realise that there was in fact a two-year interval between the death of his father and the time that Mr M had started to work. Behind this initial amnesia lay the most enormous repressed anguish and fear. Mr M slowly recalled a lengthy period when he lived in constant fear of being sent away for being a burden. Money for food was very scarce and his mother would spend many hours a day cleaning to earn small sums of money for the large family. Mr M recalled overhearing a conversation between his mother and a man friend in which he advised her to put him in a home if he was too much for her. This exacerbated his terror of putting a foot wrong and he was haunted by images of grey-clothed, very unhappy-looking rows of youngsters, of similar age to himself, out walking from a nearby orphanage.

It was evident that Mr M's worries about being abandoned by his wife and his therapist were little different in form from the intense worries he had about his mother between the ages of twelve and fourteen years. At the age of fourteen Mr M started to go out to work and would bring little pieces of meat home from the butcher's shop. He felt that he was now mother's favourite and that his place was secure, providing that he could bring home these contributions. However, Mr M was so traumatized by the preceding two years that unconsciously he could never allow himself to feel dependent again. For Mr M, emotional and financial dependency on his wife was the unavoidable and terrifying consequence of retirement that led to his breakdown.

In the second year of the treatment Mr M showed small signs of improvement. He had one or two very brief spells in which he was, for the first time in years, free of worry and able to enjoy aspects of family life. However, the panic attacks continued, and it took a number of months more for Mr M to have the confidence to allow himself to enjoy himself and his family for longer of periods of time and to disaffirm himself of his worries that the therapist was endlessly looking for an opportunity to discharge him. They were able to work out that he had similar worries about his wife—that if he were to be able to give her an impression that he could manage by himself she might feel that he had less need of her and she could then feel less guilty and go off with another man. In this way Mr M had considerable secondary gain from being ill. It is important to stress that this had been totally unconscious—and needed interpretation and not moralistic judgement.

Working in a busy NHS setting does create pressures to discharge patients as soon as possible. When working with elderly patients such as Mr M it is vital to resist these pressures. This was a crucial time in his therapy. Up until his referral, Mr M's main source of conscious pleasure and self esteem in life had been as an active provider to others of resources and he needed others to be dependent on him. The therapist was aiming for Mr M to be able to obtain some pleasure from dependency and being cared for by others, and to allow himself to retire from producing for others. Up until now, these dependent and passive states had been associated with the most terrifying torture. A crucial point in the therapy was when he was able to seriously consider that the therapist might actually be prepared to consider being available to him for as long as he needed him. It was very important for this phase of his treatment that the therapist did not enact any guilt about seeing Mr M when he came for periods of time without feeling too troubled.

It is important to emphasize that Mr M's improvement was limited. His improvement was fluctuating and there were several spells when he returned to his tortured state. However, in the last year of his treatment he felt able to begin to talk about reducing the frequency of his sessions. There was a different tone to this from similar requests of the early phase of the treatment, a greater acceptance of his situation and of the limits of what could be accomplished together. In this state of mind he was far more realistic, more sad and less persecuted, much more in depressive-position functioning than paranoid–schizoid. As the possibility of cutting down sessions was being discussed, he developed a severe back pain which turned out to be secondaries from a bowel cancer, and it was only a few weeks before he died a painful and unpleasant death.

This case illustrates a number of general points about psychodynamic therapies with the elderly:

1. The therapist or psychiatrist may be more therapeutic if paradoxically they can seriously entertain the idea that the therapy or contact with the elderly patient may not finish whilst the patient is alive. This can pose psychological problems for younger therapists who are at a different phase of personal development (Martindale 1989).

2. The leading developmental struggle in some elderly patients centres on the question of whether it is psychologically safe enough to acknowledge the possibility of being dependent materially and physically on others for the rest of one's life.

3. Unconscious secondary gains from being 'ill' can be very strong.

4. It is in the interest of the patient's mental health that the therapist should not feel too uncomfortable about seeing patients who are for a time relatively symptom-free and enjoying their therapy.

Psychoanalysis

There are a limited number of case histories in the literature of successful analyses of elderly persons. Sandler (1978) thinks that there are grounds for more optimism about outcome when the analyst is not too ambitious in their goals for the patient. She emphasises that the analyst should mainly concentrate on analysis of the developmental impasse and aim to restore the person to be able to engage with the normal developmental processes for this age group. Neither full reconstruction of the past nor complete character analysis may be indicated. King (1980) gives a number of brief illustrations of successful analyses in which she illustrates her view that the disturbance of some elderly persons is because of the reawakening of developmental challenges that are very similar to those of adolescence but in reverse. She gives examples connected with issues to do with gender, sexuality, and independence/dependence conflicts. Segal (1981) gives a very convincing account of a successful analysis lasting 18 months of a 73-year-old man who had had a psychotic breakdown treated by ECT, and was left in a chronic psychotic state with depression, hypochondria, paranoid delusions, and attacks of intense rage. The course of the analysis is described, particularly the profound splitting mechanisms that the patient used as a defence against his ageing and thoughts of dying and death, which for him were associated with intense fantasies of persecution, punishment, and starvation.

GROUP PSYCHODYNAMIC THERAPIES WITH ELDERLY PEOPLE

This approach to psychological work with the elderly has been used with success for forty years. In his pioneering studies, Linden (1953) applied psychoanalytic principles to work with groups of 'chronically senile women'. He later employed a mixture of structured methods, group associations, encouragement of mutual interpretations, and transference understandings to restore social and practical functioning. These important treatments can be used in many settings for different groups of elderly patients, and are reviewed in much greater detail by MacLennan *et al.* (1988) than is possible here. Groups for the elderly have been used in acute and chronic psychiatric hospitals, nursing and other community homes, general hospitals (for example, with patients of chronic cardiac conditions), hospices for the dying, and also with relatives and other carers of those with dementia and other chronic mental and physical illness, including alcohol-addicted persons. Successful group therapy has also been conducted with less severely ill elderly people living in the community. Benefits of group psychodynamic therapy have been reported in many areas of psychological and social functioning: improvements in reality testing, depression, loneliness, other aspects of interpersonal relatedness and caring capacities, self-esteem and personal sense of integrity, sublimation of psychosexual conflicts, maladaptive behaviour, and readiness for discharge from institutions (Tross and Blum 1988).

Psychodynamic group psychotherapy should not be regarded as a single treatment, but as a collection of therapies with some patients more likely to benefit from one type of group than another and some who will not benefit from any group. A variety of techniques have been used, sometimes utilizing a single modality, for example, concentrating on verbal expression and interpretation of psychodynamics, supportive interventions, or directive and activity-based approaches. Others have integrated differing techniques at different stages in the group's development. Whatever technique is used, the reports make clear that a sound understanding of psychodynamics is essential, as is a full awareness and control by therapists over their personal biases towards ageing persons.

It is important to differentiate the aims of varying forms of group psycho-therapy. Symptom relief is obviously important, as is the minimization of institutionalization that some groups aim for. Some therapies focus on a single problem that may well have wide-ranging and serious implications for a specific group. Other treatments are more ambitious and long-term. They aim at helping the person make a considerable change in aspects of their personality and personal relationships in order to accommodate to and make the most creative use of the reality of their ageing.

Many of the groups described focus particularly on developmental tasks specific to ageing, such as accepting and integrating dependent aspects that had previously been disowned. Other group therapists have the capacities to take a group still deeper and allow its members to work on issues that they have hidden throughout their lives and only now are in a position to benefit from personal and group insight.

Group therapy in institutional settings

Hunter (1989) gives a short account of 17 brief psychodynamic psychotherapy groups she has conducted in hospitals, homes, and in the community in the UK. In two of these groups all members suffered from senile dementia. Kelly (personal communication) has conducted a psychodynamically orientated weekly group on an acute unit for the elderly mentally ill. The participants included depressed and psychotic patients and also organically disturbed elderly patients. He describes clearly the many levels at which the patients were able to respond to problems, including the capacity of the group to address issues of loneliness and sexual rivalry with younger persons. He was surprised at the way demented patients could occasionally tune into the group atmosphere in a compelling and briefly articulate way. Like Martindale (1989), he stresses the need of the younger therapists to monitor carefully their complex countertransference reactions to the elderly. These surface more openly as the patients reveal themselves to the group and the therapists in a far less restricted way than occurs in a traditional medical setting. However, he emphasizes the gains to the therapists and the ward staff, whose morale, work quality, and satisfaction increased as they gained a fuller picture of their patients.

Goodman (1988) describes groups for the elderly in an acute general psy-chiatric unit, and the multiple psychological problems associated with ageing that can be addressed and ameliorated in such a setting even though the average number of sessions attended was only seven. She describes the various ways that the group leaders offer themselves to the group members: active, directive, friendly, supportive, empathic, humorous, encouraging independence, and using behavioural and assertive techniques and concentration on the here and now.

Weiner (1988) describes short-term open-ended groups for cardiac patients, including the terminally ill. He describes the need for preparation of the patients, the important work with the ward staff, and how he helps the group respond to depression and denial, dependency and omnipotence, family issues and sexuality, and the significance and usefulness of the group modality.

Out-patient and community groups

Selection is one of the most important and difficult factors in conducting out-patient group psychotherapy. It is a very different proposition from establishing a group within a captive population in a hospital ward, nursing home, or day hospital. The most prominent psychological problem that lies behind the psychiatric manifestations of elderly people is loss—or fear of loss—of many different types. For many, loss is felt to be a sign of being unworthy (a difference between those who are mourning and those who are depressed is the lower self-esteem of the latter). Elderly people often crave to be accepted but are frightened of the possibility of being rejected or rebuffed. Groups may therefore be a particular source of hope of acceptance, but also elicit great anxiety concerning possible rejection. In selecting elderly patients for group therapy, a considerable amount of individual preparation may be necessary, as well as individual support during the introductory phase. It may well take at least a couple of months in the group for patients to feel that they and their problems will be tolerated and accepted by the group and for a sense of belonging to begin. Although many writers (Mardoyan and Weis 1981; Wolff 1957) stress the ready acceptance of elderly group members for one another, and the ease of group cohesion (Hunter 1989), I have found this far from always being the case, certainly in out-patient settings. Intolerance of differences has often been quite pernicious and difficult to contain. Racial and sexual prejudice and severe problems with envy have led to the active and hurtful rejection of fragile newcomers to psychotherapy groups. Personality clashes can also lead to rejection. The regressive longing to be loved without having to love in return has at times contributed to groups being quite uncaring about the fate of one of their number.

Too great a heterogeneity of psychological functioning is not conducive to effective long-term group psychodynamic psychotherapy with the elderly. I refer particularly to the spectrum between (a) those who are functioning at a level that recognizes their problems as being their own, and are motivated to seek further help with themselves and others as active participants knowing that some aspects will be painful, and (b) those whose motivation to join a group treatment stems more from a hope to find in the group what is missing in their lives, such as company or a sense of belonging. Although this is a polarization of a spectrum, it is my experience that elderly patients who fit much more in one of the two categories do not last long in a group that is mainly functioning in the mode of the other category. This is especially so of patients from category (a) who will understandably and appropriately be most frustrated and so not stay in a category (b) group for long—however much they may try and challenge the defences of the group. However, after a prolonged period it may well be that a group that started off functioning at quite an unsophisticated and highly defended level (category (b)) may become a safe enough setting in which much more personal exposure and intrapersonal and interpersonal interpretation is possible. It may then be feasible to introduce category (a) members. Predicting who will engage in a particular group remains a difficult and unreliable exercise, and those who do not manage to engage should be helped to find alternative treatments.

Short-term or long-term groups?

In order to address this question a very careful appraisal is needed of the nature of the difficulties of the patients, the institutional setting, and the skills of the therapists. Short-term groups may well be useful in an institutional setting to address a particular institutional problem, to maximize the opportunity to represent the internal problems of patients in interpersonal terms, to widen the diagnostic understanding, and to evaluate the therapeutic potential of exposing particular patients to one another. Groups may cushion excessive regression and institutionalization, and challenge secondary gain. There is, however, a danger that 'having a group' or 'group meetings' can become an institutional ritual that is antitherapeutic and colludes in the perpetuation of pathological institutional functioning. Much of the potential of groups to maximize healthy functioning depends on the capacities of the group leader to allow the therapeutic potential of the members with one another to emerge (see the film *One Flew Over the Cuckoo's Nest* for a crude example of the opposite!).

Short-term analytic group psychotherapy may have similar indications to those of brief individual therapy already described, especially where, after preparation, the patient is motivated to work through his problems in a group setting. In some of the enthusiastic accounts of group psychotherapy for those with major problems (Weinstein and Khanna 1986), it is very difficult to see how substantial and lasting benefits are likely to result from the brief group therapies described. Many of these enthusiastic reports are probably either with people with good premorbid functioning, who are in a transiently decompensated state, or else the changes are temporary ones in chronically dependent persons, resulting from a briefly stimulating environment. Some authors are possibly wrongly conflating the emergence of interesting, lively, and understandable group dynamics with the capacity for therapeutic change (Hunter 1989). A similar point has been made in a discussion article on assessment of suitability for psychoanalysis (Tyson and Sandler 1971).

Activity groups

In some activity groups, patients are offered a medium through which their psychological difficulties can be evoked, expressed, and elaborated and reflected on, and their defences carefully loosened. Self-identity and integrity can be enhanced. Music, art, drama, poetry, and literature are the most commonly used media, the choice depending on the skills and training of the therapist. Music and art may both be useful for those who have difficulty expressing themselves verbally, and sometimes for those who use language excessively defensively. It should be stressed that patients need no special musical or artistic ability to make use of these media; in fact those with little experience may benefit most.

Some activity groups are explicitly diversionary. They purposively divert the attention of the elderly persons away from their specific problems and attempt to interest them in other areas of life. They are supportive in that they may awaken or maintain other capabilities of the patient and bolster self-esteem that has been damaged or bruised in other aspects. These diversionary activities can be very helpful in assisting elderly patients retain or regain some sense of community, intellectual stimulation, innocent fun, and relief from the egocentric effect of their suffering. It is important to evaluate the usefulness of these activities in the full context of a therapeutic programme. There is a risk that they may be used excessively and defensively by staff who are not properly trained to work more directly with patients' disturbances.

There are many other accounts in the literature of short-term group therapies with the elderly, and these are well summarized in the books by MacLennan *et al.* (1988), and Weinstein and Khanna (1986). Nearly all the descriptions of group treatments give considerable indications of their useful contribution to the improvement in well-being of elderly persons with very varied problems. There are many techniques, and differing emphasis is given in the various accounts. The time is ripe for these to be evaluated more objectively and to look more carefully at those patients who do not benefit or even deteriorate as a result of therapy.

Long-term group analytic psychotherapy

There would be little point in offering longer-term psychotherapy unless it accomplished far more than can be achieved in shorter-term therapies. An idea of what may be achieved in long-term analytic group psychotherapy with the elderly can perhaps best be illustrated through the example of one group that has been meeting for four years. It is composed of patients ranging in age from 60 to 87 years who have all needed psychiatric help. Some had had admissions to hospital prior to entering the group. Most became mentally ill in the context of deaths of relatives, breakdown of physical health, or in anticipation of future losses. A couple of patients had also had psychiatric admissions during their younger adult years. As well as their presenting symptoms, mainly of depression, all had major personality difficulties, principally of a narcissistic type leading to lifelong impoverishment in the quality of their interpersonal relationships. Most of the group are materially poor, but two are well-off.

The group meets weekly for an hour and a half with two therapists. In spite of the therapists being explicit about the exploratory function of the group in the assessment interviews, in the early phases there was very little tangible alliance with the therapists to explore feelings further or to understand the group and individual dynamics and defences against this task. In fact, the opposite was generally the case; there were immense group pressures to move away rapidly from any opportunity to explore the personal and interpersonal, to keep the topics very neutral, and to emphasize similarity between members with respect to topics such as television programmes and current-affairs items. The following is a striking but typical example of the strength of the group's defences against understanding or knowing of one another's pain. After many months in the group, a Jewish member referred to going to an Atonement service at the synagogue, and for the first time in the group hinted at the loss of her family in the Holocaust. At that very moment the other Jewish patient interrupted to ask her, 'Which synagogue?'. Then, seemingly suddenly animated because she recognized the place, the second patient started a conversation about the architecture. Nobody in the group (including the original speaker) took the dialogue back to the losses; in fact within a few exchanges they were animatedly discussing a science fiction film!

A few members did not stay for long. However, core members who did stay, and the newcomers, started to show quite considerable symptomatic improvement. They came to the group each week in an animated and lively fashion, which has continued more or less unabated. Dependency on the group's existence was clear, and after the first few months the attendance of the group was very high and this has generally remained so. This liveliness contrasted to some extent with what the therapists were feeling about the group's relative failure to explore personal problems and feelings, and the members' tendency to dismiss the therapists' attempts to explore the dynamics of the group.

In trying to understand the above phenomena and the feelings of the therapists, it may be helpful to recall that breakdown in provision of care and treatment for the elderly is often due to the unacknowledged transferences of the younger staff persons to their older patients, in contrast to the usual emphasis on the patient's transferences. The younger therapist is keen for the patient to develop, to get better, and *to be able to manage without the therapist*, and may make manic attempts to get patients independent against the stream of the tide of the ageing process. This is a projection into the elderly person of both normal and pathological narcissistic aspects of the younger person's own developmental stages—to master, to build and build up, to be increasingly independent, to individuate from their family, yet wanting their parents or parent substitutes to be proud of and recognize their achievements. In contrast to the developmental task of the younger therapist, the older person's development may depend on facing loss of mastery and increasing dependence. The older person now needs to receive recognition and acceptance from younger persons, rather than to give these things. Consequently, the therapist may often be threatened by fears of the potential chronic neediness of their own parents because the psychic adjustments going on in the older generation are in the opposite direction to those of the younger person and seem incompatible with the latter's own strivings.

In this group, it was vital that the therapists recognized that their interpretations at that early stage were just as much an expression in the group of their narcissistic needs as of the needs of the patients. The therapists were similar to the patients in that they needed to be heard in their own way in the group; when interpretations had a particular urging quality, they were probably an expression of the therapists' need to master and achieve.

So, if verbal interventions often seemed to be ineffective in the early stages, why was it that the group members were beginning to improve? One defence in the face of loss is retreat and isolation for fear of further losses, but this only exacerbates the underlying helplessness, alienation, misery, and futility. Many of our group had expressed their problems in this way, certainly before referral. The early fragility of the group and the dropouts were also an expression of this. It is likely that the improvement in the group was largely due to increasing signs to the patients of its continued existence, and both the group and themselves surviving. In spite of the verbal interventions being relatively ineffective, the fact that a reliable long-term meeting place was provided, with minimal pressure on the group to be better or greatly improved in a finite time, has conveyed some unconscious communication of being in touch with their deepest anxieties about the therapists not surviving. Therefore, as with individual therapy, it is absolutely vital that professionals fully recognise and understand their narcissistic needs and take the greatest care not to act out their frustrations to such an extent that elderly patients are prematurely abandoned. The most gross way in which this could happen would be to terminate the group. If this had happened within the first two years, most of the patients would soon have been back under psychiatric or some other form of institutional care. However, two years further on some of the group members have allowed themselves to be much more involved in the exploratory process, and the quality of personal relationships both within and outside of the group has deepened considerably and consistently. They are benefiting considerably from exploring in the group lifelong personality difficulties, which had cause them great difficulties in intimacy, and which they had never faced or discussed before.

The approach outlined above breaches the dichotomy usually referred to in the literature between supportive and insight-orientated approaches (Tross and Blum 1988). In a group setting, the more vulnerable elderly patients need to be able to question the prevailing expectation that their environment (the group) will not survive (support) them before they are prepared or able to look further inside themselves (insight).

I have tried to emphasize some key dynamics that are particularly prominent in groups for the elderly and specific to their developmental struggles, but it should be remembered that many other factors contribute to successful therapy in group settings, and these have been reviewed by Yalom (1985).

CONCLUSION

There is now an extensive literature discussing from a psychodynamic perspective the developmental vicissitudes of the last phases of life. Similarly, there is a growing literature on the use of psychodynamically based interventions in a wide range of psychological disturbances in the elderly. The recent literature tends to concentrate rather uncritically on the successes of these interventions, in contrast to the pessimism expressed in previous eras (Freud 1905). Treatment failures and dropouts are rarely discussed. Articles tend to concentrate on only one form of psychodynamic intervention treatment. In the next era, it is to be hoped that more units involved in the care of the elderly will have professional groups sufficiently trained so that all the major psychodynamic treatments are available. It will then be possible to match treatments to patients' evolving needs and capacities rather than matching patients to the available treatments. This should lead to much more relevant research into psychotherapies for the elderly than the current inappropriate tendency to randomly allocate patients to treatments, a tendency which ignores the heterogeneity of patients with one diagnostic feature in common (Alanen 1994).

REFERENCES

Alanen, Y. (1994) Schizophrenia and psychotherapy. In: *Early treatment for schizophrenia patients* (eds Y. Alanen, B. Armelius, K. Lehtinen, B. Rosonbaum, R. Sjostram and E. Ugelstad.), pp. 15–27. Scandinavian University Press, Oslo, Norway.

Balint, E., and Norell, J. (1975). *Six minutes for the patient*. Tavistock, London.

Balint, M. (1957). *The doctor, his patient and the illness*. Pitman Publishing, London.

Bion, W. (1988) Attacks on linking. In *Melanie Klein today. Development in theory and practice. Volume 1: Mainly Theory*. (ed. E. Spillius), pp. 87–101. Routledge, London.

Butler, R. N. (1963). The life review: an interpretation of reminiscence in the aged. *Psychiatry*, **26**, 65–76.

Deitz, J. (1991). The psychodynamics and psychotherapy of depression: contrasting the self-psychological and the classical psychoanalytic approaches. *American Journal of Psychoanalysis*, **51**, 61–70.

de Jonghe, F., Rijnierse, P., and Janssen, R. (1992). The role of support in psychoanalysis. *Journal of the American Psychoanalytic Association*, **40**, 475–500.

Erikson, E. (1959). *Identity and the life cycle*, Chapter 25, p. 98. Psychological Issues, Monograph 1. International Universities Press, New York.

Freud, S. (1905). On psychotherapy. In *Standard edition of the complete psychological works of Sigmund Freud*, Volume 7 p. 264. Hogarth Press, London.

Freud, S. (1915). Our attitude to death. In *Standard edition of the complete psychological works of Sigmund Freud*, Volume 14, pp. 289–300. Hogarth Press, London.

Goodman, R. (1988). A geriatric group in an acute care psychiatric teaching hospital: pride or prejudice? In *Group psychotherapies with the elderly* (ed. B. MacLennan *et al.*) pp. 151–6. American Group Psychotherapy Monograph 5. International Universities Press, New York.

Gutmann, D. (1977). The cross-cultural perspective: notes towards a comparative psychology of ageing. In *Handbook of the psychology of ageing* (ed. J. E. Bruhn and W. Schue), pp. 30–32. Van Nostrand, New York.

Hildebrand, H. P. (1986). Dynamic psychotherapy with the elderly. In *Psychological therapies for the elderly* (ed. I. Hanley and M. Gilhooly), pp. 22–40. Croom Helm, London.

Hunter, A. J. (1989). Reflections on psychotherapy with ageing people, individually and in groups. *British Journal of Psychiatry*, **154**, 250–2.

Jaques, E. (1965). Death and the mid-life crisis. *International Journal of Psychoanalysis*, **46**, 502–14.

King, P. (1980). The life cycle as indicated by the nature of the transference of the middle aged and elderly. *International Journal of Psychoanalysis*, **61**, 153–60.

Kelly, C. (personal communication). The workings of a psychodynamic group in an acute elderly mentally ill unit.

Linden, M. E. (1953). Group psychotherapy with institutionalized senile women: study in gerontologic group psychotherapy. *International Journal of Group Psychotherapy*, **3**, 150–70.

Luborsky, L., Crits-Christoph, P., Minty, J., and Auesbach, A. (1988). *Who will Benefit from Psychotherapy? Predicting Therapeutic Outcomes*, p. 310. Basic Books, New York.

Malan, D. H. (1976). *Toward the validation of dynamic psychotherapy*, pp. 243–55 Plenum Press, New York.

MacLennan, B., Saul, S., *et al.* (1988). *Group psychotherapies with the elderly*. American Group Psychotherapy Monograph 5. International Universities Press, New York.

Mardoyan, J. L., and Weis, D. (1981). The efficacy of group counselling with older adults. *Personnel and Guidance Journal*, **60**, 161–3.

Martindale, B. V. (1989). Becoming dependent again: The fears of some elderly patients and their younger therapists. *Psychoanalytic Psychotherapy*, **4**, 67–75.

Pincus, A. (1970). Reminiscence in aging and its implication for social work practice. *Social Work*, **15**, 47–53.

Pfeiffer, E. (1971). Psychotherapy with elderly patients. *Postgraduate Medicine*, **50**, 254–8.

Porter, R. (1991). Psychotherapy with the elderly. In *Textbook of psychotherapy in psychiatric practice* (ed. J. Holmes), pp. 469–87. Churchill Livingstone, London.

Sandler, A. M. (1978). Problems in the psychoanalysis of an ageing narcissistic patient. *Journal of Geriatric Psychiatry*, **11**, 5–16.

Segal, H. (1979). Klein. Harvester Press, Brighton.

Segal, H. (1981). Fear of death. Notes on the analysis of an old man. In *The work of Hanna Segal*, pp. 173–82. Aronson, New York.

Taylor, G. J. (1987). *Psychosomatic medicine and contemporary psychoanalysis*. Stress and Health Series, Monograph 3. International Universities Press, Madison, Connecticut.

Tross, S., and Blum, J. (1988). A review of group psychotherapy with the older adult: practice and research. In *Group psychotherapies with the elderly*. American Group Psychotherapy Monograph 5. (ed. B. MacLennan *et al.*), p. 3. International Universities Press, New York.

Tyson, R., and Sandler, J. (1971). Problems in the selection of patients for psychoanalysis: comments on the application of the concepts of 'indications', 'suitability' and 'analysability'. *British Journal of Medical Psychology*, **44**, 211–28.

Wallerstein, R. S. (1986). *42 lives in treatment*, p. 38. Guildford Press, New York.

Weiner, W. (1988). Groups for the terminally ill cardiac patient. In *Group psychotherapies with the elderly*. American Group Psychotherapy Monograph 5 (ed. B. MacLennan *et al.*), pp. 175–8. International Universities Press, New York.

Weinstein, S., and Khanna, P. (1986). Depression in the elderly: conceptual issues and psychotherapeutic interventions. *Philosophical Library*, pp. 114–33. New York.

Winnicott, D. W. (1958) Primary maternal preoccupation. In *Collected papers: through paediatrics to psycho-analysis*. Tavistock London; Basic Books, New York.

Winnicott, D. W. (1963). The development of the capacity for concern. In *The maturational processes and the facilitating environment*, International Psycho-Analytical Library No. 64. (ed. J. Suthorland), pp. 73–82. Hogarth Press, London.

Wolff, K. (1957). Group psychotherapy with geriatric patients in a mental hospital. *Journal of the American Geriatrics Society*, **5**, 13–19.

Yalom, I. (1985). *The Theory and Practice of Group Psychotherapy*, Chapter 1, pp. 3–18. Basic Books, New York.

Yorke, C., Wiseberg, S., and Freeman, T. (1989). *Development and psychopathology: studies in general psychiatry*, pp. vii-ix. Yale University Press, New Haven and London.

8

Physical treatments
SANDRA EVANS

INTRODUCTION

The disorders considered in this chapter on the physical treatment of neurosis in the elderly are the mild to moderate depressive disorders, dysthymia, anxiety disorders (including general anxiety disorder and panic) obsessional and compulsive disorders, phobias, and bereavement reactions. Although the aetiologies of these disorders differ from one another, they all have their origins in the interactions between the individual's genetic constitution and external agents in the environment, such as life events and chronic difficulties (Cooper and Sylph 1973; Murphy 1982). The expression of these genetic and environmental factors is probably mediated through a final common pathway via neurotransmitters and receptor systems in the brain, hypothalamus, and other parts of the central nervous system. There is a growing body of neurobiological evidence that suggests identifiable links between affective symptoms and biological markers (Cowen and Wood 1991). However, no one theory or model of neurosis and depression is all-encompassing, and it is important to approach their treatment from a similar stance—that of multi-treatment options. It is important to bear in mind the significance of non-specific supportive measures and confident reassurances for the distressed patient (Morgan 1984); in placebo-controlled trials in depression, active treatment produces only a further 20–30 per cent more recoveries than placebo (Paykel 1989). The formal psychotherapy of psychological disturbances in older adults is becoming increasingly acceptable, and in some centres is an established form of treatment. What is even more heartening is the growing understanding that physical and psychological treatments are not mutually exclusive, and that starting an elderly person on a course of an anxiolytic or antidepressant does not preclude them from receiving counselling or cognitive therapy in addition. Indeed, some studies suggest that combinations of treatments have a synergistic effect (Bowers 1990; Blackburn *et al.* 1981). Practically, medication may be essential to reduce anxiety symptoms to the point where the patient is able to make full use of psychological treatments. It must also be borne in mind that the extent to which specific neurotic disorders are amenable to physical treatments in old age is still a moot point. A number of studies have shown the value of drug therapy in milder affective disorders in younger patients, particularly those seen by general practitioners (Blacker and

Clare 1988; Blacker *et al.* 1988; Moon and Jessinger 1991), but evidence of their effectiveness is still lacking in the elderly population.

SPECIAL CONSIDERATIONS IN THE ELDERLY

The physical risks

The drug metabolism of elderly people is much more variable than that of the young. Furthermore, a significant proportion of elderly depressed and anxious people are also physically ill and frail, and are taking combinations of other drugs. In these circumstances, the cautious clinician might be tempted to use subtherapeutic doses of psychotropic medication, or even consider not treating with medication at all despite the fact that it is indicated (Shapiro *et al.* 1984). Unfortunately, the elderly are still prepared to put up with feeling less than well (Lindesay *et al.* 1989), and patients and clinicians alike can be convinced that the depression and anxiety is a function of advanced age and that nothing can be done. The result of this misplaced caution and therapeutic nihilism is that patients who can benefit from physical treatment are left partially or completely untreated; one study found that only 27 per cent of patients thought to be suffering from DSM-III (*Diagnostic and statistical manual of mental disorders*, third edition) generalized anxiety disorder were receiving any anti-anxiety medication (Uhlenhuth *et al.* 1983).

Clinicians concerned about the physical risks attached to the drug treatment of psychiatric disorder in the elderly need to bear in mind that, untreated, these conditions have a significant excess morbidity and mortality in their own right, both from suicide and from other causes (Barraclough 1971; McClure 1984; Murphy *et al.* 1988). However, the safety of psychotropic drugs is an important consideration, and it is true that the anticholinergic and quinidine-like effects of the older tricyclic antidepressants have limited their use in physically ill elderly patients, particularly those with cardiovascular disease. The situation has improved considerably with the introduction of newer, less toxic antidepressants, such as the SSRIs (specific serotonin re-uptake inhibitors); however, experience with these compounds is still limited, and the issue of safety in overdose of these non-tricyclic antidepressants needs clarifying. Treatment with medication is a delicate balance between the risk of over-medicating, causing additional problems, and undertreating, which may prolong an illness and possibly lead to an admission. Undertreating may reduce the patient's confidence and limit their chances of returning to independent living.

Pharmacokinetics

The altered physiology of ageing brings about a change in the way that drugs are distributed, metabolized, and excreted in the elderly individual. It is considered that 65 years and over is a reasonable age to apply the principles of age-sensitive practice. However, one cannot be dogmatic in the application of these principles as there are plenty of robust individuals over 65 years and many younger people whose sensitivity to medication has been altered by ill health and disease.

Absorption

There is a decline in the number of gastric absorbing cells, decreased gastrointestinal motility and decreased active transport across the gut with increasing age. However, most psychotropic agents are passively diffused so the rate and extent of drug absorption in the elderly is largely unaltered by age factors alone (Stevenson *et al.* 1980). Changes in the gut pH and metabolism do have some effect on the bioavailability of drugs such as L-dopa, where reduced levels of dopa-decarboxylase lead to an increase in the peripheral effects of the drug.

Distribution

By contrast, the effects of ageing on the distribution of drugs are marked, and are of great importance when considering dosage. In general the elderly are smaller in stature than younger patients and may require smaller doses to achieve therapeutic blood levels of drug (Greenblatt *et al.* 1982). Ageing increases the total proportion of body fat up to twofold or threefold. This increases the volume of distribution of lipid-soluble drugs such as the metabolites of the benzodiazepines and of trazodone (Miller *et al.* 1987). The resultant increase in drug half-life and the interval before steady-state blood levels are reached may reduce the initial response to medication.

Protein binding

Many psychotropic drugs bind to albumin, so one consequence of a reduction in serum albumin levels of 15–20 per cent in the elderly (Schumacher 1980) is a rise in the amount of free drug available for receptor binding. This may help explain the increased susceptibility of the elderly to adverse drug effects and their vulnerability to multiple drug therapy. Inconsistencies in studies of protein binding in the elderly and a number of other confounding factors such as the effect of metabolism and clearance make evaluation of the significance of protein binding in the elderly difficult (Wood and Castleden 1991).

Hepatic metabolism

The liver is the primary remover of psychotropic medication from the circulation by producing both active and inactive metabolites which are then excreted by the kidneys. Liver mass in relation to body size declines with age as does blood flow and perfusion secondary to decline in cardiac output. The prevalence of slow-acetylator status is also increased with ageing (Gachalyi *et al.* 1984), and the resultant decrease in first-pass effect enhances the bioavailability of the drugs that are most highly metabolized. The activity and affinity of microsomal oxidative enzymes are reduced in the frail elderly, causing a reduction in metabolism of those drugs which undergo hepatic microsomal oxidation. The effect of tobacco smoking on the induction of these enzymes is less in the elderly than in younger patients. Alcohol misuse or chronic use induces microsomal enzymes, increasing the rate of drug metabolism.

Despite these age-related alterations in hepatic function, it is important to bear in mind that variation between individuals at a given age can be even greater. Although hepatic blood flow in persons aged 65 and over is decreased by 40 per cent compared with those aged 25, one large study of antipyrine metabolism found that there was a sixfold variation between individuals of similar age (Vestal *et al.* 1975); only 3 per cent of the variance in hepatic metabolism could be explained by age alone. This may help explain why some elderly people tolerate, indeed require, standard doses of medication, and should encourage clinicians to use these standard doses if their patients require them.

Renal excretion

The rate of glomerular filtration may decline by as much as by 50 per cent in the elderly, but the reduction in lean body mass gives rise to lower plasma creatinine levels. The resulting impression of normal renal function may be misleading and potentially hazardous when prescribing lithium or other medication that is dependent on good renal function for clearance. These drugs should be prescribed in an incremental fashion, building up from small initial doses until therapeutic levels are obtained.

Pharmacodynamics

The effect of age on neurotransmitters and receptor sensitivity remains unclear. In theory, one might expect a reduced sensitivity to psychoactive substances, and in fact such differences do exist; for example, the elderly are more resistant to the effects of propranolol. However, other psychoactive medication has the converse effect and the elderly brain is more sensitive to the effects of compounds such as benzodiazepines. The risk of toxic states increases by six times in the over-sixties compared to younger age groups (Schmidt *et al.* 1987).

Compliance

Compliance is another important factor determining the effectiveness of drug treatments. The current cohorts of elderly people come from generations that did not see the doctor or take medicines unless absolutely necessary—medical treatment was costly and they would often do without. They can be suspicious of drug treatments for psychological problems; in particular, they have been sensitized by the media presentation of benzodiazepine dependence (Tyrer 1984). If they experience unpleasant side effects of medication they may unilaterally decide to stop treatment without informing their doctors. In a small but interesting survey of medication compliance among old-age psychiatry day-hospital attenders, Ballard *et al.* (1991) found the average compliance rate to be 72 per cent compared to an ideal standard of 90 per cent (Wandless *et al.* 1979). Of particular concern was the failure to renew prescriptions and patients continuing to take discontinued medication.

Having established the need for medication, it is important to make sure that the patient is willing to take it. It is worth spending time at the outset explaining to the patient what they can expect in the way of common side-effects, and, in the case of antidepressants, warning them that there will be a delay of some weeks before they notice any benefit. Some discretion is required here, as one does not want to frighten the patient off treatment altogether. Early follow-up to review and reassure will help to maintain compliance, as will an incremental approach to establishing the therapeutic dose if side-effects are a problem. Some patients will need help in learning to distinguish between the side-effects of their treatment and the symptoms of their disorder.

Physical causes of psychological symptoms

There are a substantial number of medical causes of anxiety symptoms in the elderly (see Chapter 3). Cardiac conditions such as angina, mitral-valve disease and arrhythmias, and airways-obstruction disorders are common in the elderly and are highly correlated with symptoms of anxiety and depression. Many drugs for physical illnesses can produce anxiety symptoms, and their frequency is increased in an ageing population with its increased sensitivity to drugs. If these conditions are treated appropriately there may be little indication for psychiatric intervention, although there is bound to be some overlap in cases where the primary physical condition leads to and potentiates a secondary psychological one.

DRUG TREATMENTS

The use of drugs in the treatment of mental disorder has a long history. Sedative preparations in the form of opiates, alcohol, and herbal remedies have been used since ancient times in the treatment of insomnia and minor psychiatric symptoms. In the early part of this century, paraldehyde, bromides, and barbiturates were widely used as tranquillizing agents, and, while they no longer have any place in the management of neurotic disorder, one still comes across the occasional elderly user of such drugs who has been collecting their repeat prescription unchallenged for many years, and it is important to know something of their effects, and how to wean patients off them. Barbiturate withdrawal in physiologically dependent individuals can be very dangerous, and needs to be covered by gradually reducing doses of phenobarbitone to prevent fits.

Benzodiazepines

The tendency to use benzodiazepines in the treatment of neurotic disorders has declined generally in recent years, although the total condemnation of their use which was prevalent for a while in the early 1980s has subsided. More recent epidemiological surveys suggest that the abuse of benzodiazepines occurs less frequently than was originally thought (Rickels and Schweizer 1987), and their limited usefulness is once again being recognized. Despite the fact that formal research evidence of the effectiveness of benzodiazepines in the elderly is very limited (Salzman 1991), they are still major recipients of these drugs; in one survey, over 50 per cent of elderly people in residential care were on a benzodiazepine hypnotic or anxiolytic (Gilbert *et al.* 1988).

Clinical indications

The benzodiazepine group of drugs replaced the once popular barbiturates and meprobamate, and have been used effectively for over thirty years (Hollister and Csernansky 1990). They are potentiators of the inhibitory GABA (gamma-aminobutyric acid) neurotransmitter systems in the brain and spinal cord, an action they share with neuroleptics and tricyclic antidepressants, although it is not clear what significance this has on their clinical effectiveness. Benzodiazepines have anxiolytic, hypnotic, muscle relaxant, and anticonvulsant properties, and have a wide margin of safety, especially in overdose. There is no doubt that their speedy onset of action and generally good safety record make them extremely useful in the short-term treatment of anxiety states and as an adjunctive hypnotic in sleep disorders. The recent widespread concern about their prolonged use and their addictive properties, with a potential for a withdrawal syndrome, has led to a reduction in their use. This is all to the good if the result has been more thoughtful prescribing.

There are numerous benzodiazepines available, and their effectiveness is quite similar. They can be classified into short-acting and longer-acting according to their plasma half-lives, and a working knowledge of one compound in each category should be sufficient for good clinical practice. Temezepam is a short-acting drug which is widely used as a hypnotic in the elderly as it has minimal hangover effects (Cook *et al.* 1983). However, it should be emphasized that treatment should be for a few weeks only as these drugs have an effect on sleep quality. Short-acting benzodiazepines are also implicated in the production of 'rebound anxiety' as part of a withdrawal syndrome. On discontinuation there is also risk of rebound insomnia. Oxazepam is another short-acting benzodiazepine that is used to treat anxiety in elderly patients.

Long-acting benzodiazepines have active metabolites, a long duration of action and are slowly eliminated from the body. Their metabolism is profoundly slowed by the physiological effects of ageing, and the resultant potential accumulation of active drug in an elderly patient may cause adverse effects. This is further complicated by the increased proportion of body fat in the elderly. Benzodiazepines are stored in body fat and delay the establishment of a steady state at the start of treatment, which may give the impression that an inadequate dose has been given, with obvious risk for the unsuspecting. Steady state requires over one week to achieve.

In the elderly the most prominent indication for short-term treatment with a long-acting benzodiazepine would be for acute stress reactions, especially if the distress is profound. Severe bereavement reactions might be an indication but the risk of provoking denial mechanisms in the patient must be considered. Tyrer and Murphy (1987) have produced an excellent and balanced review of the place of benzodiazepines in the treatment of anxiety disorders.

In more recent studies, benzodiazepines are once more being advocated for specific anxiety disorders. One drug, alprazolam, is being promoted as a treatment for panic disorder and is being compared with more established treatments such as imipramine (Cross-National Collaborative Panic Study 1992). Reports of efficacy and safety are conflicting, and there is currently some controversy between the exponents of psychological and pharmacological treatments for this condition (Marks *et al.* 1992; Tiller *et al.* 1989). Other studies have suggested that alprazolam has an antidepressant effect; this is of interest but requires further investigation (Imlah 1985).

Adverse effects of benzodiazepines

The benzodiazepine withdrawal syndrome is an unpleasant cluster of physical and psychological symptoms not unlike anxiety and panic themselves (see Chapter 10). Severe withdrawal symptoms include hyperthermia, convulsions, and psychotic symptoms of paranoia, and visual and auditory hallucinations. Withdrawal symptoms are most likely with short-acting drugs, and represent a physiological dependence upon them. The effects of benzodiazepine withdrawal on sleep include the reduction in REM (rapid eye movement) and stage IV sleep, and reduction in the subjective quality of sleep—leaving the patient feeling unrefreshed. There are a number of reports of adverse effects of benzodiazepines on short-term memory, recall, and general intellectual functioning as well as reduced motor co-ordination (Fancourt and Castleden 1986). Depression of respiratory drive is a problem in drug interactions, particularly those which potentiate the benzodiazepines; these include interactions with alcohol and the antihistamines. Drowsiness may cause unsteadiness and so increase the risk of falls and fractures. Patients with even mild diffuse brain degeneration may be more at risk of confusion with paradoxical reactions, disinhibition, or incontinence.

Duration of treatment

It is now agreed that treatment with benzodiazepines at all ages should be short-term only. The best responders to short-term anxiolytic medication are non-psychotic anxious individuals with high levels of somatic and psychic symptoms. Those with anxiety complicating depression do not do well; indeed, the benzodiazepines are likely to make them feel worse. Similarly, people with personality problems do not fare well and are arguably among the most likely to become dependent.

Anxiety symptoms commonly subside with time, and the majority of patients can probably be weaned off treatment after about six to eight weeks. Rickels *et al.* (1983) reported on a group of chronically anxious patients in which 50 per cent of those treated with diazepam remained symptom-free when blindly switched to eight weeks of placebo. In patients in whom prolonged treatment appears unavoidable, it is helpful to be aware that the maximum benefit occurs within six weeks and so it is advisable to institute intermittent treatment in which drug therapy is interrupted every few weeks for as long as possible and the patient is maintained on the lowest therapeutic dose during treatment. These patients require enormous support, and ideally should be in anxiety-management groups to help them learn to manage their symptoms in other ways.

Antidepressants

Tricyclic and related drugs

Antidepressants are indicated in a variety of neurotic disorders, in particular mild and moderate depression, mixed anxiety and depression, dysthymia, and generalized anxiety. Since Klein noted in 1964 that imipramine had a beneficial effect on panic attacks (Klein 1964), low doses of this drug have been used in the treatment of both panic disorder and generalized anxiety disorder (Johnstone *et al.* 1980; Kahn *et al.* 1986). Antidepressants such as clomipramine with serotonin re-uptake inhibiting functions in addition to adrenergic action have been used in the pharmacological treatment of obsessive–compulsive disorder (OCD) for many years (Jenike 1985). While antidepressants are effective in a range of neurotic disorders, Healy (1991) cautions us against redefining anxiety symptoms as part of a depressive picture, in case this precipitates another explosion of long-term prescribing, this time with antidepressants such as the SSRIs taking the place of the benzodiazepines as a psychiatric panacea.

Until the introduction of second-generation tricyclic antidepressants (secondary amines such as desipramine), amitriptyline and imipramine were the standards by which efficacy and side-effects were measured. Despite their relative toxicity due to a large number of potential unwanted effects, they are extremely effective both as antidepressants and as anxiolytics. These tertiary amine tricyclics are more likely to produce antimuscarinic side-effects than the secondary amines, and are consequently not well tolerated by many elderly people or those who have serious cardiac problems or suffer with urinary retention, constipation, or narrow-angle glaucoma.

Some doubts have also been raised by Kutcher *et al.* (1986) about the accepted safety of the secondary amine tricyclics in the elderly, with significant electro-cardiogram (ECG) changes in 40 per cent of patients on desipramine. Generally, all tricyclic antidepressants possess a number of side-effects that are of concern in an elderly frail population. They can cause orthostatic hypotension, giving rise to falls and fractures. They exacerbate urinary problems in prostatism, and they can be cardiotoxic and should not be used in patients with recent myocardial infarction. They are also lethal in overdose. Their use in the neurotic disorders in the elderly, apart perhaps from the specific treatment of panic, should now be second in line to the non-tricyclic and the serotonin re-uptake inhibitor antidepressants.

Lofepramine, another second-generation tricyclic, has a number of advantages over the older group. It has far fewer muscarinic side-effects than amitryptline or imipramine, is better tolerated by the elderly and is relatively safe in overdose. Dorman (1988) cites a retrospective study of 210 elderly depressives with a mean age of 75.8 years treated with the lofepramine. Seventy per cent of patients were reported to have made a satisfactory response to treatment, and the reduced toxicity was of major interest. Bucknall *et al.* (1988) report a double-blind placebo, crossover study of lofepramine's antidepressant effect in patients with coexistent heart disease. Numbers were small and both drug and placebo were comparable for paucity of cardiovascular effects. Nevertheless, caution is advised with patients receiving cardiac medication, particularly digoxin.

Trazodone is an antidepressant that blocks the re-uptake of serotonin without antimuscarinic side-effects. The tetracyclic drugs mianserin and maprotiline have recently been associated with a number of problems, mianserin in particular being responsible for a number of aplastic anaemias and hepatic conditions. It is now advisable to take a full blood count every 4 weeks in the first 3 months of treatment and thereafter to monitor regularly. The drug should be withdrawn if signs of infection develop. Maprotiline has been associated with convulsions. Although these drugs have proven efficacy in depression and are much less antimuscarinic in their side-effects profile than the tricyclics, their place in the treatment of the elderly has been superseded by trazodone and lofepramine; these are now drugs of first choice in the elderly out-patient with mild to moderate depressive symptoms, particularly if night sedation is required. Trazodone can safely be given as a once-daily dose, and both drugs are well tolerated—enabling rapid increments to therapeutic doses.

Serotonin re-uptake inhibitors

There are currently five specific serotonin re-uptake inhibitor (SSRI) antidepressants available to British prescribers, and it is difficult to evaluate differences between them except in terms of price. They are all relatively expensive drugs, particularly when used in extended courses of treatment. There have been a number of studies indicating the efficacy of the SSRIs, including comparison with the standard tricyclics (Aberg-Wistedt 1989). All SSRIs have similar side-effects, most frequently nausea, vomiting, insomnia, anxiety, sweating, and headaches. These tend to wear off as treatment progresses but, understandably, compliance can be difficult to achieve in the elderly, particularly in the case of insomnia and nausea. The SSRIs do not have anticholinergic side-effects and are relatively safe in overdose. The Guillain-Barré adverse reaction, which brought about the withdrawal of zimelidine, seems not to occur with the remaining drugs.

Evidence for the recent concern that SSRIs increase the risk of suicide is lacking; indeed Montgomery and Fineberg (1989) report a reduction in suicidal thoughts on this medication. Specific serotonin re-uptake inhibitors produce an adverse serotonergic syndrome when combined with monoamine oxidase inhibitors (MAOIs), and can also increase central nervous system toxicity to lithium, and care should be exercised if augmenting with this drug.

Monoamine oxidase inhibitors

One of the physiological concomitants of ageing is an increase in the CNS of the enzyme monoamine oxidase, which metabolizes presynaptic monoamines, and it has been hypothesized as a potential cause, or at least a complicating factor, in late-life depression. MAOIs have a considerable track record in the successful treatment of depression, particularly atypical depressions and those with mixtures of phobic and anxiety features, and symptoms of fatigue (Quitkin *et al.* 1988). Their main disadvantage is from the 'cheese reaction', particularly in the frail elderly such as those on antiparkinsonian medication. For those atypical depressives or the chronically dysthymic who do not mind the dietary restrictions, it is an effective treatment, but has tended to be prescribed less since newer, less problematic treatments have arrived. In particular, the new reversible MAOI-B drugs such as moclobamide are said to offer the advantages of the MAOIs without need for the dietary caution. How true this is remains to be seen.

The practice of combination drug treatments for severe, prolonged, and intractable depression has somewhat reduced in popularity of late. Lithium augmentation is now well established and effective practice in the elderly has been reported (Finch and Katona 1989). The augmentation of antidepressant effect by combining a tricyclic antidepressant with an MAOI, usually phenelzine, and in severe cases adding L-tryptophan or lithium, is beyond the scope of this chapter as such treatments are rarely required in neurotic disorders. They are undoubtedly powerful treatments but carry high levels of risk. The combination of SSRIs with MAOIs is particularly hazardous and should not be attempted. The use of psychostimulants, such as pemoline or thyroid hormone, either alone or in combination with other drugs should not be necessary in this group of patients.

Neuroleptics

The anxiolytic properties of some neuroleptics are well established, and in the short-term treatment of severe anxiety symptoms, low-dose neuroleptic medication may be of use (Mendels *et al.* 1986). Not all neuroleptics have this property, however, so the pharmacological effects of dopamine blockade are unlikely to be the mechanism of action. Similarly, the antihistamine and anticholinergic properties which sedate the patient do not seem to be associated with anxiolysis.

The risks of prolonged treatment in the elderly are well known, particularly the hazards of inducing extrapyramidal symptoms of parkinsonism and akathisia, which may make the patient feel more agitated. The emergence of receptor supersensitivity and the production of tardive dyskinesia increase in frequency in the elderly and are more common in women.

One thioxanthene neuroleptic, flupenthixol, is marketed as an antidepressant in low doses. It appears to have only mild antidepressant properties and clinicians would be well advised to use a regular antidepressant for established depression. Flupenthixol may have a place in the treatment of mixed anxiety and depression with judicious prescribing and regular review to reduce risk of long-term side-effects, but evidence of its effectiveness for this purpose in the elderly is lacking.

Beta blockers

Anxiety has both psychic and somatic manifestations, the latter consisting of a number of unpleasant sensations such as dryness of the mouth, tachycardia, sweating, and trembling. The affected individual may also experience difficulty in swallowing and breathing, and a sinking feeling in the stomach, which may confirm the patient's view that they are about to die. The classical vicious cycle of anticipation leading to further anxiety or panic can be quickly induced in a vulnerable individual, and it is possible that as an adjunct to anxiety management, beta blockade may be useful in assisting the reduction in this spiralling effect.

Beta blockers can be effective in reducing sympathetic components of anxiety —such as palpitations, tremulousness, and tachycardia—but they can also increase fainting and unsteadiness by lowering the heart rate and blood pressure. An elderly person already anxious about feeling giddy or unsteady may be at risk, and caution is recommended. Kathol *et al.* (1980) report that propranolol in moderate doses of 40 mg four times daily also improved some of the psychological concomitants of anxiety, including irritability and apprehension. It is essential to point out that beta blockade is contra-indicated in patients with asthma, chronic obstructive airways disease, sinus bradycardia, and heart failure. These drugs can also be associated with unpleasant dreams.

Antihistamines

Like the phenothiazine neuroleptics, the probable efficacy of antihistamines in anxiolysis is linked to their sedative properties. Drugs such as hydroxyzine have a long history and good record of safety in the elderly, and indeed have been used to quieten agitated patients with diffuse organic brain disorder. They do, however, have a number of side-effects, especially hypotension and potential for paradoxical stimulation, which means that they must be used judiciously. Neurotically anxious elderly individuals with chronic obstructive airways disease, in whom any drug with potential for depression of respiratory drive would be contra-indicated, may benefit from antihistamines as part of the therapy.

Buspirone

Buspirone is an anxiolytic belonging to a new class of drugs, the azapirones, which are structurally unrelated to the benzodiazepines and have a totally different mode of action. Buspirone has no significant action on benzodiazepine or GABA receptors but is a partial 5-HT(1A) agonist. Activation of 5-hydroxytryptamine (5-HT (1A)) autoreceptors in the limbic system by buspirone diminishes 5-HT neuronal firing and limits 5-HT release. This reduction in 5-HT neurotransmission probably underlies its anxiolytic effect while the augmentation of noradrenergic transmission increases attention and arousal (Levine 1988). The main indications for treatment with buspirone is in generalized anxiety disorder when anxiety features are chronic and refractory, when longer-term therapy is required (Feighner 1987), or when there is risk of dependence and therefore benzodiazepines are not indicated. Unlike benzodiazepines, buspirone has a slow onset of action, taking around two weeks for therapeutic effect to set in (Jacobsen *et al.* 1985). This makes it unsuitable for acute anxiety states, and it has no place in the assisted withdrawal of benzodiazepines. There is evidence that it may have some antidepressant qualities (Robinson *et al.* 1990), and because of its 5-HT properties may have some use in the treatment of obsessive–compulsive disorder. Buspirone is considered safe and well tolerated in the elderly, although caution must be taken in hepatic and renal impairment. The starting dose should be low and the data sheet suggests that a dose of 30 mg should not be exceeded in the elderly. A standard efficacious dose for most cases is 20 mg.

The unwanted effects of buspirone include nervousness, headache, and dizziness (Singh and Beer 1988), and less commonly excitement and diarrhoea. It does not cause sedation and cannot be used as an hypnotic. It does react with MAOIs as there have been reports of patients becoming hypertensive with combination treatment, but in general it appears to react little with other medications. The advantages are that it is unlikely to impair psychomotor performance, and it does not seem to have a withdrawal syndrome (Lader 1991). Given its apparent advantages it is hard to see why buspirone is not prescribed more often, particularly in elderly patients, as an effective anxiolytic and adjunct to behavioural treatments. It may be that the slow onset of response to treatment in severe anxiety disorders is problematic, giving benzodiazepines the advantage. In longer-term anxiety disorders, particularly when insomnia and low mood are commonly present, antidepressants are preferred.

When to treat—when to stop

Recently the Old Age Depression Interest Group (1993) completed a multicentre trial of dothiepin versus placebo over a 2 year period and found that the patients maintained on antidepressants had less than half the relative risk of relapse than those on placebo. They recommend that elderly patients should be maintained on antidepressants for at least 2 years. Koenig *et al.* (1989) report a trial of antidepressants in the treatment of major depression in medical in-patients aged 65 years and over. Medical illness prevented 80 per cent from completing the trial. Short-term follow-up was carried out on all subjects, including those too unwell to take part in drug therapy. Exposure to antidepressants did not predict remission at follow-up due to spontaneous remission in the untreated group.

Perhaps the safest conclusion to draw from those two examples is that not enough is yet known about the outcome of depression or neurotic disorder in general to make dogmatic statements about how long patients should be medicated. Much can change in two years in the life of an elderly individual: changes for the better or for worse in life circumstances, physical illnesses, and physical treatments for other disorders. As a general principle, patients should be withdrawn from drug treatment slowly and under supervision of their practitioner. Signs of relapse can more easily be distinguished from signs of rebound/withdrawal effects. Supportive measures and psychological treatments should continue beyond drug therapy.

REFERENCES

Aberg-Wistedt, A. (1989). The antidepressant effects of 5-HT uptake inhibitors. *British Journal of Psychiatry*, **155** (Supp. 8), 32–40.

Ballard, C. G., Mohan, R. N. C., Handy, S., and Dodwell, D. (1991). Medication compliance and dispensing among psychogeriatric patients. *Psychiatric Bulletin* **15**, 624–5.

Barraclough, B. M. (1971). Suicide in the elderly. In *Recent advances in psychogeriatrics*, (ed. D. W. K. Kay and A. Walk), pp. 87–9. Headley Bros, Ashford.

Blackburn I. M., Bishop, S., Glen, A. Whalley, L. J., and Christie, J. E. (1981). The efficacy of cognitive therapy in depression: a treatment trial using cognitive therapy and pharmacotherapy, each alone and in combination. *British Journal of Psychiatry*, **139**, 181–9.

Blacker, C. V. R., and Clare, A. W. (1988). The prevalence and treatment of depression in general practice. *Psychopharmacology*, **95**, 14–17.

Blacker, R., Shanks, N. J., Chapman, N., and Davey, A. (1988). The drug treatment of depression in general practice: a comparison of nocte administration of trazodone with mianserin, dothiepin and amitriptyline. *Psychopharmacology*, **95**, 18–24.

Bowers, W. A. (1990). Treatment of depressed inpatients. Cognitive therapy plus medication, relaxation plus medication and medication alone. *British Journal Psychiatry*, **156**, 73–8.

Bucknall, C., Brooks, D., Curry, P. V., Bridges, P. K., Bouras, N., and Ankier, S. I. (1988). Mianserin and trazodone for cardiac patients with depression. *European Journal of Clinical Pharmacology*, **33**, 565–9.

Cook, P. J., Huggett, A., Graham-Pole, R., Savage, I. T., and James, I. M. (1983). Hypnotic accumulation and hangover in elderly inpatients: a controlled double-blind study of temezepam and nitrazepam. *British Medical Journal*, **286**, 100–2.

Cooper, B., and Sylph, J. (1973). Life events and the onset of neurotic illness in general practice. *Psychological Medicine*, **13**, 421–35.

Cowen, P. J., and Wood, A. J. (1991). Biological markers of depression. *Psychological Medicine*, **21**, 825–30.

Cross-National Collaborative Panic Study, Second Phase Investigators. (1992). Drug treatment of panic disorder. Comparative efficacy of alprazolam, imipramine and placebo. *British Journal of Psychiatry*, **160**, 191–202.

Dorman, T. (1988). The management of depression and the use of lofepramine in the elderly. *British Journal of Clinical Practice*, **42**, 459–64.

Fancourt, G., and Castleden, M. (1986). The use of benzodiazepines with particular reference to the elderly. *British Journal of Hospital Medicine*, **v**, 321–5.

Feighner, J. P. (1987). Buspirone in the long term treatment of generalised anxiety disorder. *Journal of Clinical Psychiatry*, **48** (Supp.), 3–6.

Finch, E. J. L., and Katona, C. L. E. (1989). Lithium augmentation in the treatment of refractory depression in old age. *International Journal of Geriatric Psychiatry*, **4**, 41–6.

Gachalyi, B., Vas, A., Hajos, P., and Kaldor, A. (1984). Acetylator phenotypes: effect of age. *European Journal of Clinical Pharmacology*, **26**, 43–5.

Gilbert, A., Quintrell, L. N., and Owen, N. (1988). Use of benzodiazepines among residents of aged-care accommodation. *Community Health Studies*, **12**, 394–9.

Greenblatt, D. J., Sellers, E. M., and Shader, R. I. (1982). Drug disposition in old age. *New England Journal of Medicine*, **306**, 1081–8.

Healy, D. (1991). The marketing of 5-hydroxytryptamine: depression or anxiety? *British Journal of Psychiatry*, **158**, 737–42.

Hollistor, L. E. and Csernansky, J. G. (1990). *Clinical Pharmacology of Psychotherapeutic Drugs* (3rd edition). Churchill Livingstone, New York.

Imlah, N. W. (1985). An evaluation of alprazolam in the treatment of reactive or neurotic (secondary) depression. *British Journal of Psychiatry*, **146**, 515–19.

Jacobson, A. F., Dominguez, M. D., Burton, J., Goldstein, M. D., and Steinbook, R. M. (1985). Comparison of buspirone and diazepam in generalised anxiety disorder. *Pharmacotherapy*, **5**, 290–6.

Jenike, M. A. (1985). *Handbook of geriatric psychopharmacology*. PSG Publishing Company, Littleton, Massachusetts.

Johnstone, E. C., Owens, D. G., Frith, C. D., McPherson, K., Dowie, C., Riley, G., *et al.* (1980). Neurotic illness and its response to anxiolytic and antidepressant treatment. *Psychological Medicine*, **10**, 321–8.

Kahn, R. J., McNair, D. M. Lipman, R. S., Cori, L., Rickels, K., Downing, R., *et al.* (1986). Imipramine and chlordiazepoxide in depressive and anxiety disorders: 2. Efficacy in anxious outpatients. *Archives of General Psychiatry*, **43**, 79–85.

Kathol, R. G., Noyes, R., Slyman, D. J., Crowe, R. R., Clancy, J., and Kerbor, R. E. (1980). Propranolol in chronic anxiety disorders. A controlled study. *Archives of General Psychiatry*, **37**, 1361–5.

Klein, D. F. (1964). Delineation of two drug responsive anxiety syndromes. *Psychopharmacology*, **5**, 397–408.

Koenig, H. G., Goli, V., Shelp, F., Kudler, H. S., Cohen, H. J., Meador, K. G., and Blazer, D. G. (1989). Antidepressant use in elderly medical inpatients: lessons from an attempted clinical trial. *Journal of General Internal Medicine*, **4**, 498–505.

Kutcher, S. P., Reid, K., Dubbin, J. D., and Shulman, K. I. (1986). Electocardiogram changes and therapeutic desipramine and 2-hydroxy-desipramine concentrations in elderly depressives. *British Journal of Psychiatry*, **148**, 676–9.

Lader, M. (1991). Can buspirone induce rebound, dependence or abuse? *British Journal of Psychiatry*, **159** (Supp. 12), 45–51.

Levine, S. (1988). Buspirone: clinical studies in psychiatry. In *Buspirone: a new introduction to the treatment of anxiety* (ed. M. Lader). International Congress And Symposium Series No. 139. Royal Society of Medicine, London.

Lindesay, J., Briggs, K., and Murphy, E. (1989). The Guy's / Age Concern Survey. Prevalence rates of cognitive impairment, depression and anxiety in an urban elderly community. *British Journal of Psychiatry*, **155**, 317–29.

Marks, I., Greist, J. Basoglu, Noshirvani, H. and O'Sullivon, G. (1992). Comment on the Second Phase of the Cross-National Collaborative Panic Study. *British Journal of Psychiatry*, **160**, 202–5.

McClure, G. M. G. (1984). Trends in suicide for England and Wales 1975–1980. *British Journal of Psychiatry*, **144**, 119–24.

Mendels, J., Frajewski, T. F., Huffer, V., Taylor, R. J., Secunda, S., Schless, A., *et al.* (1986). Effective short term treatment of generalised anxiety disorder with trifluoperazine. *Journal of Clinical Psychiatry*, **47**, 170–4.

Miller, L. G., Greenblatt, D. J., Friedman, H., Burstein, E., Scavone, J. M., and Harmatz, J. S. (1987). Trazodone kinetics in old age. *Clinical Pharmacology and Therapeutics*, **41**, 210.

Montgomery, S. A., and Fineberg, N. (1989). Is there a relationship between serotonin receptor subtypes and selectivity of response in specific psychiatric illnesses? *British Journal of Psychiatry*, **155** (Supp. 8), 63–70.

Moon, C. A., and Jessinger, D. K. (1991). The effects of psychomotor performance of fluvoxamine versus mianserin in depressed patients in general practice. *British Journal of Clinical Practice*, **45**, 259–62.

Morgan, H. G. (1984). Do minor affective disorders need medication? *British Medical Journal*, **289**, 783.

Murphy. E. (1982). The social origins of depression in old age. *British Journal of Psychiatry*, **141**, 135–42.

Murphy, E., Smith, R., Lindesay, J., and Slattery, J. (1988). Increased mortality rates in late-life depression. *British Journal of Psychiatry*, **152**, 347–53.

Old Age Depression Interest Group (1993). How long should the elderly take antidepressants? A double-blind placebo-controlled study of continuation/prophylaxis therapy. *British Journal of Psychiatry*, **162**, 175–82.

Paykel, E. S. (1989). Treatment of depression. The relevance of research for clinical practice. *British Journal of Psychiatry*, **155**, 754–63.

Quitkin, F. M., Stewart, J. W., McGrath, P. J., Leibowitz, M. R., Harrison, W. M., Tricamo, E., *et al.* (1988). Phenelzine versus imipramine in the treatment of probable atypical depression: defining syndrome boundaries of selective MAOI responders. *American Journal of Psychiatry*, **145**, 306–11.

Rickels, K., and Schweizer, E. E. (1987). Current pharmacotherapy of anxiety and panic. In *Psychopharmacology: the third generation of progress* (ed H. Y. Meltzer), pp. 1193–1203. Raven Press, New York.

Rickels, K., Case, W. G., Downing, R. W., and Winokur, A. (1983). Long-term diazepam therapy and clinical outcome. *Journal of the American Medical Association*, **250**, 767–71.

Robinson, D. S., Rickels, K., Feighner, J., Fabre, L. F., Gommans, R. E., Shrotriya, R., *et al.* (1990). Clinical effects of the 5-HT (1A) partial agonist in depression: a composite analysis of buspirone in depression. *Journal of Clinical Psychopharmacology*, **10** (Supp. 3), 67–76.

Salzman, C. (1991). Pharmacologic treatment of the anxious elderly patient. In *Anxiety in the elderly* (ed. C. Salzman and B. D. Lebowitz), p. 14. Springer Publishing Co., New York.

Schmidt, G., Grohmann, R., Strauss, A., Spiess-Kiefer, D., Lindmeier, D., and

Mulleroerlinghausen, B. (1987). Epidemiology of toxic delirium due to psychotropic drugs in psychiatric hospitals. *Comprehensive Psychiatry*, **28**, 242–9.

Schumacher, G. E. (1980). Using pharmacokinetics in drug therapy: VII. Pharmacokinetic factors influencing drug therapy in the aged. *American Journal of Hospital Pharmacology*, **37**, 559–62.

Shapiro, S., Skinner, E. A., Kessler, L. G., Von Korff, M., and German, P. S. (1984). Utilisation of health and mental health services: three epidemiologic catchment area sites. *Archives of General Psychiatry*, **41**, 971–8.

Singh, A. N., and Beer, M. (1988). A dose range-finding study of buspirone in geriatric patients with symptoms of anxiety. *Journal of Clinical Psychopharmacology*, **8**, 67–8.

Stevenson I. H., Salem, S., O'Malley, K., Cusak, B., and Kelly, J. G. (1980). Age and drug absorption. In *Drug Absorption* (ed. L. F. Prescott and W. S. Nimmo), pp. 235–61. Adis Press, Sydney.

Tiller, J., Schweitzer, I., Maguire, K., and Davies, B. (1989). Is diazepam an antidepressant? *British Journal of Psychiatry*, **155**, 483–9.

Tyrer, P. J. (1984). Benzodiazepines on trial. *British Medical Journal*, **288**, 1101–1102.

Tyrer, P., and Murphy, S. (1987). The place of benzodiazepines in psychiatric practice. *British Journal of Psychiatry*, **151**, 719–23.

Uhlenhuth, E. H., Balter, M. B., Mellinger, G. D., Cisin, I. H., and Clinthoree, J. (1983). Symptom check-list syndromes in the general population. *Archives of General Psychiatry*, **40**, 1167–74.

Vestal, R. Norris, A., Tobin, J. D., Cohon, B. H., Shock, N. W., and Andres, R. (1975). Antipyrine metabolism in man: influence of age, alcohol, caffeine and smoking. *Clinical Pharmacology and Therapeutics*, **18**, 425–34.

Wandless, I., Mucklon, J. C., Smith, A., and Prudham, D. (1979) Compliance with prescribed medicines: a study of elderly patients in the community. *Journal of the Royal College of General Practitioners*, **29**, 391–6.

Wood, P., and Castleden, M. (1991). Psychopharmacology in the elderly. In *Psychiatry in the elderly* (ed. R. Jacoby and C. Oppenheimer), pp 339–37. Oxford University Press, Oxford.

9

Personality disorders
ROBERT C. ABRAMS

INTRODUCTION

Personality disorders are enduring patterns of dysfunctional behaviour which pervade multiple facets of a person's life. Usually there is an interpersonal focus, and always there is impairment in functioning. In this definition the aspects of pervasiveness, referring to the impact of the disorder on different domains of life, and impairment in functioning are together what make personality disorders *mental* disorders. It is their persistence over long periods and their interpersonal focus which make them disorders of personality.

Individuals with personality disorders may be suspicious, litigious, or expect to become exploited; they may be emotionally excessive, yet shallow, and have little capacity for empathy with others; they may show impulsivity and an indifference with respect to antisocial acts; they may require constant reassurance. Personality disorders can cause as much pain and suffering for people in the patient's world as the patient himself. These conditions are not easily recognized, even by physicians and the educated public, and, to an extent that has yet to be calculated, they are expensive to society.

DSM-III (*Diagnostic and statistical manual of mental disorders*, third edition) (American Psychiatric Association 1980) elaborated the Axis II personality disorders from a group of traditional personality types (Table 9.1). Fourteen years later, and into its third version (DSM-IV) (American Psychiatric Association 1994), the clinical usefulness of the personality disorder axis has been affirmed (Widiger 1991). However, theoretical and methodological problems remain. First, there is heterogeneity of symptoms within individual disorders and overlap among different disorders (Gunderson 1992). Personality disorders therefore lack convergent and discriminant properties. Moreover, their theoretical underpinnings are unclear. For example, personality disorders can be described in terms of a failure of adaptation (McGlashan 1986), pathological intrapsychic organization (Kernberg 1975), interactions of genetic and environmental influences (Fulker 1981), dysfunctional learning and information processing (Beck 1967), or dysregulation of serotonergic or dopaminergic neurotransmitter systems (Cloninger 1987). Although the DSM-III-R (revised version of DSM-III) personality disorders may be related to an underlying five-factor trait structure (neuroticism, extroversion, openness to experience,

Table 9.1. DSM-III-R Axis II personality disorders.

Cluster A
Paranoid
Schizoid
Schizotypal
Cluster B
Antisocial
Borderline
Histrionic
Narcissistic
Cluster C
Avoidant
Dependent
Obsessive–compulsive
Passive–aggressive

agreeableness, and conscientiousness) (Costa and McCrae 1990), the clustering of symptoms sometimes seems arbitrary, failing to 'cut nature at its joints'. DSM-III-R may also be culture-bound, and as Cloninger (1987) pointed out, the content of Axis II disorders has been subject to socio-political fashion.

While the multiaxial philosophy of DSM-III represented a conceptual break-through, subsequent research has shown that the Axis II diagnoses are distorted in patients with acute depression or anxiety (Hirschfield *et al.* 1983; Reich *et al.* 1987); the personality disorders often resolve with remission of the Axis I disorder. The multiaxial approach also introduced ambiguity at the boundaries of Axis I disorders, where, in an example frequently used, schizotypal personality disorder might be more closely related clinically and genetically to schizophrenia than to other personality disorders (Siever *et al.* 1991). Similarly, affective instability characterizes both low-grade affective disorders and several personality disorders, and chronic anxiety symptomatology could belong to either anxiety disorder or Cluster C personality-disorder categories. In addition, the basic Axis I / Axis II relationship is not well understood. The relationship might be: *predispositional*, in which the personality disorder predisposes to the development of an Axis I syndrome; *prodromal*, in which the personality disorder also precedes the Axis I syndrome but as a forme fruste; *pathoplastic*, in which the pre-existing personality disorder modifies the clinical expression of the Axis I disorder, or affects its prognosis; *interactional*, in which major mental disorders like schizophrenia or depression permanently alter or scar the personality; or *orthogonal*, in which the Axis I and Axis II disorders coexist by chance.

To the dismay of most researchers in this field, Axis II provides only categorical diagnoses, lacking dimensional scales or continua along which all individuals can be placed. Examination of the component trait structure of personality disorders and the measurement of change are both impeded by the absence of a dimensional component. The absence of dimensional scaling also causes problems for clinicians. One patient might meet only few criteria for a personality disorder, not sufficient to be given a full diagnosis, yet have significant impairment in social and operational functioning as a result of meeting those criteria. Neither the partial criteria nor the associated impairment in functioning are noted on Axis II.

The subtlety of boundaries with Axis I disorders, together with the fact that patients are asked to acknowledge symptomatology that has negative social implications, limits the reliability of personality-disorder diagnoses (Loranger *et al.* 1991). Even skilled clinicians cannot confidently make these diagnoses without the use of multiple observers in diverse contexts. Nevertheless, despite these shortcomings, personality disorders in close to their present form are likely to be enduring features of all psychiatric nosologies. The remainder of this chapter discusses their implications for the later stages of life.

PERSONALITY DISORDERS AND AGEING

From the inception of DSM-III Axis II, personality disorders were considered to be conditions of young adulthood. The original introduction to Axis II (American Psychiatric Association 1980) stated that '. . . personality disorders are generally recognizable by adolescence or earlier and continue throughout most of adult life, though they often become less obvious in middle or old age.' Although there have been no longitudinal studies of personality disorder tracking patients' outcome as far as senescence, personality disorder symptomatology does appear to change over the life span; the nature of age-related change may vary with the disorder. Using cross-sectional regression analysis of the relationships of different personality disorders with age, Tyrer (1988) proposed that Axis II can be divided into mature and immature disorders. The mature disorders, including obsessive–compulsive, schizotypal, schizoid, and paranoid, tend to be stable over time; in the case of schizotypal personality disorder, spectrum and genetic relationships to Axis I schizophrenia suggest that it would be a lifetime disorder (Tyrer 1988; Siever *et al.* 1991). The immature or flamboyant personality disorders, including antisocial, borderline, histrionic, narcissistic, and passive–aggressive, appear to be more evident in younger individuals and may also have younger age of onset. The mature personality disorders in this scheme are all Cluster A (odd–eccentric) disorders, with the exception of obsessive–compulsive disorder from Cluster C (anxious–fearful), while the immature disorders are all Cluster B (dramatic–emotional) disorders, with the exception of passive–aggressive disorder from Cluster C.

Support for a maturation hypothesis, especially in immature disorders such as borderline and antisocial, has been found in suicide-mortality data and in follow-up studies. The suicide-mortality data reviewed by Tyrer (1988) suggest that personality disorder patients have higher rates of completed suicide than other psychiatric patients during the first five years following diagnosis, after which time the differences are no longer significant. Frequently cited follow-up studies by McGlashan (1986) and Stone (1990) indicate a flattening, or decline in the most florid borderline symptomatology, by the second decade of follow-up. Improvement in these patients was not restricted to overt symptomatology but was also reflected occupationally and globally (McGlashan 1986). However, this does not imply uniformity of improvement across all spheres of functioning, since some of the patients in McGlashan's study who advanced in occupational or instrumental domains never developed satisfactory personal relationships.

DSM-III-R personality disorders appear to be relatively infrequent in old age (Schneider *et al.* 1992; Abrams 1991). Fogel and Westlake (1990), reviewing the triaxial diagnoses of over 2000 in-patients with major depression, found that patients over 65 years had a lower overall rate of Axis II diagnoses. In the absence of longitudinal studies, however, the reason for the paucity of personality disorders is a matter of speculation. For example, a decline in the immature personality disorders could contribute. Yet the age profile of dramatic-cluster personality disorders in the community is not linear, but rather resembles a reverse J-shaped curve in which core traits decline until the age of 60 years, then take a slight upturn (Reich *et al.* 1988).

It is also possible that DSM-III-R criteria do not address issues relevant to the lives of ageing persons and thus fail to capture personality traits in their contemporaneous context. Narcissistic pathology in the elderly may be especially poorly captured by current nosology. At times the criteria for Cluster B disorders appear to be aimed at a modal 25-year-old faced with the tasks of establishing a career and finding a life partner. Age bias could easily lead to underestimation of narcissistic pathology, with symptoms dismissed as normative for age. On the other hand, there are no clear guidelines to help the clinician take into account the impact of memory impairment, illness, loss, other negative age-related life events, or declining social supports, all of which could affect personality disorder assessment in a false-positive direction. The recent finding that elderly patients meet a relatively large number of criteria for the 'not otherwise specified' (NOS) category of Axis II, but few other personality-disorder diagnoses, suggests that personality dysfunction in the elderly is more abundant than the number of categorical diagnoses would indicate (Abrams *et al.* 1993; Kunik *et al.* 1993).

Another plausible reason for the relative scarcity of full-blown personality disorders in the elderly might be the reluctance of clinicians to make these diagnoses. Psychiatrists frequently assess geriatric patients during episodes of acute depression or while they are in a crisis, both circumstances in which the kind of information-gathering necessary to make an Axis II diagnosis is difficult. Typically, the lack of informants and the ordering of priorities during an acute illness lead clinicians to defer evaluation for personality disorders. Also, patients' self-perceptions are likely to be negatively skewed during periods of depression (Hirschfeld *et al.* 1983; Reich *et al.* 1987). Furthermore, in order to diagnose personality disorders in elderly patients the clinician must be able to establish that the pathological behaviours or relationships have been present throughout most of adult life. Geriatric clinical experience suggests that there are some individuals with mild or compensated personality dysfunction in young or middle adulthood who in old age show a marked worsening of these trends; such late-onset patients do not meet the 'characteristic of long-term functioning' requirement of Axis II and are therefore not assigned personality-disorder diagnoses. DSM-III and DSM-III-R also fail to provide for past personality disorders, those present throughout much of adult life but attenuated in old age. Thus, the time frame guidelines of DSM-III-R may serve to limit the number of diagnoses. In addition, the extent to which young adults with personality disorders commit suicide, develop major depression, or have another affective denouement by the time they reach late middle age is unknown. Finally, there may be factors unique to the present cohort of elderly persons which underlie the epidemiology of personality disorders.

What are the signs and symptoms of personality disorder in the elderly? Although there are insufficient data to justify general statements, it has been suggested that Cluster C disorders may predominate (Schneider *et al.* 1992; Kunik *et al.* 1993). However, these are impressions derived mostly from studies of recovered elderly depressives, and it is possible that residual depression led the subjects to exaggerate their avoidant and dependent tendencies. Depression is also phenomenologically related to anxious–fearful traits. Even in the absence of a depression confound, increased dependency based on realistic physical changes could be misinterpreted by patient, family, and clinician, resulting in spuriously high estimations of Cluster C symptomatology. In DSM-IV (American Psychiatric Association 1994) the criteria for avoidant and dependent personality disorders appear to focus more clearly on *internal* inhibition or restraint with anxious motives. For example, one may be avoidant because of embarrassment, shame, fear of ridicule, or feelings of inadequacy. These new criteria might help clinicians distinguish anxious avoidance from schizoid phenomena, and psychological from realistic dependency.

Since there is little information from studies using *clinical* criteria, it is reasonable to ask whether age-related personality changes are supported by studies employing trait dimensions. Increasingly, what the psychological literature shows is stability of personality traits over the life span. Originally, large-scale investigations using the Minnesota Multiphasic Personality Inventory (MMPI) (Dahlstrom *et al.* 1972; Swenson *et al.* 1973) showed that older medical patients scored higher on scales measuring introversion, concern with health, immaturity, and depression than younger adult medical patients. These data initially seemed to support the notion that a quiet, inner-directed attitude typifies the ageing personality, with disengagement as its predominant social-psychological model (Cumming and Henry 1961). Declines in sociopathy and criminality (Woodruff *et al.* 1971) with advancing age were also documented. However, the early MMPI data were cross-sectional, and have been contradicted by longitudinal MMPI data emphasizing stability within individuals over time (Leon *et al.* 1979). Dimensional scores on the Eysenck Personality Inventory psychoticism (P), extroversion (E), and neuroticism (N) subscales also showed persistence over

30 years (Eysenck and Eysenck 1985), and more recently, McCrae and Costa (1990) presented further evidence of stability using the five-factor trait model.

If underlying personality traits persist over time, why might older people have fewer or different clinical personality disorders? The possible prominence of the NOS category suggests that with ageing, personality dysfunction is not necessarily reduced but is less tied to traditional personality-disorder typologies. This hypothesis in turn raises the possibility that a new nosology of personality disorders for the second half of life, analogous to the one for children and adolescents, might be justified. For example, a 'dissatisfied' personality disorder describing a complaining, disgruntled, self-defeating, help-rejecting attitude might be one candidate for validation. This entity would comprise symptoms from current passive–aggressive, narcissistic, histrionic, dependent, and other disorders. Another possible category might be a 'depressive' personality disorder covering chronic dysthymia in the elderly. Validating such new categories might prove more interesting and useful than simply translating DSM criteria into a geriatric context.

The overall implication of these comments is that underlying personality traits appear to remain stable in individuals as they age, but the *clinical expression of those traits might change*. To understand the direction and magnitude of such changes, studies are needed which use both categorical and dimensional methodologies. In the following section personality disorders in the elderly will be considered in relation to specific clinical contexts.

PERSONALITY DISORDERS AND PSYCHIATRIC DISORDERS IN THE ELDERLY

Personality disorders and depression

It has already been noted that personality dysfunction can be closely associated with Axis I syndromes, with various aetiological, predispositional, genetic, and temporal relationships considered possible (Hirschfield *et al.* 1983) In the general psychiatric literature, these relationships have been best studied in the area of depression; patients' premorbid and postmorbid personalities have been extensively evaluated. To summarize, mixed-aged unipolar depressives have been found to have a premorbid pattern of instability, neuroticism, introversion, and rigidity; compared to normal or manic subjects, depressives have more introversion, obsessionality, neuroticism, and aggression (Hirschfield and Klerman 1979; von Zerssen 1982; Angst and Clayton 1986). In addition, associations between depression, alcoholism, and antisocial personality have been found (Woodruff *et al.* 1971). Clinical investigations using DSM-III or DSM-III-R personality disorder criteria have produced high rates of personality disorder co-morbidity in mixed-age patients with major depression, ranging from 35 per cent (Shea *et al.* 1987) to 53 per cent (Pfohl *et al.* 1984); these findings have been relatively consistent despite differences in personality assessment method,

study design, and subject populations. Among depressed out-patients with Axis
II diagnoses, personality disorders in the Cluster C (anxious–fearful) category
may be most frequent (Shea *et al.* 1987).

Associations between personality traits and depression specific to the second
half of life have historically attracted the interest of clinicians and researchers.
Titley (1936), for example, in an early study found that involutional depressives
had more lifelong anxiety, hypochondriasis, social withdrawal, and obsessional
traits than bipolar patients or normal controls. In a classic follow-up study of
92 elderly patients, Post (1972) reported that severe depression was associated
with less premorbid personality dysfunction than milder depression; this study
was probably the first to show that many depressed elderly individuals have had
considerable lifetime personality psychopathology.

The development of structured interviews to assess Axis II psychopathology
has facilitated research with geriatric subjects, and psychiatrically hospitalized
elderly depressives have been the first group to be studied. Using the Personality
Disorder Examination (PDE) (Loranger *et al.* 1987), Abrams *et al.* (1987)
assessed lifetime personality functioning according to DSM-III-R criteria in 21
recovered elderly depressives and 15 normal geriatric volunteers. In this study,
the patient group received significantly higher scores on PDE items relating
to each personality diagnosis except antisocial personality disorder, with the
largest difference between patients and controls in avoidant and dependent
disorders. However, only two subjects, both depressives, received personality
disorder diagnoses. Schneider *et al.* (1992), using a different structured interview
methodology, also found that elderly depressives had more lifetime personality
disorder symptomatology than geriatric controls, similarly with a predominance
of Cluster C criteria and few full personality disorder diagnoses. However, the
length and complexity of structured interviews limited the sample size of these
studies. More recently, Kunik *et al.* (1993) reported a larger study of depressed
geriatric inpatients using an all-sources consensus methodology to diagnose
personality disorders. These authors found that 24 per cent of subjects met
criteria for personality disorders, with NOS and dependent the most frequent
Axis II diagnoses.

The significance of possible associations between geriatric major depression
and the Cluster C disorders is unknown. As has been noted, dependent
personality disorder may be especially difficult to distinguish from depression.
These appear to be closely related, if separate dimensions; their relationships
may vary according to the subtype, severity, and chronicity of depression, with
dependent personality features perhaps more pronounced in chronic forms of
depression (Overholser 1991).

In recent years there has been an emerging conceptualization of geriatric
depression as a heterogeneous group of disorders in which later age of onset
of illness may be associated with different etiological and clinical characteristics.
Later age of depression onset appears to be related to a greater degree of
medical illness (Alexopoulos *et al.* 1988), brain changes (Eastwood and Corbin
1986; National Institutes of Health 1991), dementia (Alexopoulos *et al.* 1988),

and possibly also a higher rate of recurrence (Keller 1985), while earlier onset is more associated with family history of depression (Mendlewicz and Baron 1981). Together, these findings have suggested that late-onset depression could be a symptomatic expression of various conditions presenting in old age.

What are the implications of age at depression onset for the relationship between depression and personality disorder? One possibility is that onset of depression earlier in life would make a history of personality disorder more probable. Preliminary data of Abrams *et al.* (1993) suggest that this may be true. In the author's experience, many patients with first episode of major depression in old age have led lives remarkably free of personality dysfunction up to that time. More research in this area is needed, using larger samples and designs in which the effect of age of depression onset is not reduced to a simple dichotomy (early versus late onset).

Finally, chronic depression in the elderly may be associated with dysfunctional personality. Dysthymia, for example, a chronic low-grade depressive syndrome affecting as much as 15 per cent of the geriatric population (Blazer and Williams 1980), has been viewed both as a primary affective disorder with prominent character pathology and as a personality disorder with secondary affective features (Moore 1985); Akiskal (1983) has suggested that there may be subgroups of each, operationally defined by response to antidepressant drugs. 'Double depression', or severe recurrent major depression with incomplete remissions, is another chronic syndrome of importance in geriatric psychiatry; Post (1962, 1972) called this disorder 'depressive invalidism' to emphasize its pervasively negative effect on functioning, including personality. The term 'masked depression' refers to yet another chronic depressive syndrome, believed to be common in the elderly, in which cognitive or somatic symptoms are more prominent than dysphoric mood or neurovegetative signs (Pichot and Hassan 1973). Masked depression has also been associated with premorbid personality dysfunction (Lesse 1968).

Implications of personality disorders for outcome of geriatric major depression await more definitive data. In the study of Kunik *et al.* (1993) there were no differences between depressed patients with and without personality disorders in length of hospital stay or short-term outcomes of depression. However, it is not possible to extrapolate from these findings to the longer-term outlook. For example, it has been suggested on the basis of family interviews that a high percentage of completed geriatric suicides have personality disorders (Loebel 1990). Also, as has been noted, dependent traits and symptoms might predict chronicity of depression.

Personality disorders and cognitive impairment: the problem of organicity

Behavioural change can occur in the context of acute and chronic organic brain pathology; such changes are commonly observed in elderly medical and psychiatric patients. However, it is uncertain whether this behaviour should be regarded as dysfunctional personality change or organic pathology. The strategy of DSM-III-R was to categorize organic symptoms concerned with the quality of affect and its regulation as an 'organic personality syndrome', while reserving the more purely cognitive symptomatology for the diagnosis of dementia. One early proposal for DSM-IV involved eliminating the term 'organic' (Spitzer *et al.* 1989). In this proposal, dementia, delirium, and amnestic disorder would be grouped together in a 'cognitive impairment disorders' category, while the other presently labelled organic disorders—including personality, mood, and anxiety disorder—would be termed 'secondary'. The nosological reclassification of organic personality disorder to secondary personality disorder in Axis II would emphasize the personality aspect by listing this entity according to phenomenology rather than etiology.

But how should such secondary personality phenomena be studied? Demented patients' impairments in memory and judgement greatly reduce the value of their responses on self-report instruments. In both clinical practice and research, one frequently taken approach has been to rely on family members or other informants who have known the cognitively impaired individual over a long period of time. However, responses may vary according to who is the informant. Also, most of the DSM-III-R personality disorder criteria are irrelevant to the present circumstances of persons who have even a moderate degree of dementia. The task is rather to determine if there have been any changes in the underlying trait structure. A schedule of observed behaviours, focusing on dimensions such as aggression, passivity, agitation, self-centredness, and suspiciousness was used by Rubin *et al.* (1987) to characterize the progression of personality changes in Alzheimer's disease. In another study, coarsened and immature behaviour as well as loss of energy and enthusiasm distinguished demented from non-demented men (Petry *et al.* 1988). Demented elderly men may also have more agitated and assaultive behaviours than women with the same disorder (Souder *et al.* 1993). However, at least some of these behaviours are not clearly personality phenomena, and would probably be viewed by Spitzer *et al.* (1989) as symptoms of cognitive impairment disorder. Experimental paradigms for assessing true personality change in dementia, for example exploratory behaviour (Young *et al.* 1986), are heuristically interesting, but lie outside of the language and concepts of the clinician.

Observational paradigms for various traits or disorders may eventually facilitate the study of personality in dementia. Cognitive–experimental self-theory suggests that individuals consciously or unconsciously hold particular views of the world and basic, unchallenged assumptions about themselves ('self-postulates'), which in turn determine their characteristic coping styles; pathological coping techniques and their maladaptive self-postulates constitute personality disorders (Epstein 1991). Demented patients may retain vestiges of their former coping styles and self-postulates. Thus, some personality disorder criteria might be reliably assessed by care-givers who know the patients intimately, even if non-verbally, in the way that many mothers can subtly describe the personalities of their pre-verbal infants. It is clear that new and creative assessment methodologies will be required to advance understanding of personality functioning in dementia.

Personality disorders and late-onset functional psychoses

Late-onset schizophrenia has been an officially recognized disorder since 1987, when DSM-III-R used the term to describe patients in whom the onset of schizophrenic symptoms occurred after the age of 44 years. Before that, the entity of psychotic symptoms developing in the second half of life had occupied various other nosological niches, from Kraeplin's paraphrenia to atypical psychosis in DSM-III, which restricted schizophrenic diagnoses to patients whose symptoms began before the age of 45 years. Of interest here is that a substantial number of these patients appear to have had paranoid or schizoid premorbid traits (Jeste *et al.* 1991), some of which probably represented personality disorders. Late-onset schizophrenics have been considered by others to be eccentric and socially isolated long before the occurrence of frank psychotic symptoms, but compared to earlier-onset schizophrenics they were more likely to have worked, married, and had children (Jeste *et al.* 1991; Jeste *et al.* 1988).

The importance of Cluster A personality disorders in relation to late-onset schizophrenia lies mainly in their prognostic implications. Young adults with these personality disorders are more likely than the general population to develop schizophrenic symptoms in middle or old age. These premorbid personality disorders are sometimes difficult to distinguish from a prodromal phase of the schizophrenic illness itself. The distinction made by DSM-III-R is that the prodrome represents a *decline* in the patient's overall functioning, while premorbid personality disorder reflects a level of impaired functioning which is *stable* over a long period.

The entity of late-life delusional disorder is the present-day successor to Kraepelin's paranoia (distinguished from paraphrenia by the complete absence of hallucinations) and the DSM-III category of paranoid disorder. DSM-III-R suggests that delusional disorder in general is more likely to occur in individuals with avoidant, paranoid, or schizoid personality disorders (American Psychiatric Association 1987). Data from geriatric populations, however, are lacking.

PERSONALITY AND ADAPTATION IN OLD AGE

Personality traits are meaningful not only in relation to the Axis I psychiatric syndromes of old age, but as indicators of the quality of life. Global well-being, satisfaction with life, and capacity to cope with illness and loss have seemed to some authors to be the important outcomes to evaluate in studies of personality and ageing (Malatesta 1981; Costa *et al.* 1987). Research using large samples suggests that overall well-being tends to be stable over time, perhaps because the frequency and intensity of both positive and negative emotions tend to decline with age (Costa *et al.* 1987). However, on an individual level, elderly people must be able to cope with a succession of crises which increasingly threaten well-being. Personality traits may be among the critical factors in adaptation to these negative life events of old age (Neugarten 1977; Murphy 1982).

Since there may be relatively few categorical personality disorders in the elderly population, research on personality and adaptation to age-related stresses must rely on dimensional trait measurements. However, adaptation in old age also has clinical implications. For example, who succumbs to invalidism in reaction to illness, loss, and loneliness? Who does not? Lyness *et al.* (1993) have recently shown that the functional status of depressed patients was more closely related to medical and psychiatric *disability* than to symptom severity, supporting clinical observations that patients with similar illnesses can present very differently with respect to overall functioning. Personality traits may well contribute to these differences.

In recent years, psychoanalytic theorists and clinicians have argued that growth and change are continuous throughout the life cycle (Colarusso and Nemiroff 1987), whether or not a person's underlying trait structure remains stable. Freud's early ideas about the declining plasticity of the personality (Freud 1906) have given way to developmental theories of the second half of life. In most of these theories, the concept of adaptation to changing circumstances and roles is central. Some authors, such as Cath and Sadavoy (1991), have viewed the ageing person as faced with a number of developmental tasks which, to be faced successfully, demand high levels of psychological integration and adaptive strength. One such task is disengagement, which refers here to the gradual relinquishing of active involvement in many social and occupational roles and the loss of relationships; this must be achieved without despair or excessive envy of younger persons. Additional related tasks suggested by Cath and Sadavoy include the maintenance of self-identity and self-esteem. Reminiscing (Butler 1963; Coleman 1974), sometimes glossing over failures and disappointments of the past (Erikson *et al.* 1986), and involvement in new roles and relationships (Cath 1975) are all thought to facilitate achievement of these tasks. Mourning for one's own eventual death may be another task to be faced. However, as a central aspect of the midlife crisis, emotional preparation for death may be more correctly viewed as a task of middle age than of old age (Cath and Sadavoy 1991). Also, there is evidence that the fear of death may recede as death itself approaches (Lieberman and Tobin, 1983).

Other developmental theorists emphasize adaptation to general phases or stages of life rather than to specific tasks. Erikson developed a well-known sequence of human development involving psychological, sexual, and social aspects of functioning (Erikson 1959; Erikson *et al.* 1986). His stages each involve challenges or crises, and are epigenetic in that successful resolution of crises of preceding stages will facilitate the confrontation of succeeding ones. Thus, the final achievement of integrity in old age reflects to some degree the outcome of earlier crises in the stages of intimacy and generativity, as well as those of childhood. Vaillant and Vaillant (1990), on the basis of a longitudinal sample of Harvard alumni, proposed that unfolding adulthood is characterized by use of progressively more mature forms of psychological defence. They found that personality traits more prominently manifested recently better predict psychological functioning in late middle or old age than traits evident in young adulthood; with increasing age, 'the detrimental effects of personality disorder become less apparent' (Vaillant and Vaillant 1990). Other authors, such as Gould (1972) and Levinson *et al.* (1978), have also proposed schemata of adult psychological development in which a process of maturation is implicit. Neugarten (1964) described a final stage of compensatory social introversion, called 'interiority' in which elderly people gradually withdraw from a world in which they play less active roles and turn inward for a final consolidation of the sense of self. In all of these conceptualizations, versatile personalities redirect their energies towards sources of self-esteem and integrity to cope with mounting losses and waning physical vigour.

It is evident, however, that the contribution of personality traits to adaptation and coping in old age have not yet been addressed directly. To be fair, what is adaptive in old age is not always clear. Should one face inevitable death unblinkingly, or with a cognitive distancing? The level of risk taking and preference for environmental stimuli found in a 20-year-old would probably not be adaptive for an 80-year-old, but *some* excitement should optimally appeal to the older person. Clearly, the study of personality and adaptation to ageing has just begun.

MANAGEMENT

In recent years there has been a growing body of writings on the psychothera-peutic treatment of elderly patients (Myers 1984; Sadavoy and Leszcz 1987). The general tone is optimistic, and the clinical experience from which these articles are derived suggests that elderly people may be amenable, if not eager, to resolve lifelong conquests, mourn old and recent losses, and seek new meaning from the totality of their lives. An exception to this optimism, however, is the treatment of the severely narcissistic older person.

While the importance of Cluster C disorders in the elderly has been empha-sized thus far, old age also encourages the expression of narcissistic traits and defences, possibly as a protection against experiences of humiliation (Sadavoy 1987). In its more severe forms, narcissism represents a malignant entity characterized by pathological internal object relations and the absence of an internalized value system ('the grandiose self') (Kernberg 1976). Thus, the severely narcissistic person has few inner resources upon which to rely when confronted with the same demands upon adaptation as his elderly peers. In old age there may be no happier past over which to reminisce.

In the author's clinical experience there are several observable hallmarks of severe narcissism in old age. The first, perhaps the most frequent, is chronic envy. As used here, envy refers not to transient feelings of jealously of others' youth, wealth, or success, but to a more pervasive orientation in which, for example, the accomplishments of one's children cannot be unambivalently enjoyed. Individuals with chronic envy view others' successes as diminishing their own and look upon the progress of peers, younger colleagues, and children with fear and alarm. Another clinical feature of severe narcissism is chronic anger. In the elderly this sometimes takes the form of feuds with friends or family members, resulting in the destruction of the relationship or in a harshly unforgiving hostility; often a narcissistic injury is at the core of the estrangement.

An exceptionally rigid refusal to accept the limitations imposed by ageing can also be seen in some individuals. Severely narcissistic persons frequently deny the implications of ageing to an extent which can be revealed in the complete refusal to seek medical care, in an exaggerated response to minor ailments, or if seriously ill, in the belief that they are unique in the degree of their suffering. Also, memories of significant business reversals or disappointments recur painfully, since there is an inadequate sense of self-worth to compensate for misfortunes of judgement or circumstance; the narcissistic businessman who lost his business cannot, even if he accepts responsibility, be consoled. Finally, the patient in hospital or long-term care settings who immobilizes the staff with conflicts over their care is likely to have some of the powerful splitting operations of the borderline personality organization of pathological narcissism; this is well beyond the level of narcissism inherent in the 'dissatisfied' personality syndrome.

Despite the suffering inherent in severe narcissism, elderly people with this symptomatic constellation do not readily seek treatment on their own. For these patients, the psychotherapeutic relationship is experienced more as a challenge than a validator of self-esteem, and the mourning of losses and disappointments becomes too global and painful to undertake. Realistically, psychotherapy with the narcissistic patient in old age cannot be expected to resolve a lifetime of failed relationships and missed opportunities.

However, some clinicians have focused on the creative use of institutional supports for these patients (Sadavoy 1987; Tobin 1989). Group living, whether in retirement communities, adult homes, or nursing homes, may not only protect against loneliness and the ravages of self-neglect, but can as well provide a watchful social setting to supplant some of the patient's deficient internal resources. Sadavoy (1987) describes how a psychotherapist might function in a nursing-home setting by working not only with the patient, but also with the staff in order to fashion the milieu into a force against the destructiveness of the narcissistic patient. A comprehensive treatment plan would include the involvement of family members to help the treatment team establish goals consistent with the patient's long-term functioning. For some, institutionalization offers the best opportunity for treatment.

The general principles of psychiatric treatment of the elderly also apply to patients with personality psychopathology. The first is that careful assessment should precede any psychotherapeutic intervention. In the case of personality disorders, which are most frequently found in the setting of Axis I disorders, accurate multiaxial diagnosis is especially important. If present, concurrent Axis I conditions, particularly affective or anxiety disorders, should be optimally treated with medication or other means before planning overly ambitious psychotherapy aimed at fundamental personality change. Similarly, medical conditions should be investigated as fully as possible and the facts known by the psychotherapist at the outset. Again, a collaterally informed picture of the patient's long-term functioning is essential for the setting of achievable goals.

As already indicated, treatment more often than not involves family members or care-givers. For this reason scrupulous attention should be paid to rules and principles of doctor–patient confidentiality. Possible reasons for breaking these rules should be anticipated and discussed with the patient at the start of treatment. The conduct of psychotherapy with elderly patients is discussed more fully elsewhere in this volume, but it can be suggested here that the therapist in individual psychotherapy generally finds it helpful to abandon strict neutrality and speak from the position of a real person in the patient's life, even in the most psychoanalytically orientated of treatments. Further, psychotherapy with elderly people differs in the length of the time-frame covered; transference issues continue to be directed from childhood sources and early parental relationships, but will also contain contributions from more recent experience. Group therapies may be useful in both in-patient and out-patient settings (Thompson *et al.* 1987), particularly with personality disorder patients.

Pharmacotherapy is most often dictated by the presence or absence of an Axis I disorder; use of medication has not been studied in geriatric personality disorders. The literature about younger personality-disorder patients focuses mainly on borderline personality disorder. Findings from these studies suggest that psychotic-spectrum symptomatology is more effectively treated by neuroleptic medication than placebo (Goldberg *et al.* 1986), and amitriptyline may be more effective than placebo but no more effective than haloperidol in antidepressant effect (Soloff *et al.* 1987). Lithium, carbamazepine, and monoamine oxidase inhibitors (MAOIs) may be useful in specific situations. However, at the present state of knowledge, there is no clear guidance for the clinician.

REFERENCES

Abrams, R. C. (1991). The ageing personality (editorial). *International Journal of Geriatric Psychiatry*, **6**, 1–3.
Abrams, R. C. Alexopoulos, G. S., and Young, R. C. (1987). Geriatrics depression and DSM-III-R personality disorder criteria. *Journal of the American Geriatrics Society*, **35**, 383–6.
Abrams, R. C., Rosendahl, E., and Alexopoulos, G. S. (1993). Personality disorders in geriatric depression. In *New research abstracts, Annual Meeting of The American Psychiatric Association, San Francisco*, p. 233. American Psychiatric Association, Washington.
Akiskal, H. S. (1983). Dysthymic disorder: psychopathology of proposed depressive subtypes. *American Journal of Psychiatry*, **140**, 11–20.
Alexopoulos, G. S., Young, R. C., Meyers, B. S., Abrams, R. C., and Shamoian, C. A. (1988). Late-onset depression. *Psychiatric Clinics of North America*, **11**, 101–15.
American Psychiatric Association (1980). *Diagnostic and statistical manual of mental disorders* (3rd edn). American Psychiatric Association, Washington.

American Psychiatric Association (1987). *Diagnostic and statistical manual of mental disorders* (3rd edn, revised). American Psychiatric Association, Washington.

American Psychiatric Association (1994). *Diagnostic and Statistical Manual of Mental Disorders* (4th edition). American Psychiatric Association, Washington.

Angst, J., and Clayton, P. J. (1986). Premorbid personality of depressed, bipolar and schizophrenic patients with special reference to suicidal issues. *Comprehensive Psychiatry*, **27**, 511–32.

Beck, A. T. (1967). *Depression: clinical, experimental, and theoretical aspects*, pp. 3–87. Harper and Row, New York.

Blazer, D., and Williams, C. D. (1980). Epidemiology of dysphoria and depression in an elderly population. *American Journal of Psychiatry*, **137**, 439–44.

Butler, R. (1963). The life review: an interpretation of reminiscence in the aged. *Psychiatry*, **26**, 65–70.

Cath, S. H. (1975). Some dynamics of middle-later years: a study in depletion and restitution. In *Geriatric psychiatary: grief, loss, and emotional disorder in the ageing process*, (ed. M. Berezin and S. H. Cath), pp. 21–72. International Universities Press, New York.

Cath, S. H., and Sadavoy, J. (1991). The ageing process: psychological aspects. In *Comprehensive review of geriatric psychiatry* (ed. J. Sadavoy, L. W. Lazarus, and L. F. Jarvik), pp. 79–98. American Psychiatric Press, Washington.

Cloninger, C. R. (1987). A systematic method for clinical description and classification of personality variants. *Archives of General Psychiatry*, **44**, 573–88.

Colarusso, C. A., and Nemiroff, R. A. (1987). Clinical implications of adult development theory. *American Journal of Psychiatry*, **144**, 1263–70.

Coleman, P. G. (1974). Measuring reminiscence characteristics from conversations as adaptive features in old age. *International Journal of Ageing and Human Development*, **5**, 281–94.

Costa, P. T., and McCrae, R. R. (1990). Personality disorders and the five-factor model of personality. *Journal of Psychiatry*, **4**, 362–71.

Costa, P. T., Zonderman, A. N., McCrae, R. R., Cornoni-Huntley, J., Locke, B. Z., and Barbano, H. E. (1987). Longitudinal analyses of psychological well-being in a national sample: stability of mean bands. *Journal of Gerontology*, **42**, 50–5.

Cumming, E., and Henry, W. E. (1961). *Growing old*. Basic Books, New York.

Dahlstrom, W. G., Welsh, G. S., and Dahlstrom, L. E. (1972). *An MMPI handbook. Volume 1: Clinical interpretation*. University of Minnesota Press, Minneapolis.

Eastwood, M. R., and Corbin, S. W. (1986). The relationship between physical illness and depression in old age. In *Affective disorders in the elderly* (ed. E. Murphy), pp. 177–86. Churchill Livingstone, New York.

Epstein, S. (1991). Cognitive–experimental self-theory: implications for developmental psychology. In *Minnesota Symposium in Child Psychology*, pp. 79–123. Erlbaum, Newark, New Jersey.

Erikson, E. H. (1959). *Identity and the life-cycle: Selected Papers*, p. 5. International Universities Press, New York.

Eysenck, H. J., and Eysenck, M. W. (1985). *Personality and individual differences*, pp. 3–342. Plenum Press, New York.

Erikson, E. H., Erikson, J. M., and Kivnick, H. Q. (1986). *Vital involvement in old age*, pp. 54–238. W. W. Norton, New York.

Fogel, B. S., and Westlake, R. (1990). Personality disorder diagnoses and age in inpatients with major depression. *Journal of Clinical Psychiatry*, **51**, 232–5.

Freud, S. (1906). On psychotherapy. In *Collected papers*, Vol. 1 (ed. J. Riviere), pp. 249–6. Hogarth Press, London.

Fulker, D. W. (1981). The genetic and environmental architecture of psychoticism, extroversion, and neuroticism. In *A model for personality* (ed. H. J. Eysenck), pp. 88–122. Springer-Verlag, New York.

Goldberg, S. C., Schultz, S. C., Schultz, P. M., Resnick, R. J., Hamer, D. M., and Friedel, R. O. (1986). Borderline and schizotypal personality disorders treated with low-dose thiothixene vs. placebo. *Archives of General Psychiatry*, **43**, 680–6.

Gould, R. L. (1972). The phases of adult life: a study in developmental psychology. *American Journal of Psychiatry*, **129**, 521–31.

Gunderson, J. G. (1992). Controversies about diagnosis of personality disorders. In *Review of psychiatry*, Vol. 11 (ed. A. Tasman), pp. 9–24. American Psychiatric Press. Washington.

Hirschfield, R. M. A., and Klerman, G. L. (1979). Personality attributes and affective disorders. *American Journal of Psychiatry*, **136**, 67–70.

Hirschfield, R. M. A., Klerman G. L., Clayton, P. J., Keller, M. B., McDonald-Scott, M. A., and Larkin, B. H. (1983). Assessing personality: effects of the depressive state on trait measurement. *American Journal of Psychiatry*, **140**, 695–9.

Jeste, D. V., Harris, M. J., Pearlson, G. D., Rabins, P., Lesser, I. M., Miller, B., et al. (1988). Late-onset schizophrenia: studying clinical validity. *Psychiatric Clinics of North America*, **11**, 1–14.

Jeste, D. V., Manley, M., and Harris, M. J. (1991). Psychiatric disorders: psychoses. In *Comprehensive review of geriatric psychiatry*, (ed. J. Sadavoy, L. W. Lazarus, and L. F. Jarvik), pp. 353–68. American Psychiatric Press, Washington.

Keller, M. B. (1985). Chronic and recurrent affective disorders: incidence, course, and influencing factors. In *Chronic treatments in neuropsychiatry* (ed. D. Kemali and C. Racagni), pp. 111–120. Raven Press, New York.

Kernberg, O. F. (1975). *Borderline conditions and pathological narcissism*, pp. 227–62. Jason Aronson, New York.

Kunik, M. E., Mulsant, B. H., Rifai, A. H., Sweet, R., Pasternak, R., Rosen, J., et al. (1993). Personality disorders in elderly inpatients with major depression. *The American Journal of Geriatric Psychiatry*, **1**, 38–45.

Leon, G. R., Gillum, B., Gillum, R., and Gouze, M. (1979). Personality stability and change over a 30-year period middle-age to old age. *Journal of Consulting and Clinical Psychology*, **47**, 517–24.

Lesse, S. (1968). The multivariant masks of depression. *American Journal of Psychiatry*, **124** (Supp. 1), 35–40.

Levinson, D. J., Darrow, C. N., Klein, E. B. Levinson, M. L., and Mckee, B. (1978). *The seasons of a man's life*. Knopf, New York.

Lieberman, M. A., and Tobin, S. S. (1983). *The experience of old age*. Basic Books, New York.

Loebel, J. P. (1990). Completed suicide in the elderly. In *Abstracts of the Third Annual Meeting and Symposium, American Association for Geriatric Psychiatry, San Diego, California*, p. 2. AAGD, Greenbelt, MA.

Loranger, A. W., Susman, V. L., Oldham, J. M., and Russakoff, L. M. (1987). The personality disorder examination: a preliminary report. *Journal of Personality Disorders*, **1**, 1–13.

Loranger, A. W., Lenzenweger, M. F., Gartner, A. F., Lehmann Susman, V., Herzig, J., Zammit, et al. (1991). Trait-state artifacts and the diagnosis of personality disorders. *Archives of General Psychiatry*, **48**, 720–8.

Lyness, J. M., Carrie, E. D., Conwell, Y., King, D. A., and Cox, C. (1993). Depressive symptoms, medical illness and functional status in depressed psychiatric inpatients. *American Journal of Psychiatry*, **150**, 910–15.

Malatesta, C. Z. (1981). Affecting growth over the lifespan: involution or growth? *Merrill-Palmer Quarterly*, **27**, 143–73.

McCrae, R. R., and Costa, P. T. (1990). *Personality in adulthood*. The Guilford Press, New York.

McGlashan, T. H. (1986). The Chestnut Lodge follow-up study III. Long-term outcome of borderline personalities. *Archives of General Psychiatry*, **43**, 20–30.

Mendlewicz, J., and Baron, M. (1981). Morbidity risks in sub-types of unipolar depressive illness: differences between early and late onset forms. *British Journal of Psychiatry*, **139**, 463–6.

Moore, J. T. (1985). Dysthymia in the elderly. *Journal of Affective Disorders*, Supp. 1, 515–21.

Murphy, E. (1982) Social origins of depression in old age, *British Journal of Psychiatry*, **141**, 135–42.

Myers, W. A. (1984). *Dynamic therapy of the older patient*. Jason Aronson, New York.

National Institutes of Health (1991). *Diagnosis and treatment of depression in late life*. Reprinted from National Institutes of Health Consensus Development Conference Consensus Statement, 9 (3), U.S. Department of Health and Human Services, Public Health Service, National Institutes of Health. Bethesda, MA.

Neugarten, B. L. (1964). *Personality in middle and late life*, pp. 192–7. Atherton Press, New York.

Neugarten, B. (1977). Personality and ageing. In *Handbook of the psychology of ageing* (ed. J. E. Birren and K. W. Schaie), pp. 626–49. Van Nostrand Reinhold, New York.

Overholser, J. C. (1991). Categorical assessment of the dependent personality disorder in depressed patients. *Journal of Personality Disorders*, **5**, 243–55.

Petry, S. Cummings, J. L., Hill, M. A., and Shapiro, J. (1988). Personality alterations in dementia of the Alzheimer type. *Archives of Neurology*, **45**, 1187–90.

Pfohl, B., Stangl, D., and Zimmerman, M. (1984). The implications of DSM-III personality disorder for patients with major depression. *Journal of Affective Disorders*, **7**, 309–18.

Pichot, P., and Hassan, J. (1973). Masked depressions and depressive equivalents—problems of definitions and diagnosis. In *Masked depression: an international symposium*. (ed. P. Kielholz), pp. 61–76. Hans Huber, Berne.

Post, F. (1962). *The significance of affective symptoms in old age*, p. 70. Maudsley Monographs, 10. Oxford University Press, London.

Post, F. (1972). The management and nature of depressive illness in late life: a follow-through study. *British Journal of Psychiatry*, **121**, 393–404.

Reich, J., Nduaguba, M., and Yates, W. (1988). Age and sex distribution of DSM-III personality cluster traits in community population. *Comprehensive Psychiatry*, **29**, 298–303.

Reich, J., Noyes, R., Hirschfeld, R., Coryell, W., and O'Gorman, T. (1987). State and personality in depressed and panic patients. *American Journal of Psychiatry*, **144**, 181–7.

Rubin, E. H., Morris, J. C., Storandt, M., and Berg, L. (1987). Behavioural changes in patients with mild senile dementia of the Alzheimer's type. *Psychiatry Research*, **21**, 55–62.

Sadavoy, J. (1987). Character disorders in the elderly: an overview. In *Treating the elderly with psychotherapy: the scope for change in later life* (ed. J. Sadavoy and M. Leszcz), pp. 175–229. International Universities Press, Madison, Conneticut.

Sadavoy, J., and Leszcz, M. (ed.) (1987). *Treating the elderly with psychotherapy: The scope for change in later life.* International Universities Press, Madison, Connecticut.

Schneider, L. S., Zemansky, M. F., Berden, M., and Sloane, R. B. (1992). Personality in recovered depressed elderly. *International Psychiatrics*, **4**, 177–85.

Shea, M. T., Glass, D. R., Pilkonis, P. A., Watkins, J., and Docherty, J. P. (1987). Frequency and implications of personality disorders in a sample of depressed outpatients. *Journal of Personality Disorders*, **1**, 27–42.

Siever, L. J., Bernstein, D. P., and Silverman, J. M. (1991). Schizotypal personality disorder: a review of its current status. *Journal of Personality Disorders*, **5**, 178–93.

Soloff, P. H., George, A., Nathan, R. S., Schulz, P. M., Cornelius, J. R., and Perel, J. M. (1987). Amitriptyline versus haloperidol in borderlines. In *Abstracts, Annual Meeting of the American Psychiatric Association, Chicago*, pp. 217–8. American Psychiatric Association, Washington.

Souder, E., Wiseman, E. J., Liem, P., and Hazelwood, M. (1993). Aggression in dementia: gender differences. In *New research abstracts, Annual Meeting of the American Psychiatric Association, San Francisco*, p. 235. American Psychiatric Association, Washington.

Spitzer, R. L., Williams, J. B., First, M., and Kendler, K. (1989). A proposal for DSM-IV: solving the 'organic/non-organic' problem. *Journal of Neuropsychiatry and Clinical Neuroscience*, **1**, 126–7.

Stone, M. H. (1990). *The fate of borderline patients: successful outcome and psychiatric practice*, pp. 22–85. Guilford Press, New York.

Swenson, W. M., Pearson, J. S., and Osborne, D. (1973). *An MMPI source book: basic item, scale, and pattern data on 50,000 medical patients.* University of Minnesota Press, Minneapolis.

Thompson, L. W., Gallagher, D., and Breckenridge, J. S. (1987). Comparative effectiveness of psychotherapies for depressed elders. *Journal of Consulting and Clinical Psychology*, **55**, 385–90.

Titley, W. (1936). Prepsychotic personality of patients with involutional melancholia. *Archives of Neurology and Psychiatry*, **36**, 19–33.

Tobin, S. S. (1989). Issues of care in long-term settings. In *Psychiatric consequences of brain disease in the elderly* (ed. D. Conn, A. Grek, and J. Sadavoy), pp. 163–87. Plenum Press, New York.

Tyrer, P. (1988). *Personality disorders: diagnosis, management, and course.* Wright, London.

Vaillant, G., and Vaillant, C. O. (1990). Natural history of male psychological health. XII: A 45-year history of predictions of successful ageing at age 65. *American Journal of Psychiatry*, **147**, 31–7.

von Zerssen, D. (1982). Personality and affective disorders. In *Handbook of affective disorders* (ed. E. S. Paykel), pp. 212–28. The Guilford Press, New York.

Widiger, T. A. (1991). DSM-IV reviews of the personality disorders: introduction to special series. *Journal of Personality Disorders*, **5**, 122–34.

Woodruff, R. A., Guze, S. E., and Clayton, P. J. (1971). The medical and psychiatric implications of antisocial personality (sociopathy). *Diseases of the Nervous System.* **32**, 712–14.

Young, R. C., Abrams, R. C., Alexopoulos, G. S., and Smith, G. P. (1986). Investigatory behaviour in geriatric affective disorder. In *Abstracts of the Annual Meeting of the Gerontological Society of America*, p. 978. AAGP, Greenbelt, MA.

10

Alcohol and drug abuse
STEPHEN TICEHURST

INTRODUCTION

The world's elderly population has increased rapidly during the second half of this century, and in most countries this trend will continue well into the next century. More elderly people will abuse alcohol and other substances simply because of this demographic change. Like many aspects of ageing, substance abuse in the elderly has been relatively neglected and underestimated. The literature that does exist contains contradictions and conflicting opinions. This chapter will review the evidence and examine areas of contemporary debate concerning substance abuse in the elderly.

ALCOHOL

Drinking patterns in the elderly

Overall, older people drink less than younger adults. Daily drinkers represent 10–22 per cent of the elderly population (Liberto et al. 1992). Abstinence increases from 22 per cent in the fourth decade of life to 47 per cent in the seventh decade and around 80 per cent in the ninth decade (Busby et al. 1988; Christopherson et al. 1984; Benshoff and Roberto 1987; Jensen and Bellecci 1987; Saunders et al. 1989). Not only do fewer elderly people drink regularly, but those who do are more moderate in their consumption (Wattis 1983). Aged male drinkers consume an average of one to three drinks daily. Women drinkers consume less, averaging one drink per day (Bridgewater et al. 1987; Glynn et al. 1984). Heavy drinking is relatively rare in the aged, with only three out of 475 women (0.7 per cent) in rural New Zealand reporting drinking more than 50 ml of alcohol daily. In men, the figure was 5.7 per cent (Busby et al. 1988). The decline in drinking with age is most marked in heavy drinkers and in men (Saunders et al. 1989; Cahalan and Cisin 1968), and has been shown in longitudinal as well as cross-sectional studies (Adams et al. 1990).

Older people, especially women, drink less in public and more when alone or with their families. Common reasons given for drinking relate to social occasions and meals. Regular and heavy drinkers are more likely to report drinking to improve their mood. Compared with younger age groups, few elderly people admit drinking to help cope with social situations (Busby *et al.* 1988; Cahalan and Cisin 1968).

Some writers suggest that the elderly tend to under-report their alcohol consumption, and that families and professionals may collude to minimise reporting (Chatham 1984; Wattis 1981). While there is some evidence to support this view, this phenomenon is by no means unique to the elderly.

Reasons for altered consumption with age

One half of elderly drinkers attribute their declining intake to a decreasing ability to tolerate alcohol (Nordstrom and Berglund 1987). Physiological changes with ageing and an increased frequency of pathological processes combine to make the elderly person more vulnerable to the effects of alcohol. The elderly have a decreased volume of distribution which potentiates the effect of alcohol (Zimberg 1984; Atkinson 1987). Prolonged storage times may be related to increased body fat relative to muscle. Target organ cell loss, for example in the brain, also acts to potentiate the effects of alcohol. With increasing age, the pleasant effects of alcohol may occur over a narrower dose range, with a lower threshold for unpleasant effects. The excitatory phase is shorter with a more rapid entry into the sedative phase, especially for elderly women (Jolley and Hodgson 1985). Age is also related to a decline in the development of tolerance, although the healthy ageing liver remains as capable of metabolizing ethanol as at younger ages (Ritzmann and Melchior 1984). Alcohol-induced peripheral vasodilation can result in an increased risk of hypothermia in the elderly (Gambert 1992).

A variety of social and psychological factors may also contribute to the decrease in alcohol intake with age. Reduced opportunities for social activity are a major reason given by both sexes for drinking less (Busby *et al.* 1988; Mishara and Kastenbaum 1980). Other reasons are financial stringency, retirement from or loss of alcohol-related jobs, decreased drive, and increasing maturity (Post 1982). Many American women give religious or moral reasons for abstinence (Cahalan and Cisin 1968).

Despite the general trend towards decreased consumption with age, 7 per cent of men and 11 per cent of women report drinking more in old age (Busby *et al.* 1988). The most common reasons given for this increase are having more time available, more money to spend, and changes in family circumstances. Many authors have suggested reasons why the elderly may increase their alcohol intake. These include the multiple losses of ageing, changing social roles, lowered self-esteem, and awareness of death (Brody 1982; Blose 1978). This reflects society's negative perception of ageing.

Prevalence of alcohol-related problems and disorders

Difficulties in measuring the problem

Defining the problem   There is a lack of consensus as to when a person's substance use becomes a disorder or a disease. Operational criteria may enable us to communicate better, but the issue of classifying substance abuse and dependence remains problematic. The *Diagnostic and statistical manual of mental disorders* (third edition, revised) (DSM-III-R) of the American Psychiatric Association (1987) has moved away from strict physiological criteria for dependence, with an increasing emphasis on the importance of social, psychological, and behavioural components of the syndrome.

DSM-III-R delineates substance abuse and dependence in a way which can be summarized as follows:

Abuse is a maladaptive pattern of psychoactive substance use with one of the following:

(1) continued use despite knowledge of having a persistent or recurrent social, occupational, psychological, or physical problem that is caused or exacerbated by use;

(2) recurrent use in hazardous situations.

Symptoms may persist for longer than a month or occur repeatedly over a longer period of time.

Dependence requires at least three of the following over a period of at least one month:

(1) use in larger amounts or over longer time than is intended;

(2) persistent desire or unsuccessful attempts to cut down;

(3) a great deal of time spent procuring the substance or recovering from its effects;

(4) intoxication at times when major roles are expected to be met or when it is hazardous to be intoxicated;

(5) reduced social, occupational, or recreational activities due to substance abuse;

(6) continued use despite persistent or recurrent related social, psychological, or physical problems;

(7) marked tolerance;

(8) withdrawal;

(9) frequent ingestion to relieve or avoid withdrawal symptoms.

Dependence takes precedence over abuse as a diagnosis.

The ICD-10 (*International Classification of diseases*, tenth revision) classification of mental and behavioural disorders (World Health Organization 1992) has a section entitled 'Mental and behavioural disorders due to psychoactive substance abuse'. First the drug or drugs involved is/are specified, and then the syndrome is refined using further clinical descriptors. These include acute intoxication, harmful use, dependence syndrome, and withdrawal state. 'Harmful use' is analogous to 'abuse' in DSM-III-R. However, harmful use specifically excludes social harm or disapproval as being grounds alone for making the diagnosis. The 'dependence syndrome' of ICD-10 stresses that substance use takes on a higher priority than other behaviours that once had greater value for the affected individual.

It can be seen that the terms 'alcoholism' and 'addiction' have fallen from use in current classification systems.

Methodological problems   As definitions of alcohol-related problems have changed markedly in the past few decades, it is often difficult to directly compare results from different studies. Many of the criteria developed in younger patients may not be valid for the elderly. For example, the physiological changes of ageing suggest that 'total consumption' criteria may need to be adjusted downward to remain valid measures of dangerous intake in the elderly. In addition, some of the items on alcohol-problem inventories are less relevant in the aged, for example work absenteeism and driving under the influence.

Methodological issues such as questionnaire design and sample selection cloud the interpretation of results from single surveys. Studies that use self-report alone have an inherent bias towards underestimating problem drinking. However, service providers can also fail to appreciate the extent of the problem; one survey revealed under-reporting by a factor of between four and nine (Edwards *et al.* 1973).

Drinking behaviour and related problems are also strongly influenced by cultural, ethnic, and socio-economic factors (Seymour and Wattis 1992); in particular, social-class differences may account for much of the difference between studies, with high socio-economic status increasing the availability of alcohol (Livingston and King 1993).

Prevalence in different settings

The community   Cross-sectional studies show that alcohol-related problems decline with age. This pattern exists for both sexes in community, out-patient, and in-patient settings (Cahalan and Cisin 1968; Drew 1968; Hagnall and Tunving 1972; Myers *et al.* 1984; Reifler *et al.* 1982). Liberto *et al.* (1992) provide a comprehensive review of community prevalence surveys.

Using the Diagnostic Interview Schedule, the 6 month prevalence of alcohol abuse/dependence in the United States Epidemiologic Catchment Area study (ECA) was 3 per cent in men over the age of 65 and 1 per cent in women (Myers *et al.* 1984). For men aged 65 years and above, this was the third most common psychiatric diagnosis identified. A United Kingdom study (Saunders *et al.* 1989) found that 1 per cent of an elderly community sample had problem drinking as defined by the Geriatric Mental State. Using different criteria, between 20 per cent and 30 per cent of elderly males in some communities have been said to be heavy drinkers (Cahalan and Cisin 1968; Bridgewater *et al.* 1987).

As well as differences between countries, regional variations within countries have been noted (Myers *et al.* 1984), as has significant change over time in the same geographical area (Hagnall and Tunving 1972; Ojesjo 1980).

Hospitals Elderly patients who abuse alcohol tend to be concentrated in general medical rather than psychiatric or generic alcohol-treatment settings (Ticehurst 1990). In the United States, over three-quarters of elderly patients with alcohol-related problems are treated in general Veterans Administration Hospitals. Younger drinkers in contrast are usually treated in state mental hospitals (Mishara and Kastenbaum 1980). This difference may reflect the predominance of physical rather than behavioural complications of alcohol abuse in the elderly.

Curtis *et al.* (1989) found 21 per cent of elderly in-patients of a general hospital suffered from 'alcoholism'. Only 37 per cent of these were recognized as having a problem by house staff. Younger patients were twice as likely to be recognized. Speckens *et al.* (1991) found 9 per cent of elderly in-patients had self-reported alcohol problems. However, only 0.5 per cent of elderly patients received an alcohol-related diagnosis at discharge. Adams *et al.* (1992) found that 14 per cent of elderly emergency department patients had current alcohol abuse. In a study of admissions to a hospital unit for the elderly mentally ill, Mears and Spice (1993) found that 19 per cent were problem drinkers, one-third of whom had not been detected during routine medical assessment.

Other treatment settings Alcohol abuse is the third most common mental disorder in geriatric and psychogeriatric outreach programmes, affecting 6 to 10 per cent of patients (Reifler *et al.* 1982; Wattis 1981). In one study, the local doctor was aware of the situation in only half the cases (Malcolm 1984). A general-practice survey of elderly patients reported that 4 per cent of elderly men drank more than 21 units per week and 3 per cent of elderly women consumed more than 14 units per week (Iliffe *et al.* 1991). In 1992, a National Census of Clients of Drug and Alcohol Treatment Service Agencies in Australia showed that less than 4 per cent of 5730 clients were aged over 60 years, and less than 1 per cent were over 70 years. Eighty-two per cent of these elderly clients reported problems with alcohol, and 7 per cent each with tobacco and benzodiazepines (Stinziani, personal communication).

Aetiology

Drug use is a pervasive historical and cultural phenomenon. Some people abuse rather than use psychoactive substances for reasons that remain obscure. There is little specific information regarding the causes of such abuse in the elderly. Rates of alcohol abuse and dependence in the general population are related to the levels of alcohol consumption by the community as a whole, which are related in turn to disposable income. Therefore, as more affluent cohorts enter old age, we may expect to see an increase in the size of the abusing minority. Alcohol dependence has also been attibuted to genetic factors, although these are less important in late-onset cases (Goodwin 1985).

Psychiatric disorder and personality attributes also predispose to alcohol abuse. About one in ten patients admitted for alcohol abuse/dependence are also depressed, but which condition occurs first is often unclear (Finlayson *et al.* 1988). Agoraphobia and social phobia may predispose to the abuse of alcohol. With regard to personality, older alcohol abusers tend to be more psychologically stable than their younger counterparts (Glatt 1978). They display fewer authority conflicts and greater social bonding, but are less psychologically minded. They bring more stoicism, less regression and fewer crises to treatment (Kofoed *et al.* 1984). They score lower on Minnesota Multiphasic Personality Inventory scales of psychopathic deviance, paranoia and hypomania (McGinnis and Ryan 1965; Penk *et al.* 1982). Female elderly patients admitted to an in-patient addiction unit are less likely to report problems with coping and psychosocial problems than younger clients (Blankfield and Maritz 1990).

Late-onset alcohol abuse

A significant proportion of elderly alcohol abusers take up heavy drinking in old age. Rates of such late-onset drinking vary between 7 per cent and 40 per cent (Holzer *et al.* 1984; Finlayson *et al.* 1988). The aetiology, homogeneity, and clinical features of this group have been widely debated.

Rosin and Glatt (1971) identified two groups of elderly alcoholics. Two-thirds were habitual drinkers who continued into old age. The other third were 'late-onset alcoholics', whose previously innocuous drinking had been 'exacerbated by the physical, mental and environmental effects of ageing'. Reactive factors thought to be operating in the latter group included bereavement, retirement, loneliness, physical infirmity, and marital stress. Convincing differences between the groups were only demonstrated for bereavement and retirement. Other studies have failed to find a consistent relationship between elderly drinking and either marital status (Finlayson *et al.* 1988; Saunders *et al.* 1989) or retirement (Ekerdt *et al.* 1989). Other factors found to be associated with late-onset alcohol abuse include higher socio-economic class, less family alcoholism (Penick *et al.* 1987), being female, and psychological stability (Atkinson *et al.* 1985).

Not all authors agree with the utility of the late-onset concept (Caracci and Miller 1991). Most older persons do not drink excessively despite the stresses of ageing, and not all late-onset drinkers report stress as the reason for their drinking. Some studies have criticized the concept on methodological grounds, while others have questioned the supposed better prognosis and response of late-onset cases to simple intervention strategies (Mishara and Kastenbaum 1980; Brody 1982; Atkinson *et al.* 1985). Further evidence is required to clarify whether late-onset drinking is unique to the elderly, or simply represents the movement in and out of problem drinking apparent at younger ages (Glynn *et al.* 1984; Vaillant 1983).

Clinical presentation

Diagnosis of alcohol abuse in the elderly can be difficult because the manifestations may be atypical, unsuspected, or masked by coexisting disorders
(Zimberg 1984). It may be recognized as a problem in only half of elderly
patients later found to have major alcohol difficulties (Rosin and Glatt 1971).
Elderly problem drinkers may fail to reveal their predicament in over 50 per cent
of cases (Saunders *et al.* 1989). Clinical suspicion should be aroused when elderly
patients present with any of the following symptoms:

Medical

In general medical settings, the elderly alcohol abuser may present with
incontinence, malnutrition, hypothermia, hypoglycaemia, trauma, seizures,
polyneuropathy, peptic ulceration, vomiting, impotence, osteomalacia, cardio-
myopathy, anaemia, diarrhoea, pancreatitis, or liver disease (Wattis 1981; Glatt
1978; Harris *et al.* 1987; Schuckit and Pastor 1978). The clinical impression that
falls occur more commonly amongst elderly alcohol abusers has been questioned
by Nelson *et al.* (1992). However, it remains wise to consider alcohol abuse
when an elderly patient presents with unexplained falls. Patients found to have
macrocytosis, diminished serum albumin, elevated liver enzymes, or increased
uric acid require investigation of their alcohol use (Hurt *et al.* 1988). Problems
with establishing therapeutic levels of drugs such as phenytoin and anticoagulants
may be a sign of alcohol abuse in the elderly.

Neuropsychiatric

Alcohol abusers can suffer from a wide range of neuropsychiatric complications.
Conditions causing cognitive impairment include transitory Korsakoff-like states,
delirium, permanent amnestic syndromes, and dementia (Wattis 1983; Lishman
1987). Patients may present with problems due to mixed intoxication with
benzodiazepines and other drugs, drug interactions, or unrecognised combined withdrawal states (Finlayson 1984; Finlayson *et al.* 1988). In the elderly,
intoxication may also be complicated by subdural haematoma following a fall
(Marco and Kelen 1990), or by underlying brain disease, such as dementia.
Another atypical presentation of alcohol dependence in the elderly is 'interval delirium' several days following hospital admission, or post-operatively
(Millar 1984).

Alcohol abuse is also associated with functional psychiatric disorder, notably
depression (Schuckit and Pastor 1978). The consequences of abuse can potentiate
the direct depressive effects of alcohol. Alternatively, drinking may arise from
pre-existing depression, personality difficulties, anxiety disorders, or other
major psychiatric disorders. Attempted suicide by an isolated widower may
be a dramatic presentation of alcohol abuse. Morbid jealousy, hallucinosis,
and withdrawal states may mimic other psychiatric disorders. Other possible
presentations include grief and loneliness (Mishara and Kastenbaum 1980). In
one geriatric-mental-health team, depression, confusion, and suspicion were the

most common presenting symptoms in patients whose alcohol problems were unrecognized (Reifler *et al.* 1982).

Forensic

Up to one-third of elderly persons who break the law suffer from alcohol abuse or dependence. More elderly offenders (20 per cent) were under the influence of alcohol at the time of the offence than their younger counterparts (Taylor and Parrott 1988). This is even more likely if the alleged crime involved violence, when up to 75 per cent of offenders used alcohol (Rosner *et al.* 1991). Nearly 60 per cent of arrests of elderly American males are either for drunkenness or driving under the influence (Glynn *et al.* 1984).

Social

The behaviour associated with alcohol abuse, and society's response to this, is often a valuable pointer to the problem. For example, alcohol abuse is often easier to diagnose in the patient's home than in clinical settings, because of the evidence of bottles, glasses, and the smell of alcohol (Seymour and Wattis 1992). More seriously, the features of the 'senile recluse syndrome' (Post 1984), self-neglect, aggression, and behaviour that precipitates family quarrels, may be the presenting features of an underlying alcohol problem. Alcohol abuse can also lead to social opprobrium and isolation; friends, relatives, accommodation facilities, and treatment agencies may all avoid the elderly alcohol abuser, leading to a cycle of loneliness and further drinking.

Clinical course and prognosis

There is little information regarding the natual course of alcohol abuse and dependence in the elderly. Many variations in clinical course have been documented in younger people (Vaillant 1983). At one extreme, unremitting consumption from an early age militates against survival into old age (Drew 1968); at the other extreme, however, there is some evidence that light to moderate use of alcohol is associated with a decreased mortality rate, even in the elderly (Scherr *et al.* 1992). Most alcohol abusers moderate their consumption with age, but some elderly people take up drinking after a break of years or months and some start *de novo*. Others gradually escalate their consumption in old age and present after years of 'silent drinking', when brain damage or social breakdown intervenes. Saunders *et al.* (1991) showed that a past drinking history was related to presentation with depression and dementia in later life. Cook *et al.* (1991) found that depression in such ex-drinkers was more likely to be less severe and of the 'neurotic–reactive' type.

Blow *et al.* (1992) have demonstrated the importance of co-morbidity in determining the level of impairment associated with alcohol abuse. Their war-veteran patients showed escalating levels of organic brain syndromes with age. This peaked in the over-seventy group, of whom 18 per cent had an organic diagnosis. Depression and anxiety remained important co-morbid diagnoses throughout the life span, with major depression also reaching its peak (11.8 per cent) in the over-seventy group. Meanwhile, the numbers of patients with alcohol problems in addition to schizophrenia, personality disorders, and other substance abuse all fell with increasing age.

Screening at-risk groups

Identifying who is at risk of alcohol and other substance abuse in late life is still a rather speculative exercise. A past history of heavy, silent alcohol use may indicate patients vulnerable to stress. Elderly persons following a life event such as bereavement, those with insomnia, and those in chronic pain may be at risk of developing alcohol problems. Patients who have previously been dependent on alcohol are more likely to become dependent on benzodiazepines. Depression and dementia (King 1986) may be risk factors for substance abuse.

As most screening tools such as the CAGE questionnaire (Mayfield *et al.* 1974) have been developed for younger alcohol abusers, their validity may be limited in the elderly, particularly those with cognitive impairment. However, Willenbring *et al.* (1987) have validated the Michigan Alcoholism Screening Test (MAST) in a small group of elderly patients, and Atkinson (1991) has reported the development of a geriatric version of MAST (MAST-G) by Blow and colleagues in Ann Arbor. In their study of elderly mentally ill in-patients, Mears and Spice (1993) found that consumption of 14 or more units per week was associated with problem drinking in both sexes, with a high degree of specificity and sensitivity.

Treatment

Management of the individual patient

The initial difficulty with the treatment of alcohol abuse is recognition by both the patient and the health services that the problem exists (Zimberg 1978). Under-reporting and the reluctance of professionals to acknowledge excess drinking are major barriers to treatment. When patients are recognized, they are often seen as somebody else's problem and so fall between services. When elderly patients present, direct questioning on alcohol usage is essential. An attempt should be made to obtain a corroborative history. A home visit can often be invaluable in identifying and confronting the issue of alcohol (Jolley and Hodgson 1985).

Once alcohol dependence or abuse is recognized, hospital admission is usually needed. Such an admission breaks the alcoholic routine and allows for a complete assessment of the patient's physical and mental state as well as for management of withdrawal. Arguments have been put for placing treatment facilities in geriatric, psychogeriatric (Jolley and Hodgson 1985), traditional alcohol (Glatt 1978), and age-specific alcohol units (Kofoed *et al.* 1987). A combination of all these facilities would allow flexibility and maximize patient acceptance, although this runs the risk of diluting the available expertise.

Once the patient has been admitted, a longer-term management plan then needs to be formulated. Whether total abstinence or controlled drinking is the most appropriate goal in treatment remains controversial (Post 1982; Jolley and Hodgson 1985). Elderly patients who abuse alcohol can and do moderate their drinking. However, patients who present with a picture of dependence should be encouraged to accept abstinence as their goal. A variety of methods aimed at preventing the re-emergence of damaging drinking have been advocated. Some patients do well at home, others repeatedly fail there but achieve abstinence in an institutional residential setting. Amelioration of the underlying social stressors backed by psychotherapeutic interventions, more emphasis on group socialization, family casework, medical treatment, and treatment of depression have all been suggested. As with younger abusers, some elderly people find Alcoholics Anonymous suitable (Droller 1964). Disulfiram is not recommended in the elderly because of increasing risks involved with ingesting alcohol whilst taking the drug (Dunne and Schipperheijn 1989).

Because of individual differences, a flexible treatment approach is needed in dealing with alcohol dependent patients. The elderly respond better to supportive social intervention than intensive confrontation (Kashner *et al.* 1992; Zimberg, 1984). Environmental manipulation and day hospital care are also useful adjuncts to treatment (Rosin and Glatt 1971). Group therapy may become fragmented when significant numbers of elderly clients are included in general treatment programmes, as they may have difficulty identifying with the problems of younger drinkers. The group process in specific treatment programmes for the elderly is slower paced than in younger groups (Kofoed *et al.* 1984). Behavioural modification packages using a self-management philosophy have been used. This approach looks at antecedents, behaviour during drinking, and consequences of drinking, as well as providing general problem-solving skills (Dupree *et al.* 1984). Patients with frontal-lobe impairment may do better in a structured environment (Moos and Finney 1984). However, there is no agreement as to whether brain damage or psychopathology alter treatment outcome (Mishara and Kastenbaum 1980; Helzer *et al.* 1984). The possible use of the therapeutic-community concept in nursing homes has been suggested to deal with alcohol-related problems (Wattis 1981).

In summary, the treatment of the elderly alcohol abuser revolves around adapting treatment regimens evolved with younger patients to the particular medical, psychological, and social aspects of ageing. An eclectic approach based on flexibility to maximize compliance should be the underlying theme. A community approach to the prevention of substance abuse will have a far greater impact in the long term than individual treatment.

Alcohol withdrawal and its management

Alcohol withdrawal is usually characterized by tremor, tachycardia, hypertension, anxiety, nausea, and insomnia. Withdrawal symptoms become more severe with age, and detoxification becomes more likely to be complicated by intercurrent illness (Liskow *et al.* 1989). Seizures usually occur within the first 24 hours of withdrawal if they are to occur. The withdrawing patient should be nursed in a calm, well-lit environment by confident and supportive staff. If sedation is necessary, shorter-acting benzodiazepines and chlormethiazole are preferred.

Intramuscular thiamine (50–100 mg) for three days is necessary in patients with poor oral intake or cognitive impairment. Oral supplements may suffice in other patients, but glucose loads should not be given before adequate thiamine stores are ensured. In cases of Wernicke's encephalopathy, thiamine should be given intravenously.

Given that the half-life of benzodiazepines may be prolonged in the elderly, care should be taken that they do not accumulate. Benzodiazepine dosage should be empirically determined with the aim of reduction in distressing symptoms over a period of no more than a week. Dosage for patients over the age of 70 years should begin as much as two-thirds lower than for a fit younger patient. One approach is to give 5–10 mg of diazepam and monitor the response. This dose can be repeated every two hours, repeated until withdrawal symptoms are controlled. Despite this initial caution, Liskow *et al.* (1989) found older patients (average age 64 years) in an in-patient unit required higher doses of chlordiazepoxide for control of withdrawal symptoms than a younger group (average age 28 years). However, the older group had a high rate of past delirium tremens (30 per cent) and may have been a particularly heavily dependent group. Any regimen is only a guide, as differences in alcohol consumption and individual variations in metabolism ensure wide variations in the dosage of benzodiazepine required.

Anxiolytics are rarely needed after the third day of withdrawal. In severe withdrawal, delirium tremens can supervene with hallucinations and cardiovascular decompensation (Foy 1986). Such patients must be managed in an in-patient medical setting due to the high mortality rate.

Intervention studies

Most published studies comparing older alcohol abusers with younger groups show at least as good a response to treatment (Janick and Dunham 1983). Groups of elderly subjects have also been studied in age-specific treatment programmes, but sample sizes have been small and patients highly selected (Kofoed *et al.* 1984). Retrospective methods and inadequate controls further limit conclusions that can be drawn from presently available studies. Co-morbidity with other psychiatric, personality, and medical disorders also complicates the picture. Generally, response rates to treatment have been disappointing (Wattis 1981). Continued drinking is the norm, with a significant minority of drinkers achieving abstinence and a smaller group returning to moderate drinking.

As with younger patients, the majority of elderly patients with problem drinking reject or fail to complete treatment programmes (Dupree *et al.* 1984; Atkinson 1990), although one study has found that elderly women were less likely to discharge themselves from treatment (Blankfield and Maritz 1990). Results for those who do complete treatment are generally good, whether abstinence or modified drinking is the goal. Those who continued in the study of Dupree *et al.* (1984) were socially isolated, late-onset drinkers, often widowed or highly motivated. Dropouts had a lower expectation of success at commencement, were more depressed, drank more, and had a more external locus of control than those who stayed in treatment. One factor associated with improvement was an expansion in the social network of those who completed therapy. Kashner *et al.* (1992) randomly allocated older alchohol abusers to elder-specific supportive therapy and traditional therapy with confrontational techniques. The elder-specific treatment used reminiscence, promoted self-esteem, and peer group relationships and was tolerant of failure and respectful of age. Both techniques included in-patient care and out-patient treatment. Patients in the elder-specific regimen were two to three times more likely to be abstinent at 6 and 12 months post-discharge. This finding was statistically significant. Unfortunately there was no untreated control group, and it remains possible that the difference in outcome was due to a negative effect of confrontational therapy. Carstensen *et al.* (1985) followed up 16 male veterans (aged 65–70) for 2 to 4 years after a behavioural treatment programme which entailed a 28-day in-patient treatment on a social-learning model. One half reported abstinence in the 6 month period prior to follow-up. Another 12 per cent reported significant modification of their drinking. However, the abstinent group represented less than one-third of the original group. Again, there was no control group. The small numbers involved make it difficult to generalize from this retrospective study.

Ethical and medicolegal problems

Despite proponents of the disease model of alcoholism, most legislatures place the responsibility for substance abuse and dependence firmly with the sufferer. In many patients, however, dependence undermines free will and impacts adversely upon others. This creates dilemmas for clinicians and law-makers alike. In the elderly it is particularly common for substance abuse to become linked with self-destructive consequences, often cerebral in nature. Subtle frontal-lobe and memory impairment can impair judgement, and a point may come when the abuser can no longer make an informed decision concerning drinking. The point at which intervention without consent becomes possible is rarely clear-cut, and clinicians and families are often forced to look on helplessly as this process of deterioration unfolds. Legislation is determined more by social attitudes than by clinical variables. In the United Kingdom, the 1983 Mental Health Act forbids compulsory admission and treatment for alcohol abuse alone, but this is possible if another mental disorder (including that due to brain disease) is present.

Future Trends

Each new generation of elderly people will have different attitudes to alcohol. However, evidence on recent cohort changes in consumption is inconclusive

(Mishara and Kastenbaum 1980; Glynn *et al.* 1984; Hilton and Clark 1987; Smart and Adlaf 1988; Adams *et al.* 1990). The most likely explanation for observed trends is that successive cohorts are continuing to decrease their consumption with age, but from a higher base level. Because of this trend, future drinking patterns look likely to increase amongst the elderly. This will combine with a rapidly increasing elderly population to accentuate alcohol problems in this age group.

OTHER SUBSTANCE ABUSE

As with alcohol, the extent to which elderly people abuse prescribed drugs and other substances is not known with any certainty, although we can be sure that it has been underestimated. While most attention has been paid to dependence upon psychotropic drugs in recent years, it should not be forgotten that other classes of drug, such as analgesics and laxatives, also have considerable potential for abuse in this age group (Higgitt 1992).

Benzodiazepines

Elderly people in developed countries are heavy users of psychotropic medi-cation, particularly benzodiazepines, and the use of these drugs appears to be declining less in this age group than in younger adults (Beardsley *et al.* 1988; Sullivan *et al.* 1988; Mant *et al.* 1988). Benzodiazepine anxiolytics and hypnotics are prescribed more frequently for elderly women than elderly men, and often for complaints far removed from anxiety or insomnia; for example, Lyndon and Russell (1990) found that elderly patients taking benzodiazepines were no more likely to suffer from anxiety or depression than controls. Elderly residents in nursing homes are a group who are particularly liable to be prescribed psychotropic medication for a wide range of disturbed behaviours. Whilst this practice does not necessarily constitute abuse, it may lead to deleterious side-effects and dependency, and has generated a great deal of controversy since there is little evidence that non-antipsychotic medication is useful in the management of disturbed behavior in dementing patients (Risse and Barnes 1986).

Elderly people are more vulnerable to the side-effects of benzodiazepine use (Kruse 1990), which include ataxia, loss of spontaneity, drowsiness, depressed mood, memory impairment, paradoxical excitement, and delirium. While dependence is usually associated with long-term use, Higgitt (1992) presents evidence for tolerance and withdrawal developing within 2 to 6 weeks. Many elderly patients are initially prescribed benzodiazepines for insomnia, often precipitated by a life event, such as illness or bereavement. This prescription is often continued for years afterwards, despite the hypnotic effect waning within weeks. Despite this, 90 per cent of patients wanted to continue taking the medication and 64 per cent said they would have trouble coping without it.

Although the short-acting benzodiazepines are more likely to cause withdrawal reactions, it appears that potency is more important in this regard, since some agents with short elimination half-lives such as lorazepam are much more troublesome than others, such as oxazepam (Higgitt 1992). The longer-acting agents are prone to accumulate in the elderly and cause a hangover effect the next day. The half-life of these drugs is increased by as much as fourfold (Higgitt 1988).

Education for doctors, nurses, and patients is a vital part of any strategy to reduce the inappropriate prescription of benzodiazepines. Home visits provide an opportunity to detect multiple packets of benzodiazepines from multiple doctors. Tablets left can be checked against prescription date and dosage to monitor over-use. Intervention can be effective, as Salzman *et al.* (1992) demonstrated in a study in which more than half of the patients withdrawn from benzodiazepines remained medication-free at twelve months follow-up. Higgitt (1988) maintains there is a strong case against long-term benzodiazepine use in the elderly. Short-term use should be limited to four weeks with appropriate alternative strategies for the medium and long term.

Benzodiazepine withdrawal and its management

The treatment of withdrawal in the elderly remains largely empirical. Untreated, withdrawal symptoms may last from two to eight weeks. Initial symptoms resemble an exaggerated recurrence of anxiety and insomnia. More serious withdrawal reactions are reported to include hyperacusis, confusional states, fits, and psychotic symptoms such as hallucinations (Foy *et al.* 1986). These reactions are best avoided by gradual dose reduction. All withdrawal regimes need to be flexible and tailored to the individual, but the general principles of tapering proposed by the American Psychiatric Association (1990) are a useful guideline. These suggest that the first 50 per cent of the daily dose can be reduced fairly quickly. The next 25 per cent is reduced more slowly, and the final 25 per cent very slowly. It may be preferable to substitute long-acting benzodiazepines for withdrawal. In the elderly, it is often the time taken to taper that is lengthened, despite the patient being on a relatively low dose. The process may take several weeks or months, particularly for out-patients. The rebound anxiety symptoms and insomnia must be monitored closely and the patient and their family need a great deal of reassurance.

Other prescribed drugs

Barbiturate abuse has almost disappeared in most countries, although a small number of elderly long-term users of barbiturates continue to be prescribed these drugs for sedative purposes. Whenever they encounter health services the opportunity should be taken to wean them on to a less dangerous tranquillizer. Other sedatives such as chlormethiazole and chloral hydrate are likely to be associated with abuse and dependence, although there is little information concerning these agents in the elderly. Prescribed analgesics such as opiates may lead to dependence and problems with sudden withdrawal, but abuse of these drugs does not yet appear to be a major clinical problem in the elderly. Indeed, elderly patients with chronically painful physical illnesses are probably more likely to be denied adequate amounts of analgesic medication because of misguided concerns that they may become addicted (Lander 1990). Prescription agents of all kinds can be used by patients in a manner different from that which the doctor has intended. The management of withdrawal should follow the general principles of benzodiazepine reduction. Ongoing education is the best approach to prevention of the problem.

Over-the-counter preparations – medicinal and otherwise

There is little direct evidence concerning abuse of and dependence on over-the-counter substances, such as analgesics, cough remedies, and laxatives, by the elderly. However, two-thirds of American elders take over-the-counter substances and this proportion increases with age, particularly among women (Miller, 1991). Some of these preparations may be taken in response to symptoms of anxiety and depression, or to assuage personal needs that are not being met elsewhere. Some of the medication can have psychiatric side-effects caused by anticholinergic and antihistaminic ingredients, and others have addictive potential because they contain small doses of caffeine (Abrams and Alexopoulos 1988). Chronic use of laxatives can constitute abuse, and may result in colonic atonia. The management of problems arising from over-the-counter medication is probably best addressed by family physicians routinely enquiring about their use and providing information on the possible dangers of such substances.

It is worth emphasizing that tobacco is the most commonly abused substance in the elderly and is a greater cause of physical ill health than any other substance in this age group. Health services should reinforce the negative health consequences of continued smoking and the proven benefit to health of cessation at any age.

Illicit substances

Access to and abuse of illicit drugs are rare in present cohorts of elderly people. Only 2 or 3 per cent of American veterans aged over 60 years with an alcohol problem were found by Blow *et al.* (1992) to be also abusing other substances. This co-morbidity is ten times less common than for young adult males. The tendency for antisocial personality disorder to diminish with age may partly explain this decline in illicit drug abuse with age, as may a growing disinclination to seek novelty with the passing of the years. Until recently, the harmfulness of many illicit drugs and the lifestyle associated with their use has probably also militated against longevity for chronic abusers. It is possible that increasing numbers of opiate abusers are now surviving into old age, although such patients remain little studied.

CONCLUSIONS

Although alcohol abuse among the elderly is less common than at younger ages, it is probably under-recognized, undertreated and on the increase. Failure to address this problem has implications in terms of increased physical, psychiatric and social complications. The elderly alcohol abuser ofter presents atypically and not to traditional alcohol treatment services. As a result, treatment agencies need to be able to respond in the community, general hospitals, and the legal system. Geriatric, psychogeriatric, and alcohol treatment teams should establish guidelines on a regional basis to prevent patients from falling between services. Education of workers in geriatric care and social support settings is needed to improve identification of problems of alcohol and other substance abuse in the elderly.

Even though it is not yet clearly established that treatment helps elderly substance abusers, age-specific programmes may be of benefit. Modified styles of treatment with less confrontation and more peer support have been proposed. Therapy aimed at managing primary social and psychological problems such as bereavement, loneliness, and isolation is particularly important for the late-onset substance abuser. Because of the synergistic effect of advancing years and physical damage, any person presenting with alcohol problems in old age should have a thorough medical assessment.

After tobacco and alcohol, benzodiazepine consumption is associated with the greatest risk of abuse and dependence in the elderly. In most cases, heightened care when prescribing these agents for insomnia or anxiety at times of crisis would lead to fewer problems in the long run.

REFERENCES

Abrams, R. C., and Alexopoulos, G. S. (1988). Substance abuse in the elderly: over-the-counter and illegal drugs. *Hospital and Community Psychiatry*, **39**, 822–9.

Adams, W. L., Garry, P. J., Rhyne, R., Hunt, W. C., and Goodwin, J. S. (1990). Alcohol intake in the healthy elderly. Changes with age in a cross-section and longitudinal study. *Journal of the American Geriatrics Society*, **38**, 211–16.

Adams, W. L., Magruder-Habib, K., Trued, S., and Broome, H. L. (1992). Alcohol abuse in elderly emergency department patients. *Journal of the American Geriatrics Society*, **40**, 1236–40.

American Psychiatric Association (1987). *Diagnostic and statistical manual of mental disorders*, (3rd edn, revised). American Psychiatric Association, Washington.

American Psychiatric Association (1990). *Benzodiazepine dependence, toxicity and abuse*, pp. 35–38. American Psychiatric Press, Washington.

Atkinson, R. M. (1987). Alcohol problems of the elderly. *Alcohol and Alcoholism*, **22**, 415–17.

Atkinson, R. M. (1990). Aging and alcohol use disorders: diagnostic issues in the elderly. *International Psychogeriatrics*, **2**, 55–72.

Atkinson, R. M. (1991). Alcohol and drug abuse in the elderly. In *Psychiatry and the elderly* (ed. R. Jacoby and C. Oppenheimer), pp. 819–51. Oxford University Press, Oxford.

Atkinson, R. M., Turner, J. A., Kofoed, L. L., and Tolson, R. L. (1985). Early versus late onset alcoholism in older persons: preliminary findings. *Alcoholism : Clinical and Experimental Research*, **9**, 513–15.

Beardsley, R. S., Gardocki, G. L., Larson, D. B., and Hidalgo, J. (1988). Prescribing of psychotropic medication by primary care physicians and psychiatrists. *Archives of General Psychiatry*, **47**, 1117–19.

Benshoff, J. J., and Roberto, K. A. (1987). Alcoholism in the elderly: clinical issues. *Clinical Gerontologist*, **7**, 3–14.

Blankfield, A., and Maritz, J. S. (1990). Female alcoholics. IV: Admission problems and patterns. *Acta Psychiatrica Scandinavica*, **82**, 445–50.

Blose, I. L. (1978). The relationship of alcohol to aging and the elderly. *Alcoholism: Clinical and Experimental Research*, **2**, 17–29.

Blow, F. C., Cook, C. A. L., Booth, B. M., Falcon, S. P., and Friedman, M. J. (1992). Age related psychiatric comorbidities and level of functioning in alcoholic veterans seeking outpatient treatment. *Hospital and Community Psychiatry*, **43**, 990–5.

Bridgewater, R., Leigh, S., James, O. F. W., and Potter, J. F. (1987). Alcohol consumption and dependence in elderly patients in an urban community. *British Medical Journal*, **295**, 884–5.

Brody, J. A. (1982). Aging and alcohol abuse. *Journal of the American Geriatrics Society*, **30**, 123–6.

Busby, W. J. Campbell, A. J., Borrie, M. J., and Spears, G. F. S. (1988). Alcohol use in a community-based sample of subjects aged 70 years and older. *Journal of the American Geriatrics Society*, **36**, 301–5.

Cahalan, D., and Cisin, I. H. (1968). American drinking practices: summary of findings from a national probability sample. I. Extent of drinking by population subgroups. *Quarterly Journal of Studies on Alcohol*, **29**, 130–51.

Caracci, G., and Miller, S. (1991). Epidemiology and diagnosis of alcoholism in the elderly (a review). *International Journal of Geriatric Psychiatry*, **6**, 511–15.

Carstensen, L. L., Rychtarik, R. G., and Prue, D. M. (1985). Behavioral treatment of the geriatric alcohol abuser: a long term follow-up study. *Addictive Behaviors*, **10**, 307–11.

Chatham, L. R. (1984). Greetings. In *Nature and extent of alcohol problems among the elderly* (ed. G. Maddox, L. N. Robins, and N. Rosenburg), pp. 5–6. Springer, New York.

Christopherson, V. A., Escher, M. C., and Bainton, B. R. (1984). Reasons for drinking among the elderly in rural Arizona. *Journal of Studies on Alcohol*, **45**, 417–23.

Cook, B. L., Winokur, G., Garvey, M., and Beach, V. (1991). Depression and previous alcoholism in the elderly. *British Journal of Psychiatry*, **158**, 72–5.

Curtis, J. R., Geller, G., Stokes, E. J., Levice, D. M., and Moore, R. D. (1989). Characteristics, diagnosis and treatment of alcoholism in elderly patients. *Journal of the American Geriatrics Society*, **29**, 956–67.

Drew, L. R. H. (1968). Alcoholism as a self-limiting disease. *Quarterly Journal of Studies on Alcohol*, **29**, 956–67.

Droller, H. (1964). Some aspects of alcoholism in the elderly. *Lancet*, **2**, 137.

Dunne, F. J., and Schipperheijn, J. A. M. (1989). Alcohol and the elderly. *British Medical Journal*, **298**, 1660–1.

Dupree, L. W., Broskowski, H., and Schonfeld, L. (1984). The Gerontology Alcohol

Project: a behavioral treatment program for elderly alcohol abusers. *The Gerontologist*, **24**, 510–16.

Edwards, G., Hawker, A., Hensman, C., Peto, J., and Williamson, V. (1973). Alcoholics known or unknown to agencies: epidemiological studies in a London suburb. *British Journal of Psychiatry*, **123**, 169–83.

Ekerdt, D. J., De Labry, L. O., Glynn, R. J., and Davis, R. W. (1989). Changes in drinking behaviors with retirement: findings from the Normative Aging Study. *Journal of Studies on Alcohol*, **50**, 347–53.

Finlayson, R. E. (1984). Prescription drug abuse in older persons. In *Alcohol and drug abuse in old age*, (ed. R. M. Atkinson), pp. 61–70. American Psychiatric Press, Washington.

Finlayson, R. E., Hurt, R. D., Davis, L. J., and Morse, R. M. (1988). Alcoholism in elderly persons: a study of the psychiatric and psychological features of 216 inpatients. *Mayo Clinic Proceedings*, **63**, 761–8.

Foy, A. (1986). The management of alcohol withdrawal. *The Medical Journal of Australia*, **145**, 24–7.

Foy, A., Drinkwater, V., March, S., and Mearrick, P. (1986). Confusion after admission to hospital in elderly patients using benzodiazepines. *British Medical Journal*, **293**, 1072.

Gambert, S. R. (1992). Substance abuse in the elderly. In *Substance abuse. A comprehensive textbook* (2nd edn) (ed. J. H. Lowinson, P. Ruiz, R. B. Millman, and J. G. Langrod), pp. 843–51. Williams and Wilkins, Baltimore.

Glatt, M. M. (1978). Experiences with elderly alcoholics in England. *Alcoholism: Clinical and Experimental Research*, **2**, 23–6.

Glynn, R. J., Bouchard, G. R., Locastro, J. S., and Hermos, J. A. (1984). Changes in alcohol consumption behaviors among men in the Normative Aging Study. In *Nature and extent of alcohol problems among the elderly* (ed. G. Maddox, L. N. Robins, and N Rosenburg), pp. 101–16. Springer, New York.

Hagnall, O., and Tunving, K. (1972). Prevalence and nature of alcoholism in a total population. *Social Psychiatry*, **7**, 190–201.

Harris, M., Sutherland, D., Cutter, G., and Ballangarry, L. (1987). Alcohol related hospital admissions in a country town. *Australian Drug and Alcohol Review*, **6**, 195–8.

Helzer, J. E., Carey, K. E., and Miller, R. H. (1984). Predictors and correlates of recovery in older versus younger alcoholics. In *Nature and extent of alcohol problems among the elderly* (ed. G. Maddox, L. N. Robins, and N. Rosenberg), pp. 83–100. Springer, New York.

Higgitt, A. C. (1988). Indications for benzodiazepine prescriptions in the elderly. *International Journal of Geriatric Psychiatry*, **3**, 239–43.

Higgitt, A. C. (1992). Dependency on prescribed drugs. *Reviews in Clinical Gerontology*, **2**, 151–5.

Hilton, M., and Clark, W. B. (1987). Changes in American drinking patterns and problems, 1967–1984. *Journal of Studies on Alcohol*, **48**, 515–22.

Holzer, C. E., Robins, L. N., Myers, J. K., Weissman, M. M., Tischler, G. L., Leaf, P. J., *et al.* (1984). Antecedents and correlates of alcohol abuse and dependence in the elderly. In *Nature and extent of alcohol problems among the elderly* (ed. G. Maddox, L. N. Robins, and N. Rosenberg), pp. 217–44. Springer, New York.

Hurt, R. D., Finlayson, R. E., Morse, R. M., and Davis, L. J. (1988). Alcoholism in elderly persons: medical aspects and prognosis of 216 inpatients. *Mayo Clinic Proceedings*, **63**, 753–60.

Iliffe, S., Haines, A., Booroff, A., Goldenberg, E., Morgan, P., and Gallivan, S. (1991). Alcohol consumption by elderly people: a general practice survey. *Age and Ageing*, **44**, 307–17.

Janik, S. W., and Dunham, R. G. (1983). A nationwide examination of the need for specific alcoholism treatment programs for the elderly. *Journal of Studies on Alcohol*, **22**, 193–8.

Jensen, G. D., and Bellecci, P. (1987). Alcohol and the elderly: relationships to illness and smoking. *Alcohol and Alcoholism*, **22**, 193–8.

Jolley, D., and Hodgson, S. (1985). Alcoholism in the elderly: a tale of women and our times. In *Recent advances in geriatric medicine 3* (ed. B. Isaacs), pp. 113–22. Churchill Livingstone, Edinburgh.

Kashner, T. M., Rodell, D. E., Ogden, S. R., Guggenheim, F. G., and Karson, C. N. (1992). Outcomes and costs of two VA inpatient treatment programs for older alcoholic patients. *Hospital and Community Psychiatry*, **43**, 985–9.

King, M. B. (1986). Alcohol abuse and dementia. *International Journal of Geriatric Psychiatry*, **1**, 31–6.

Kofoed, L. L., Tolson, R. L., Atkinson, R. M., Turner, R. L., and Toth, R. F. (1984) Elderly groups in an alcoholism clinic. In: *Alcohol and drug abuse in old age* (ed. R. M. Atkinson), pp. 35–49. American Psychiatric Press, Washington.

Kofoed, L. L., Tolson, R. L., Atkinson, R. M., Toth, R. F., and Turner, R. L. (1987). Treatment compliance of older alcoholics: an elder specific approach is superior to 'mainstreaming'. *Journal of Studies on Alcohol*, **48**, 47–51.

Kruse, W. H. (1990). Problems and pitfalls in the use of benzodiazepines in the elderly. *Drug Safety*, **5**, 328–44.

Lander, J. (1990). Fallacies and phobias about addiction and pain. *British Journal of Addiction*, **85**, 803–9.

Liberto, J. G., Oslin, D. W., and Ruskin, P. E. (1992). Alcoholism in older persons: a review of the literature. *Hospital and Community Psychiatry*, **43**, 975–84.

Lishman, W. A. (1987). *The psychological consequences of cerebral disorder* (2nd edn), p. 32. Blackwell Scientific Publications, Oxford.

Liskow, B. I., Rinck, C., Campbell, J., and De Souza, C. (1989). Alcohol withdrawal in the elderly. *Journal of Studies on Alcohol*, **50**, 414–21.

Livingston, G., and King, M. (1993). Alcohol abuse in an inner city elderly population: the Gospel Oak survey. *International Journal of Geriatric Psychiatry*, **8**, 511–14.

Lyndon, R. W., and Russell, J. D. (1990). Can overuse of psychotropic drugs in the elderly be prevented? *Australian and New Zealand Journal of Psychiatry*, **24**, 77–81.

Malcolm, M. T. (1984). Alcohol and drug use in the elderly visited at home. *The International Journal of the Addictions*, **19**, 411–18.

Mant, A., Duncan-Jones, P., Saltman, D., Bridges-Webb, C., Kehoe, L., Lansbury, G., and Chancellor, A. H. B. (1988). Development of long-term use of psychotropic drugs by general practice patients. *British Medical Journal*, **296**, 251–4.

Marco, C. A., and Kelen, G. D. (1990). Acute intoxication. *Emergency Medicine Clinics of North America*, **8**, 731–48.

Mayfield, D., McLeod, G., and Hall, P. (1974). The CAGE questionnaire: validation of a new alcoholism screening instrument. *American Journal of Psychiatry*, **131**, 1121–3.

McGinnis, C., and Ryan, C. (1965). The influence of age on MMPI scores of chronic alcoholics. *Journal of Clinical Psychology*, **21**, 271–2.

Mears, H. J., and Spice, C. (1993). Screening for problem drinking in the elderly: a study in the elderly mentally ill. *International Journal of Geriatric Psychiatry*, **8**, 319–326.

Millar, H. R. (1984). Acute confusional and other symptomatic states. In *Handbook of studies on psychiatry of old age* (ed. D. W. K. Kay and G. D. Burrows), pp. 217–34. Elsevier, Amsterdam.

Miller, N. S. (1991). Alcohol and drug dependence. In *Comprehensive review of geriatric psychiatry*, (1st edn) (ed. J. Sadavoy, L. W. Lazarus, and L. Jarvik), pp. 387–401. American Psychiatric Press, Washington.

Mishara, B. L., and Kastenbaum, R. (1980). *Alcohol and old age*. Grune and Stratton, New York.

Moos, R. H., and Finney, J. W. (1984). A systems perspective on problem drinking among older adults. In *Nature and extent of alcohol problems among the elderly* (ed. G. Maddox, L. N. Robins, and N. Rosenberg), pp. 151–72. Springer, New York.

Myers, J. K., Weissman, M. M., Tischler, G. L., Holzer, G. L., Leaf, P. J., Orvaschel, H., *et al.* (1984). Six month prevalence of psychiatric disorders in three communities. *Archives of General Psychiatry*, **41**, 959–67.

Nelson, D. E., Sattin, R. W, Langlois, J. A., De Vito, C. A., and Stevens, J. A. (1992). Alcohol as a risk factor for fall injury events among elderly persons living in the community. *Journal of the American Geriatrics Society*, **40**, 658–61.

Nordstrom, G., and Berglund, M. (1987). Ageing and recovery from alcoholism. *British Journal of Psychiatry*, **151**, 382–8.

Ojesjo, L. (1980). Prevalence of known and hidden alcoholism in the revisited Lundby population. *Social Psychiatry*, **15**, 81–90.

Penick, E. C., Powell, B. J., Bingham, S. F., Liskow, B. I., Miller, N. S., and Read, M. R. (1987). A comparative study of familial alcoholism. *Journal of Studies on Alcohol*, **48**, 1136–45.

Penk, W. E., Charles, H. L., Patterson, E. T., Roberts, W. R., Dolan, M. P., and Brown, A. S. (1982). Chronological age differences in MMPI scores. *Journal of Consulting and Clinical Psychology*, **50**, 322–24.

Post, F. (1982). Functional disorders. 1. Description, incidence and recognition. In *The psychiatry of late life*, (ed. R. Levy and F. Post), pp. 176–96. Blackwell Scientific Publications, Oxford.

Post, F. (1984). Schizophrenic and paranoid psychoses. In: *Handbook of studies on psychiatry of old age*. (ed. D. W. Kay and E. D. Burrows), pp. 291–302, Elsevier, Amsterdam.

Reifler, B., Raskind, M., and Kethley, A. (1982). Psychiatric diagnoses among geriatric patients seen in an outreach program. *Journal of the American Geriatrics Society*, **30**, 368–76.

Risse, S. C., and Barnes, R. (1986). Pharmacologic treatment of agitation associated with dementia. *Journal of the American Geriatrics Society*, **34**, 368–76.

Ritzmann, R. F., and Melchior, C. L. (1984). Age and development of tolerance to and physical dependence on alcohol. In *Alcoholism in the elderly* (ed. J. T. Hartford and T. Samorajski), pp. 117–38. Raven Press, New York.

Rosin, A. J., and Glatt, M. M. (1971). Alcohol excess in the elderly. *Quarterly Journal of Studies on Alcohol*, **32**, 53–9.

Rosner, R., Wiederlight, M., Harmon, M., and Cahn, D. J. (1991). Geriatric offenders examined at a forensic psychiatry clinic. *Journal of Forensic Sciences*, **36**, 1722–31.

Salzman, C., Fisher, J., Nobel, K., Glassman, R., Wolfson, A., and Kelley, M. (1992).

Cognitive impairment following benzodiazepine discontinuation in elderly nursing home residents. *International Journal of Geriatric Psychiatry*, **7**, 89–93.

Saunders, P. A., Copeland, J. R. M., Dewey, M. E., Davidson, I. A., McWilliam, C., Sharma, V. K., *et al.* (1989). Alcohol use and abuse in the elderly: findings from the Liverpool Longitudinal Study of continuing health in the community. *International Journal of Geriatric Psychiatry*, **4**, 103–8.

Saunders, P. A., Copeland, J. R. M., Dewey, M. E., Davidson, I. A., McWilliam, C., Sharma, V. K., and Sullivan, C. (1991). Heavy drinking as a risk factor for depression and dementia in elderly men. Findings from the Liverpool longitudinal community study. *British Journal of Psychiatry*, **159**, 213–16.

Scherr, P. A., LaCroix, A. Z., Wallace, R. B., Berkman, L., Curb, K. D., Cornoni-Huntley, J., *et al.* (1992). Light to moderate alcohol consumption and mortality in the elderly. *Journal of the American Geriatrics Society*, **40**, 651–7.

Schuckit, M. A., and Pastor, P. A. (1978). The elderly as a unique population: alcoholism. *Alcoholism: Clinical and Experimental Research*, **2**, 31–8.

Seymour, J., and Wattis, J. P. (1992). Alcohol abuse in the elderly. *Reviews in Clinical Gerontology*, **2**, 141–50.

Smart, R. G., and Adlaf, E. M. (1988). Alcohol and drug use among the elderly: trends in use and characteristics of users. *Canadian Journal of Public Health*, **79**, 236–42.

Speckens, A. E., Herren, T. J., and Rooijmans, H. G. (1991). Alcohol abuse among elderly patients in a general hospital as identified by the Munich Alcoholism Test. *Acta Psychiatrica Scandinavica*, **83**, 460–2.

Sullivan, C. F., Copeland, J. R. M., Dewey, M. E., Davidson, I. A., McWilliam, C., Saunders, P. A., *et al.* (1988). Benzodiazepine usage among the elderly: findings of the Liverpool community study. *International Journal of Geriatric Psychiatry*, **3**, 289–292.

Taylor, J., and Parrott, J. M. (1988). Elderly offenders. *British Journal of Psychiatry*, **152**, 340–6.

Ticehurst, S. (1990). Alcohol and the elderly. *Australian and New Zealand Journal of Psychiatry*, **24**, 252–60.

Vaillant, G. E. (1983). *The natural history of alcoholism*, p. 160. Harvard University Press, Cambridge.

Wattis, J. P. (1981). Alcohol problems in the elderly. *Journal of the American Geriatrics Society*, **24**, 131–4.

Wattis, J. P. (1983). Alcohol and old people. *British Journal of Psychiatry*, **143**, 306–7.

Willenbring, M. L., Christensen, K. J., Spring, W. D., and Rasmussen, R. (1987). Alcoholism screening in the elderly. *Journal of the American Geriatrics Society*, **35**, 864–9.

World Health Organization, (1992). *The ICD-10 Classification of mental and behavioural disorders. Clinical descriptions and diagnostic guidelines*, pp. 72–83. World Health Organization, Geneva.

Zimberg, S. (1978). Diagnosis and treatment of the elderly alcoholic. *Alcoholism: Clinical and Experimental Research*, **2**, 27–9.

Zimberg, S. (1984). Diagnosis and management of the elderly alcoholic. In *Alcohol and drug abuse in old age* (ed. R. M. Atkinson), pp. 23–4. Americal Psychiatric Press, Washington.

11

Eating disorders
CLARE BOWLER

INTRODUCTION

Although anorexia and bulimia nervosa are usually considered to be psychiatric disorders of young people, there has in recent years been increasing awareness of and interest in these conditions in the elderly. In the literature on eating disorders, 'older patients' are usually those in their late teens and early twenties, and the diagnosis of these disorders in elderly patients was initially regarded with some scepticism. However, a number of published case reports have established that both anorexia and bulimia nervosa can afflict people aged 65 years and above (Launer 1978; Price *et al.* 1985; Nagaratnam and Ghougassian 1988; Ramell and Brown 1988; Hsu and Zimmer 1988; Gower and Crisp 1990). This literature has recently been reviewed in detail by Cosford and Arnold (1992) (Tables 11.1 and 11.2).

Although anorexia nervosa was first described in post-menopausal women in the 1930s (Berkman 1930; Ryle 1936; Carrier 1939), most modern psychiatric nosologies preclude diagnoses of eating disorders in the elderly by including an upper age limit in the diagnostic criteria. For example, the Feighner criteria explicitly exclude the diagnosis of anorexia nervosa if the onset is over the age of 25 years (Feighner *et al.* 1972). DSM-III-R (*Diagnostic and statistical manual of mental disorders*, third edition, revised) describes eating disorders as beginning in adolescence with rare cases commencing as late as the early thirties (American Psychiatric Association 1987), and ICD-10 (*International Classification of diseases*, tenth revision) similarly states that anorexia nervosa affects older women only 'up to the menopause' (World Health Organization 1992). This definitional problem has hindered the recognition of the older eating-disordered patient. Dally and Gomez (1979) have stated that an upper age limit of 35 years is necessary for a diagnosis of primary anorexia nervosa, but they described a variant occurring above this age which they named 'anorexia tardive' and which they consider to be a secondary syndrome.

SYMPTOMATOLOGY

The elderly cases of eating disorders described in the recent literature have many of the classical clinical features found in younger patients. Severe self-induced

Table 11.1. Reports of eating disorders occurring for the first time over the age of 50 years. (Reprinted from Cosford and Arnold (1992), with permission.)

Author	Age	Duration	Diagnosis	Clinical features*	Past history	Concurrent illness	Treatment	Outcome
Kellet et al. (1976)	54	2 years	Anorexia nervosa	1. Fear of fatness and distorted body image 2. Marked weight loss 3. No bulimia 4. Laxative abuse and self-induced vomiting	Depression Abnormal grief reaction Daughter left home just prior to onset	None	Behavioural programme	Initial moderate improvement Subsequent ongoing weight loss
Launer (1978)	70	3 weeks	Anorexia nervosa	1. Fear of fatness and distorted body image 2. Marked weight loss 3. No bulimia 4. Laxative abuse	Abnormal eating attitudes and obsessional personality (for 40 years)	Obsessional personality	Behavioural programme Chlorpromazine Clomipramine	Good weight gain, not sustained on discharge
Jonas et al. (1984)	56	3 months	Bulimia	1. 'Overconcerned' with weight 2. No weight loss 3. Episodes of overeating 4. Self-induced vomiting	Rapid-cycling bipolar affective disorder (for 18 years)	Severe depressive episodes	Imipramine Phenelzine	Bulimic features disappeared with treatment of depressive episodes
Price et al. (1985)	68	1 year	Anorexia nervosa	1. Distorted body image, denial of weight loss 2. Marked weight loss 3. No bulimia 4. Laxative abuse	Husband died 2 years before (normal grief reaction)	None	Behavioural programme	Good recovery over 9 months Lost to follow-up
Rammell and Brown (1988)	67	5 years	Anorexia nervosa	1. Fear of weight gain and distorted body image 2. Marked weight loss 3. No bulimia 4. Self-induced vomiting	Multiple bereavement 7 years before followed by episodes of depression	None	Group therapy Antidepressants Chlorpromazine Insulin	No improvement over 4 years Rapid improvement, sustained 6 months later

Table 11.1. (cont.)

Author	Age	Duration	Diagnosis	Clinical features*	Past history	Concurrent illness	Treatment	Outcome
Hsu and Zimmer (1988) (case 1)	67	5 years	Bulimia nervosa	1. Preoccupation with weight 2. No weight loss 3. Binge eating 4. Self-induced vomiting	Chronic depression (for 25 years)	Depression, on diazepam, trazodone and dexamphetamine	Cognitive behavioural therapy	Alleviation of bulimic symptoms
Hsu and Zimmer (1988) (case 2)	64	2 years	Anorexia nervosa	1. Fear of fatness 2. Marked weight loss 3. Binge eating	Death of husband 1 year prior to onset	Depression	Amitriptyline	Depression alleviated Refused treatment of eating disorder
Hsu and Zimmer (1988) (case 3)	57	2 years	Bulimia	1. No fear of fatness 2. Weight gain 3. Binge eating	Depression (for 30 years)	Depression	Cognitive therapy Tranylcypromine	No benefit Depression and binge eating alleviated

*Clinical features are divided into four categories: 1, psychopathology; 2, change in body weight; 3, episodes of overeating (bulimia); 4, methods used to avoid fattening effect of food.

Table 11.2. Reports of eating disorders persisting beyond the age of 50 years. (Reprinted from Cosford and Arnold (1992), with permission.)

Author	Age	Age of first onset	Diagnosis	Clinical features*	Past history	Concurrent illness	Treatment	Outcome
Theander (1985) (case 1)	60	18	Anorexia nervosa of bulimic type	2. Marked weight loss (weight 30 kg) Other features not described†	Continuously unwell for 45 years Many hospital admissions	None described	Not described	Not described
Theander (1985) (case 2)	60	19	Anorexia nervosa	2. Marked weight loss (weight 33 kg) Other features not described†	Continuously unwell for 30 years Many hospital admissions	None described	Not described	Not described
Hsu and Zimmer (1988) (case 4)	59	18	Anorexia nervosa	1. Distorted body image 2. Marked weight loss 3. Binge eating 4. Self-induced vomiting	3 previous, episodes. mixed anorectic and bulimic symptoms	Depression	Cognitive behaviour therapy Doxepin	Initial improvement, soon refused further treatment
Hsu and Zimmer (1988) (case 5)	72	18	Anorexia nervosa	1. Distorted body image 2. Marked weight loss 3. No bulimia	2 prior episodes, recent relapse after retirement and daughter's marriage	None	Behaviour modification	Initial improvement Rapid relapse
Gower and Crisp (1990)	80	15	Anorexia nervosa	1. Phobic avoidance of normal weight 2. Marked weight loss 3. No bulimia 4. Laxative abuse	Relapse after husband's death 15 years ago Overdose 15 years years ago	None	None	No follow-up reported
Cosford and Arnold (1991)	73	20	Anorexia nervosa	1. Fear of fatness and distorted body image 2. Marked weight loss 3. No bulimia	Single former episode Persistent abnormal eating attitudes between episodes	None	Behavioural programme	Substantial weight gain sustained 6 months later

*Clinical features are divided into four categories: 1, psychopathology; 2, change in body weight; 3, episodes of overeating (bulimia); 4, methods used to avoid fattening effect of food.

weight loss is a core clinical feature of anorexia nervosa at all ages; in young women this is associated with amenorrhoea, but in the elderly this is obviously not applicable as a symptom. Generally, patients with anorexia nervosa maintain their appetite, but consider themselves as overeating on meagre quantities of food. In bulimia nervosa, first described by Russell in 1979, there are episodes of binge eating with the use of abnormal weight control mechanisms. Binge eating involves the consumption of large quantities of food, usually high-calorie carbo-hydrate, which the patient has actively been avoiding. A key clinical feature is that the patient feels overwhelmed by feelings of loss of control over their eating. The episode of binge eating is usually terminated by self-induced vomiting or exhaustion. Weight-control mechanisms used in eating disorders are self-induced vomiting, abuse of laxatives and diuretics, and excessive exercise. More unusual mechanisms are chewing food and spitting it out without swallowing it, abuse of amphetamines, thyroxine, and insulin and other diabetic drugs, particularly in diabetics.

Anorectic attitudes are a core feature of both anorexia and bulimia nervosa, and they are essential for the diagnosis of either of these conditions. There is a preoccupation with weight, with excessive fear of fatness—so-called 'weight phobia'. There is distortion of the body image, with patients feeling that they are fat even when they are painfully emaciated, and there is body-image disparagement with an intense loathing of one's body and body parts. Anorexia and bulimia nervosa are related conditions, and an individual may move over time from one diagnostic category to the other or fulfil the criteria for both at the same time. Approximately half of the cases of bulimia nervosa are predated by an episode of anorexia nervosa. Some clinicians considers patients with bulimia nervosa predated by an episode of anorexia nervosa to be inherently different to those where this does not occur. Young patients with bulimia nervosa tend to be older than those with anorexia nervosa, but this may not be the case in the elderly.

While many features of the psychopathology of eating disorders occur in elderly cases, it may be that the clinical picture is in some respects atypical in the elderly because of the pathoplastic effects of age. Dally and Gomez (1979) divide their category of 'anorexia tardive' into two subcategories. The first consists of 'women who pursue thinness at all costs and are prepared to use virtually any means available to achieve this'. They are usually energetic despite their emaciated appearance. The second category includes women who are anorectic and 'have sparrows' appetites, being afraid to eat too much'. They rarely vomit or use excessive amounts of laxatives. This second group of patients are usually inactive and spend their time lying down, or are bedridden. They are more prevalent and difficult to treat. These patients are passive, in contrast to the aggression inherent in the first type. The second category often have a history of chronic pain and minor illness.

Eating disorders are associated with an appreciable mortality, and while older eating-disordered patients may in one sense be regarded as 'survivors' of their illness, particularly if it is chronic, they are nevertheless particularly susceptible to severe starvation and the effects of abnormal weight control. The principal medical complications of anorexia nervosa are cardiac failure and arrhythmias with bradycardia and hypotension. Seizures, gastrointestinal problems—such as acute gastric dilatation, constipation and pancreatitis—as well as osteoporosis, dehydration, and hypothermia are additional complications. Blood tests may show leucopenia and relative lymphocytosis, metabolic alkalosis, hypokalaemia, and possibly hypoglycaemia. It is important that elderly eating-disordered patients are physically examined and laboratory tests performed on a regular basis, particularly if the patients are vomiting or abusing laxatives or diuretics. In these cases the potassium level may be sufficiently low to precipitate a fatal cardiac arrhythmia.

Of particular interest are late-onset cases whose first onset of eating disorder is in old age (Table 11.1). Some of these cases will have been totally symptom-free when younger with no prior evidence of any psychopathology of eating disorders. Other individuals may have had minimal symptoms and behaviour not amounting to a formal disorder when younger; for example, they may have been unduly weight concerned throughout their lives, whether obese or not, and perhaps dieted previously. While those with more pronounced symptoms may have suffered from subclinical anorexia or bulimia nervosa, others would have been indistinguishable from the general population, as worries about being overweight and dieting behaviour were probably as common in the past as they are today.

Another group of older individuals with eating disorders will have been symptomatic for many years (Table 11.2). Some of these cases are chronic, with an onset of the disorder in youth and persistence of their symptomatology to varying degrees throughout their lives. In follow-up studies of younger patients, 25 per cent of cases of anorexia nervosa in fact became chronic (Ratnasuriya *et al.* 1991). Alternatively, some elderly cases represent a recurrence of the eating disorder in late life, sometimes after having been symptom-free for many years. It is important to differentiate between eating disorders of late onset occurring for the first time in late life, and chronic or recurrent disorders, as they may differ in clinically important respects.

EPIDEMIOLOGY

The prevalence and incidence of eating disorders in the elderly is unknown. At all ages, morbidity rates of these conditions are difficult to establish, since individuals with anorexia and bulimia nervosa often deny their symptoms. In addition, the traditional association of eating disorders with youth no doubt contributes to cases of anorexia and bulimia nervosa in older people going unrecognized and untreated.

Although hard data are lacking, eating disorders are thought to be on the increase in all age groups, including the elderly (Hsu and Zimmer 1988). If true, it is probably due in part to improved recognition of these disorders, and in part to an actual increase in their prevalence, particularly in the young. It may be that anorexia and bulimia nervosa will figure more prominently in future psychogeriatric practice as the present young cohorts grow old, although it is not known to what extent the rates of anorexia and bulimia in a cohort's youth predict those at greater ages.

The oldest case described in the literature to date is a woman aged 94 years who was diagnosed as suffering from anorexia nervosa, although her good response to ECT suggests she may have in fact had a depressive illness (Bernstein 1972). Gower and Crisp (1990) have described anorexia nervosa in an 80-year-old woman. Elderly cases reported in the literature have the same sex distribution as younger cases, with the majority being female. Across the age spectrum one in ten cases are male, with Nagaratnam and Ghougassain (1988) describing a case of possible anorexia nervosa in a 70-year-old man. The upper-social-class bias traditionally associated with anorexia nervosa in young patients is not apparent in the published elderly case studies, although the small numbers make it difficult to comment on the association between any socio-demographic or culture-specific variables and eating disorders in this age group. Since chronic lifelong anorexia nervosa can hinder personality development, the ability to form and maintain relationships, and fertility and desire for children, individuals with a chronic disorder may be less likely to be married, in a long-term relationship, or to have had children. In these respects, they may differ from late-onset elderly patients who were free from the disorder during their formative and fertile years, but clear evidence on this is not available.

AETIOLOGY

The origins of eating disorders in younger people are multifactorial, involving psychological, psychiatric, physical, and social causes; this is doubtless true also of episodes occurring in old age. Adolescents may have difficulties coping with their developing sexuality and increased autonomy, and for a few anorexia nervosa provides a regression to a pre-pubertal state and an escape from these issues (Crisp 1980). Growing old is, like adolescence, a time of biological upheaval and social transition. At both these times of life issues surrounding dependency and autonomy are prominent. In some respects, adolescence may be considered the converse of old age; in adolescence increased autonomy is desirable whilst in old age it may be appropriate and necessary to be dependent on others. Following bereavement, an elderly person may have unwanted independence and social isolation forced upon them, and if they have had lifelong difficulty negotiating dependency, being fearful of increased reliance on others, then they may be susceptible to developing an eating disorder. Autonomy may never have been successfully negotiated in adolescence, dependency being transferred from parents directly to spouse and children; indeed, this new dependency may have been the way out of an eating disorder in youth. In older patients whose eating disorder recurs after many years of good health, it has been suggested that they rediscover previous maladaptive coping strategies of anorexia and bulimia at times of personal stress.

Depressive illness has also been implicated as having a major aetiological role, particularly in late-onset eating disorders. The relationship between these conditions is complex, since depressive symptoms are an integral feature of the eating disorders. In anorexia nervosa, depressed mood is associated with starvation and the precarious anorectic position, where the patient is fighting to maintain their low weight. Anorexia nervosa also causes sleep disturbance. It is important to establish the temporal relationship between the eating disorder and the depressed mood; if the onset of the depressive illness predates that of the anorexia or bulimia nervosa and is clearly associated with its time course, then depression may well be the cause of the eating disorder. Similarly, if the symptoms of an eating disorder occur only during episodes of formal depressive illness and remit when the depressive illness resolves, then the diagnosis of a secondary eating disorder is most likely (King 1963). This is demonstrated in the case study reported by Jonas *et al.* (1984) of a woman aged 56 years whose bulimic symptoms occurred along with severe bipolar affective disorder and were directly related to the depressive episodes, disappearing when these remitted.

It has been suggested that late-onset anorexia nervosa is an attempt by a predisposed individual to establish control during a period of increasing personal uncertainty. Cosford and Arnold (1992) propose that external losses may be sufficient to precipitate an eating disorder; for example, bereavement has been reported to precipitate anorexia nervosa in case studies of elderly people (Hsu and Zimmer 1988; Gower and Crisp 1990). Individuals appear to be susceptible in stressful situations if they have abnormal premorbid eating attitudes with undue weight concern, premorbid obesity, and obsessional personality traits with perfectionist tendencies. This leads to reliance on objective criteria such as appearance and weight to judge self-worth (Garfinkel and Garner 1982). Eating disorders are thought to be more common in Western societies where being thin is valued (Rodin *et al.* 1984). Hsu and Zimmer (1988) consider that even older women are succumbing to this social pressure—Crisp (1980) states that late-onset anorexia nervosa is associated with a significant degree of premorbid obesity.

Some authors have proposed that there is an underlying physical cause for eating disorders, although the evidence indicates that most abnormalities found in anorectic patients are secondary to weight loss. Anorexia nervosa may have a genetic component (Holland *et al.* 1984), and there was a strong family history in the late-onset case described by Gower and Crisp (1990). A number of possible mechanisms have been proposed, including pituitary insufficiency, hypothalamic lesions, and, more recently, dysfunction of cerebral serotonergic neurotransmission. This system has a role in appetite and satiety control, and Treasure and Tiller (1993) have suggested that anorexia nervosa is related to an increase in serotonergic activity, and bulimia nervosa to decreased activity. In addition, dopaminergic systems and both centrally and peripherally acting peptides have been implicated in the development of eating disorders (Goodall *et al.* 1987).

DIFFERENTIAL DIAGNOSIS

Since clinicians do not expect to encounter eating disorders in their elderly patients, it is likely that cases are missed, or given alternative diagnoses. In particular, general physicians may be unaware that an eating disorder is a viable diagnosis in the elderly. The relationship between eating disorders and depression has already been discussed; while both may coexist it should be borne in mind that depressive cognitions are an inherent part of eating disorders alone. Conversely, self-starvation in a depressed elderly patient may occur in response to nihilistic delusions, or be a form of disguised suicide; as such, it does not represent an eating disorder unless the patient also holds other anorectic attitudes. In young patients, anorexia and bulimia nervosa often occur with other neurotic disorders, notably anxiety states and obsessive–compulsive disorder. Holden (1990) has pointed out that the persistent intrusive thoughts regarding food and the urges to avoid eating have similarities with obsessive and compulsive symptoms. Many anorectic patients avoid social eating, and may be misdiagnosed as suffering from social phobia; however, this is a very rare form of phobic disorder in elderly people (Lindesay 1991). Bulimia nervosa may coexist with alcohol abuse, particularly alcoholic binges. Sometimes, the anorectic beliefs are so bizarre and are held with such conviction that they may be correctly described as a delusional idea, and the patient diagnosed as suffering from a psychotic disorder.

Other eating disorders unrelated to anorexia and bulimia nervosa may need to be considered in the differential diagnosis in an elderly patient. Pica is the persistent eating of non-nutritional substances, and usually occurs as a symptom in global disorders such as dementia or mental handicap. A number of specific neuropsychiatric disorders also affect eating and weight, for example hypothalamic tumours and the Kleine–Levin and Kluver-Bucy syndromes.

TREATMENT AND PROGNOSIS

As yet there are no published trials that specifically concern treatment of eating disorders in the elderly. Most of the case reports suggest that patients have been treated according to the principles generally applied to younger patients (Cosford and Arnold 1992). Specific treatment trials and the establishment of prognostic indicators will require the identification of more elderly patients with eating disorders.

The case reports in the literature show that older patients respond to conventional treatment. With anorexia nervosa the primary aim is weight restoration. A refeeding programme often requires in-patient management, particularly if the patient's weight is dangerously low, if their medical condition necessitates hospital admission, or if out-patient treatment has proven unsuccessful. Behavioural principles are sometimes employed alongside cognitive and dynamic psychotherapy. The patient agrees for privileges to be removed and restored to reward the weight gain. If the patient's weight loss is so severe as to pose an immediate threat to life and the patient cannot be persuaded to enter hospital, then compulsory admission may be required. Successful treatment is dependent on the patient's desire to move out of their anorectic position and their compliance with treatment, which means that compulsorily detained physical complications can be attributed to the eating disorder, the patient may be more willing to bring about change. Refeeding causes an increase in cardiac output, an expanded cardiac volume and an accelerated metabolic rate (Palla and Little 1988); cardiac failure can be precipitated, so particular care is needed with the refeeding of elderly patients.

The most widely used psychological treatment for bulimia nervosa is cognitive behavioural therapy. Patients attend on an out-patient basis and keep a diary of their food intake, episodes of vomiting, and use of abnormal weight-control mechanisms. The patient attempts to identify and master environmental stimuli that precipitate the binge eating. Treatment of coexisting depressive illness may be needed, and the specific serotonin re-uptake inhibitors (SSRIs), as well as being effective antidepressants and safe in the elderly, are considered to have an anti-bulimic action (Tiller *et al.* 1993).

In the early stages of the disorder, anorexia and bulimia nervosa run a fluctuating course with exacerbations and periods of partial remission. Long-term outcome studies of younger patients have found that many patients die either as a direct result of the disorder or from suicide. Theander (1985) found 18 per cent had died in a long-term follow-up study of primarily younger patients. As the rate for completed suicide increases with advancing age, the elderly eating-disorder patient may be a particular risk in this respect.

Late age of onset has been considered a poor prognostic feature (Morgan and Russell 1975; Hsu *et al.* 1979), although 'late onset' in most follow-up studies to date refers to onset in the twenties and thirties. The length of illness at presentation is the best-established predictive factor of outcome, with chronic, intractable cases having the poorest prognosis. These patients have formed an anorectic identity and are either treatment failures or else have never sought or received treatment. It may be that the prognosis for elderly chronic cases is better than for their younger counterparts. When they were young, bulimia had yet to be described and there were no specialist psychiatric services available for these conditions. Also, they are a survivor population, and so may have had a less severe illness with less life-threatening behaviours such as ingestion of dangerously large amounts of laxatives as a weight-control mechanism.

CONCLUSIONS

The developing awareness by professionals of eating disorders in older patients should allow for greater recognition and successful treatment. Establishing the existence of larger numbers of older patients with anorexia and bulimia nervosa will enable further investigation of the characteristics of eating disorders in this age group. They may differ from eating disorders in younger people in important and theoretically interesting ways. It may also be that late-onset cases of anorexia and bulimia nervosa differ from chronic and recurrent cases in old age, and this distinction needs to be recognized. The likely increase in rates of eating disorders in the elderly population in the future means that psychogeriatric services need to be alert and prepared for this.

REFERENCES

American Psychiatric Association (1987). *Diagnostic and statistical manual of mental disorders* (3rd edn, revised). American Psychiatric Association, Washington.

Berkman, J. M. (1930). Anorexia nervosa, anorexia, inanition and low metabolic rate. *American Journal of Medical Science*, **180**, 411.

Bernstein, I. (1972). Anorexia nervosa. 94 year old woman treated with electroshock treatment. *Minnesota Medicine*, **55**, 552–3.

Carrier, J. (1939). *L'anorexie mentale—trouble instictivo-affectif.* Thèse, Lyon.

Cosford, P., and Arnold, E. (1991) Anorexia nervosa in the elderly. *British Journal of Psychiatry*, **158**, 286.

Cosford, P., and Arnold, E. (1992). Eating disorders in late life: a review. *International Journal of Geriatric Psychiatry*, **7**, 491–8.

Crisp, A. H. (1980). *Anorexia nervosa: let me be*, pp. 42–74. Academic Press, London.

Dally, P., and Gomez, J. (1979). *Anorexia nervosa*, William Heinemann Medical Books, London. pp. 152–157.

Feighner, J. P., Robins, E., Guze, S. B., Woodraff, R. A., Winokur, G., and Munoz, R. (1972). Diagnostic criteria for use in psychiatric research. *Archives of General Psychiatry*, **26**, 57–63.

Garfinkel, P. E., and Garner, D. M. (1982). *Anorexia nervosa: a multi-dimensional perspective.* Brunner/Mazel, New York.

Goodall, E., Trenchard, E., and Silverstone, T. (1987). Receptor-blocking drugs and amphetamine anorexia in human subjects. *Psychopharmacology*, **97**, 484–90.

Gowers, S. G., and Crisp, A. H. (1990). Anorexia nervosa in an 80 year old woman. *British Journal of Psychiatry*, **157**, 754–7.

Holden, N. L. (1990). Is anorexia nervosa an obsessive compulsive disorder? *British Journal of Psychiatry*, **157**, 1–5.

Holland, A. J., Hall, A., Murray, R., Russell, G. F. M., and Crisp, A. H. (1984). Anorexia nervosa: a study of 34 twin pairs and one set of triplets. *British Journal of Psychiatry*, **145**, 414.

Hsu, L. K. G., and Zimmer, N. (1988). Eating disorders in old age. *International Journal of Eating Disorders*, **7**, 133–8.

Hsu, L. K. G., Crisp, A. H., and Harding, B. (1979). Outcome of anorexia nervosa. *Lancet*, **i**, 61–5.

Jonas, J. M., Pope, H. G., Hudson, J. I., and Satlin, A. (1984). Undiagnosed vomiting in an older woman: unsuspected bulimia. *American Journal of Psychiatry*, **141**, 7.

Kellett, J., Trimble, M., and Thorley, A. (1976). Anorexia nervosa after the menopause. *British Journal of Psychiatry*, **128**, 555–8.

King, A. (1963). Primary and secondary anorexia nervosa. *British Journal of Psychiatry*, **109**, 470–9.

Launer, M. A. (1978). Anorexia nervosa in late life. *British Journal of Medical Psychology*, **51**, 375–7.

Lindesay, J. (1991). Phobic disorders in the elderly. *British Journal of Psychiatry*, **159**, 531–41.

Morgan, H. G., and Russell, G. F. M. (1975). Value of family background and clinical features as predictors of long term outcome in anorexia nervosa. *Psychological Medicine*, **5**, 355–71.

Nagaratnam, N., and Ghougassian, D. F. (1988). Anorexia nervosa in a 70 year old man. *British Medical Journal*, **296**, 1443–4.

Palla, B., and Little, I. F. (1988). Medical complications of eating disorders in adolescents. *Pediatrics*, **81**, 613–23.

Price, W. A., Giannini, A. J., and Colella, J. (1985). Anorexia nervosa in the elderly. *Journal American Geriatrics Society*, **33**, 3.

Ramell, M. D., and Brown, N. (1988). Anorexia nervosa in a 67 year old woman. *Postgraduate Medical Journal*, **64**, 48–9.

Ratnasuriya, R. H., Eisler, I. Szmukler, G. I., and Russell, G. F. M. (1991). Anorexia nervosa: outcome and prognostic factors after 20 years. *British Journal of Psychiatry*, **158**, 495–502.

Rodin, T., Silberstein, L., and Striegel-Moore, R. (1984). Women in weight: a normative discontent. In *Psychology and gender: Nebraska Symposium on Motivation* (ed. T. B. Soderegger). University of Nebraska Press, Lincoln.

Russell, G. F. M. (1979). Bulimia nervosa: an ominous variant of anorexia nervosa. *Psychological Medicine*, **9**, 429.

Ryle, J. A. (1936). Anorexia nervosa. *Lancet*, **ii**, 893–9.

Theander, S. (1970) Anorexia nervosa. A psychiatric investigation of 94 female patients. *Acta Psychiatrica Scandinavica*, Supp. 214.

Theander, S. (1985). Outcome and prognosis in anorexia nervosa and bulimia: some results of previous investigations, compared with those of a long term Swedish study. *Journal of Psychiatric Research*, **19**, 493–508.

Tiller, J., Schmidt, U., and Treasure, J. (1993). Treatment of bulimia nervosa. *International Review of Psychiatry*, **5**, 75–86.

Treasure J., and Tiller, J. (1993). The aetiology of eating disorders—its biological basis. *International Review of Psychiatry*, **5**, 23–32.

World Health Organization (1992). *International classification of diseases* (10th revision). World Health Organization, Geneva.

12

Sex and its disorders
JOHN KELLETT

INTRODUCTION

In 1988 the expectation of life at birth was 73.0 years for a man, and 78.5 years for a woman. At the age of 60 years, the expectation was that men would survive a further 17.2 years and women a further 21.4 years (Office of Population Censuses and Surveys 1994). Clearly, there is a long time during which coitus is not for procreation, and this should remind us that its most important function in *Homo sapiens* may be to reinforce the bond between the couple by means of intimate grooming, and by the imprinting of orgasm which causes the physical characteristics of the partner to become associated with erotic stimulation and affection. The marital bond becomes increasingly vulnerable as its child-rearing function is lost and the need for partners to care for each other arises. Morris *et al.* (1988) have shown that husbands are better at caring for dependent wives if the sexual bond remains. The emphasis on the grooming and bonding functions of sexual behaviour can help us to understand the changes that occur with ageing, so that a loss of genital function is not perceived as a catastrophe but as an invitation to increase manual and oral contact, thus extending and even increasing the pleasures of intimacy.

SEXUAL ACTIVITY IN OLD AGE

We are dependent upon cross-sectional surveys for most of our information on this subject, where it is assumed that differences between age groups are due to age rather than life experience. As sexual behaviour in old age is peculiarly susceptible to cultural influences, this assumption is unlikely to be justified. The first cross-sectional surveys of the sexual behaviour of men and women were carried out by Kinsey and his colleagues (Kinsey *et al.* 1948, 1953) shortly after the Second World War. Although they had large samples of the young (2866 males and 1211 females aged 21–25 years), the samples of those aged 60 years and older were much smaller: only 87 White and 39 Black males, and 56 females. Their finding that three-quarters of males aged eighty years were impotent was based on a sample of four.

Table 12.1. Sexual activity in men by age and marital status (Kinsey *et al.* 1948).

	21–25 years				41–45 years				56–60 years	
	Single 1535		Married 751		Single 56		Married 272		Married 67	
N	%	x	%	x	%	x	%	x	%	x
Total outlets to orgasm	99	(2.7)	100	(3.9)	96	(1.9)	100	(2.0)	99	(1.1)
Masturbation	81	(1.4)	48	(0.5)	61	(1.0)	33	(0.3)	19	(0.2)
Total intercourse	61	(1.2)	100	(3.5)	66	(1.1)	99	(1.9)	97	(1.1)
Marital intercourse	—		100	(3.2)	—		99	(1.6)	94	(0.9)
Intercourse with prostitutes	29	(0.4)	13	(0.2)	39	(0.5)	9	(0.2)	8	(0.3)
Non-marital intercourse (excluding prostitutes)	59	(1.3)	24	(1.3)	52	(0.8)	24	(0.5)	22	(0.7)
Homosexual outlets to orgasm	15	(1.1)	8	(0.4)	38	(1.2)	2	(0.8)	—	
Nocturnal emissions	81	(0.4)	59	(0.2)	48	(0.2)	54	(0.2)	28	(0.1)

N = Sample size
% = percentage of those reporting activity; x = mean number of outlets per week for the active population.

According to Kinsey *et al.* (1948), there is a decline in the activity of men in all sexual outlets except intercourse with prostitutes and other non-marital partners (Table 12.1). Table 12.2 shows a similar decline in women (Kinsey *et al.* 1953), in whom an increase in masturbation is responsible for 14 per cent of orgasms in the twenties and 26 per cent in those aged 51–55 years. Unlike single men, single women were markedly less active than their married sisters. Total outlets give a clearer picture (Table 12.3), and in case the reader is puzzled by the disparity between men and women, this is largely accounted for by higher rates of male masturbation and homosexuality.

As a rule, more information can be obtained by sampling over a smaller age range. Hallstrom (1977) sampled 800 women from Gothenburg in the four age strata 38, 46, 50, and 54 years. He noted an age-related decline in sexual interest and activity but this was not significant when the effect of the menopause was controlled, suggesting that this was the crucial influence. The observed decline was much greater in the lower social classes, and Hallstrom agrees with Masters and Johnson (1966) that 'the psyche plays a part at least equal to, if not greater than that of an unbalanced endocrine system in determining the sex drive of women during the post-menopausal period of their lives'. Cutler *et al.* (1987) also found a decline in sexual activity in perimenopausal women with the lowest levels of oestrogen. However, Riley (1991), in a comprehensive review of the subject, states that 'reduced levels of vaginal lubrication and hence dyspareunia are the only features . . . that have been confirmed to be associated with decreased oestrogen levels'.

Persson (1980) studied a random sample of 166 men and 226 women aged 70 years resident in Gothenburg, and compared the characteristics of married subjects (66 men (52 per cent) and 33 women (32 per cent)) who had had intercourse in the preceding three months with the characteristics of those who had not had intercourse. Not surprisingly, the sexually active of both sexes were more likely to approve of sexual activity in old age, and the active older women were more likely to have had premarital sex and to have enjoyed intercourse. Physical health did not relate to activity except worsening of symptoms in women, though poorer mental health was found in those who were inactive. Women with younger husbands were more sexually active, which supports the view of Pfeiffer and Davis (1972) that activity is usually governed by the male—alternatively, more sexually active women may select younger male partners! Pfeiffer *et al.* (1968) had earlier sought factors related to continued sexual activity in a non-random longitudinal study. In men, age was by far the most important factor, though enjoyment and interest were increased in those with higher incomes, higher social class, and better physical health. The findings were similar for women, though higher education took the place of social class. Reduction in frequency of intercourse is not the only measure of sexuality; Weizman and Hart (1987) found that healthy married men in Israel aged 66–71 years had intercourse less often but masturbated more often than those aged 60–65 years.

Obviously, cross-sectional studies do not have the strength of longitudinal

Table 12.2. Sexual activity in women by age and marital status (Kinsey *et al.* 1953).

	21–25 years				41–45 years				56–60 years			
	Single 2810		Married 1654		Single 179		Married 497		Single 27		Married 49	
N	%	n	%	n	%	n	%	n	%	n	%	n
Total outlets to orgasm	60	(1.1)	88	(2.8)	68	(1.6)	93	(2.0)	44	(0.9)	82	(0.8)
Masturbation	35	(0.9)	27	(0.6)	50	(1.0)	36	(0.6)	35	(0.2)	—	
Marital intercourse (with or without orgasm)	—		99	(3.0)	—		94	(1.8)	—		80	(1.3)
Homosexual outlets to orgasm	5	(1.0)	1	(0.9)	—		—		—		—	
Dreams to orgasm	11	(0.2)	15	(0.2)	18	(0.1)	31	(0.1)	—		29	(0.2)

N = sample size
% = percentage of those reporting activity; n = mean number per week of those active.

Table 12.3. Outlets per week by age and sex (Kinsey *et al.* 1948, 1953).

Age	Sex	N	%	Mean
16–20	Male	3750	99	2.9
	Female	5649	50	1.1
41–45	Male	440	99	2.0
	Female	810	87	1.9
61–65	Male	58	81	1.0
	Female	53	47	0.5
71–75	Male	12	42	0.3
	Female	10	30	0.3

N = Sample size
% = Percentage active
Mean = mean of those active.

ones in determining the effect of ageing on sexual interest and activity. The first longitudinal study of sexual behaviour in older adults, carried out over six years at Duke University (Pfeiffer *et al.* 1968), showed that despite strong correlations of decline with age, 14 per cent showed an increase in sexual interest and intercourse. The median age for stopping intercourse was 68 years for men and 60 years for women, usually initiated by the male. Hallstrom followed up his sample for six years (Hallstrom and Samuelsson 1990). Two-thirds reported no change in desire. Loss of desire was associated with deterioration in relationships, and an increase with resolution of these problems. Social class had no effect.

Though every cross-sectional and longitudinal study shows a decline in sexual activity with age, a second longitudinal study from Duke University by George and Weiler (1981) indicated that the effect of ageing was only a quarter of that expected from the cross-sectional data of the males, and one-seventh that expected from the females. This implies that cross-sectional studies have been exaggerating the effects of ageing by attributing the different activity of different generations to age rather than upbringing.

This conclusion is reinforced by the study of Bretschneider and McCoy (1988) who surveyed the sexual activity of residents in retirement facilities in California. Subjects were selected for good physical health, but were aged 80 to 102 years. The sample of 100 men and 102 women, who had volunteered out of 600 possible respondents, reported frequent sexual activity. The rates for males were twice those for females, which probably reflects the sex ratio in the homes of one man to six women. Overall, 88 per cent of men and 71 per cent of women stated that they had sexual fantasies, whilst 70 per cent and 30 per cent still had intercourse at least once in the previous year.

Inevitably, in studies of a sensitive topic such as sex, there are concerns about the reliability of the data. All of these studies are based on interviews or questionnaires, and depend upon the honesty of the informant. One might predict that men would exaggerate and women minimize their ratings. However, Pfeiffer's survey (Pfeiffer *et al.* 1968) included 54 paired ratings from 31 couples where the data had been obtained from separate interviews. There was a correlation of 0.87 between the reported frequency of sexual intercourse (5 categories) of husbands and wives. Where there were differences, in eight cases it was the husband and in three the wife who reported higher activity. Bearing in mind that some discrepancy might have been due to extramarital liaisons, the level of agreement is reassuring. Similarly, Kinsey *et al.* (1948, 1953) found high rates of inter-rater and re-interview reliability in their surveys.

Bald statistics of the frequency of sexual acts tell us relatively little about the quality and intensity of sexual union in elderly people. For information about this, the reader is referred to Brecher (1988), a fascinating 'Hite report' for the elderly.

CLASSIFICATION OF SEXUAL DYSFUNCTIONS

Table 12.4 lists the sexual dysfunctions recognized by modern psychiatric nosologies such as DSM-IV (*Diagnostic and statistical manual of mental disorders*, fourth edition) and ICD-10 (*International classification of diseases*, tenth revision) which are likely to be encountered in the elderly population. They are far from being discrete and independent entities; for example, a low libido can lead to erectile failure, and repeated anorgasmia through premature ejaculation by her partner can cause a woman to lose her libido, though this may be specific to the partner. Each sexual dysfunction has both organic and psychological causes, and all can be made worse by performance anxiety. Often the attempt to separate the organic from the psychological leads to a false dichotomy (Kellett 1990; Gregoire 1990), especially in the elderly where organic causes almost always play some part in the problem. In any condition, however, it is important to establish whether it is a primary or secondary dysfunction, and whether it is general or situational: at one extreme, the venous leak syndrome will prevent any full erection from infancy, whereas at the other, erectile failure due to an argument will be limited to that partner at that time.

SEXUAL DYSFUNCTION IN THE ELDERLY

Some decline in erectile potency with age ultimately affects the majority of the male population, but this is not necessarily classifiable as 'sexual dysfunction'. Dysfunction, like disease, is defined by the patient whose expectations are not fulfilled. A loss of interest by both partners which coincides with a loss

Table 12.4. ICD-10 and DSM-IV classifications of sexual disorders.

ICD-10	DSM-IV
F52: *Sexual disorders not caused by organic disorder or disease*	*Sexual dysfunctions*
	Sexual desire disorders
F52.0: Lack or loss of sexual desire	302.71: Hypoactive sexual desire disorder
F52.1: Sexual aversion and lack of sexual enjoyment	302.79: Sexual aversion disorder
	Sexual arousal disorders
F52.2: Failure of genital response	302.72: Female sexual arousal disorder
F52.3: Orgasmic dysfunction	302.72: Male erectile disorder
F52.4: Premature ejaculation	Orgasm disorders
F52.5: Non-organic vaginismus	302.73: Female orgasmic disorder
F52.6: Non-organic dyspareunia	302.74: Male orgasmic disorder
F52.7: Excessive sexual drive	302.75: Premature ejaculation
	Sexual pain disorders
	302.76: Dyspareunia
	306.51: Vaginismus
F64: *Gender identity disorders*	*Gender identity disorders*
F64.0: Transsexualism	302.85: Gender identity disorder in adolescents/adults
F64.1: Dual-role transvestism	
F65: *Disorders of sexual preference*	*Paraphilias*
F65.0: Fetishism	302.40: Exhibitionism
F65.1: Fetishistic transvestism	302.81: Fetishism
F65.2: Exhibitionism	302.85: Frotteurism
F65.3: Voyeurism	302.20: Paedophilia
F65.4: Paedophilia	302.83: Sexual sadism
F65.5: Sadomasochism	302.84: Voyeurism
F65.6: Multiple disorders of sexual preference	302.30: Transvestic fetishism
F66: *Psychological and behavioural disorders associated with sexual development and orientation*	
F66.0: Sexual maturation disorder	
F66.1: Egodystonic sexual orientation	
F66.2: Sexual relationship disorder	

of erections will lead to cessation of coitus without distress. Sexual dysfunction in the elderly can therefore be caused as much by unrealistic expectations as by a decline in function. Osborn *et al.* (1988) surveyed 600 women aged between 35 and 59 years, stratified into five-year age bands. Half of those aged 50–59 years had operationally defined sexual problems (compared to only 14 per cent aged

35–39 years), but only 21 per cent complained of it. However, the discrepancy between having and recognizing a problem was related to age, with only just over one-fifth of those with objective problems making a complaint.

Case 1

An 80-year-old widower, admitted to a residential home, found himself surrounded by female residents and care assistants after ten years of social isolation. He presented complaining of erectile difficulties, but after reassurance and yohimbine his confidence was restored.

Physical changes

These have been detailed by Masters and Johnson (1966), who, as part of their large investigation of human sexual response, studied 34 female volunteers aged 51–80 years and 39 males aged 51–90 years. A summary of their findings is given in Tables 12.5 and 12.6. In both sexes there were a few exceptions to the general picture of reduction and loss of function, who maintained regular and frequent

Table 12.5. Changes in sexual response with age in the male (Masters and Johnson 1966).

Retained but reduced

Excitement phase

    Penile erection (often only complete at orgasm)

Plateau phase

    Nipple erection
    Testicular elevation

Orgasmic phase

    Ejaculatory power
    Rectal and ejaculatory contractions

Lost

Plateau phase

    Sexual flush
    Re-erection
    Scrotal vasocongestion

Orgasmic phase

    Ejaculatory inevitability
    Prostatic contractions

Table 12.6. Changes in sexual response with age in the female (Masters and Johnson 1966).

Retained

Excitement phase

  Nipple erection
  Clitoral tumescence (delayed if no direct stimulation)

Plateau phase

  Clitoral retraction

Retained but reduced

Excitement phase

  Vasocongestion of labia minora
  Vaginal lubrication
  Expansion of inner two-thirds of vagina
    (moves from excitement to plateau phase)
  Uterine elevation

Plateau phase

  Engorgement of areola
  Secretion from Bartholin's glands
  Orgasmic platform

Orgasmic phase

  Rectal and orgasmic contractions

Lost

Excitement phase

  Breast engorgement
  Sexual flush
  Swelling of labia majora

---

sexual contact, and whose psychological reactions were also closer to younger age groups.

The cause of this decline in the physical aspects of the sexual response is unknown. There is a gradual reduction in levels of free testosterone with age in males, but Davidson *et al.* (1983) found that it only accounted for 4 per cent of the variance in sexual activity to orgasm, while age accounted for 12 per cent. It has been suggested that despite normal levels of testosterone, ageing causes a loss of receptor sensitivity, from which one would predict that increasing levels above normal would restore function (Riley, personal communication). Weizman *et al.* (1983) have proposed a rise in prolactin as the cause of decreased sexual desire in men. In their sample of 28 men aged 60–64 years and 44 aged 65–70 years, they found a significant negative correlation with frequency of sexual intercourse, but the effect on libido was only apparent in the older cohort. Though 27 had erectile failure, there was only a trend for prolactin to be higher in this group. As prolactin levels are increased by stress, it could be argued that it is the primary stressors that are more important in impairing sexual response.

Penile engorgement requires a quadrupling of blood supply, and is dependent on a lack of atheromatous narrowing of the pudendal arteries. This increased flow is initiated by the parasympathetic nervous system, the activity of which is known to decline with age (O'Brien *et al.* 1986). The rigidity of the collagenous sacs may also decline with age, leading to loss of rigidity in the engorged penis. Though erectile failure at any age may represent true malfunction, it is noteworthy that the variation in frequency of intercourse in sexually active men fits a curve of normal distribution (Vallery Masson *et al.* 1981), which implies that the causes of decline, if not loss, are multifactorial.

Most of the above refers to male function. Though there are changes in the female, these would seem to be more the result than the cause of abstinence. Clearly, the dramatic fall in levels of oestrogen at the menopause does not stop activity, and hormone replacement therapy keeps the genitalia healthy without having much effect on libido. Sherwin and Gelford (1987) have shown that testosterone restores sexual drive to normal levels after oophorectomy, but its role in the natural menopause is unclear (Dow *et al.* 1983).

Medical factors

Chronic physical illness and disability tend to suppress libido, but they may encourage sexual activity in some cases by promoting dependency and intimacy. Most of the epidemiological studies, except that of Pfeiffer *et al.* (1968), show little effect of illness on sexual activity. Nevertheless, if the disease does not affect sexuality, the treatment may. Some opiate drugs such as coproxamol so saturate the endorphin receptors that orgasmic endorphins have little effect. Other psychotropic drugs like the benzodiazepines cause a dose-related reduction in sexual arousal (Riley and Riley 1986). Taylor Segraves (1989) has recently reviewed the mechanisms by which neuroleptics and antidepressants affect sexual function. Dopamine is probably the essential intermediary neurotransmitter between testosterone and libido (Hyppa *et al.* 1970), and libido is suppressed by dopamine-blocking drugs, such as the neuroleptics. Drugs that increase serotonergic neurotransmission, such as the new class of selective serotonin re-uptake inhibitor (SSRI) antidepressants, decrease libido, although in practice this effect needs to be weighed against the impact of depression on sexual interest and activity (see p. 217). Other peripherally acting drugs, such as thiazides and beta blockers, can inhibit engorgement, whilst some like clonidine, clomipramine, and phenelzine inhibit orgasm. Clearly, drugs that counter testosterone reduce libido in men; examples include progestogens, cyproterone acetate, and luteinizing hormone releasing

Table 12.7. Physical examination of the male with erectile failure.

Pulse and blood pressure testing for sinus arrhythmia, and pulse on Valsalva manouvre
Signs of general disease:
  Clubbing
  Pallor
  Dyspnoea
  Lymphadenopathy
  Hepatosplenomegaly, etc.
Peripheral pulses in the legs
Limitation of straight-leg raising
Spinal tenderness
Tendon reflexes in legs
Appearance of external genitalia, constistency and size of testes and other scrotal masses
Sensation of light touch and pinprick over feet and genitalia
Fundoscopy
Urine or blood test for glucose

hormone (LHRH) analogues like goserelin (whose effect may be increased by antagonism to the libido-enhancing qualities of LHRH itself). Though this may be seen as a relatively short list of drugs affecting sexual function, they are are very widely used; for example, Morgan *et al.* (1988) found that 16 per cent of those over 65 years were taking benzodiazepine hypnotics, and Cartwright and Smith (1988) found that 40 per cent of those over 80 years were on diuretics.

Diabetes mellitus is common in the elderly and can present with almost any sexual dysfunction, though erectile failure is the commonest (Fairburn *et al.* 1982). Sexual dysfunction precedes as well as follows myocardial infarction, though the cause for the former is unknown (Kellett 1987). Some of the latter results from a misinterpretation of the breathlessness of orgasm as a strain on the heart, rather than a physiological over-breathing. In practice, once the patient can climb a flight of stairs he or she can resume coitus.

Neurological disease can affect sexuality in several ways. Any form of paralysis or paresis makes coitus difficult. Spinal and neuropathic disorders affect neural control over the physical processes of arousal and orgasm. The parasympathetic outflow is at S2, at which level orgasm is sensed. Ejaculation is caused by the sympathetic outflow at L2. A lesion above L2 will allow reflex responses without sensation, whilst lower lesions affect erections. Cortical dementias may cause a loss of libido associated with a reduction in LHRH (Oram *et al.* 1981; Zeiss *et al.* 1990). Individuals with subcortical dementia retain their libido, but coarsened behaviour and impaired judgement may lead to deviant and problematic sexual activity. Poorly controlled temporal-lobe epilepsy is also a cause of lower libido

(Spark *et al.* 1984), though it is not inevitable with other forms of epilepsy (Jensen *et al.* 1990).

Other diseases associated with sexual dysfunction include myxoedema, sickle-cell disease, hypertension, neurofibromatosis, and motor-neurone disease.

Surgical factors

Many diseases that lead to surgery are likely to cause sexual dysfunction if not so treated. Examples include spinal-cord compression, rectal carcinoma, and ulcerative colitis. Sometimes, trauma from the surgery itself can be the final straw. The parasympathetic plexus supplying the penis is closely related to the rectum and the prostate, so that operations on either can damage these nerves. Major surgery inevitably has effects on the body image, but the effects on sexual function may have been exaggerated. The high incidence of dysfunction after total mastectomy was blamed on this, but, when this operation was compared to lumpectomy, loss of sexual interest was complained of by 28 per cent of the mastectomy group and 32 per cent of the lumpectomy (Fallowfield *et al.* 1990). The authors concluded that fear of cancer is the predominant factor causing loss of desire.

Surgery requires admission to hospital, which may separate a couple for the first time. The return home, often with stitches in place and a scar, leaves the couple in doubt if and when to resume coitus, particularly if dressings, a catheter, or an ileostomy bag directly interfere with intercourse. These doubts will be reinforced if the issue is not addressed; silence from the surgeon and nurses about sexual contact will convey the message that further sexual activity is unmentionable and beyond the pale.

Case 2

A 60-year-old woman who had had a lumpectomy and radiotherapy for breast cancer, and who was being treated with tamoxifen, complained of loss of libido from dyspareunia. Treatment with vaginal oestrogen suppositories resolved the problem without compromising the effect of the anti-oestrogen.

Gynaecological factors

Perhaps because gynaecology is usually combined with obstetrics, there is a tendency for this specialty to regard female genitalia as a device for childbirth rather than a source of erotic pleasure. The loss of oestrogen secretion at the menopause leads to a reduction and delay of vaginal lubrication and thinning of the mucosa, leading to cystitis. The oestrogen-deficient vagina is also more prone to infection. As a result, older women can find intercourse painful, but this can be eased by artificial lubricants, prolonged petting, and hormone replacement.

Obesity, and weakness of the muscles of the pelvic floor can lead to prolapse of the bladder into the anterior wall of the vagina, leading to discomfort on coitus and stress incontinence. Though surgical repair is usually through the vagina, sexual function is usually not affected, provided the couple are advised when to resume coitus. Rectal prolapse repair is more likely to lead to narrowing of the vagina (Francis and Jeffcoate 1966), though subsequent problems are rare.

More serious conditions like cancer may present with sexual dysfunction. Anderson *et al.* (1986) found that 75 per cent of patients had developed sexual problems *before* the diagnosis was made, even though they were no different from the normal population before the onset of symptom. The emphasis on feminine beauty makes a woman more vulnerable to these physical insults than her partner. Clearly, the imperative with cancer therapy is to save life, but awareness of the sexual function of the patient's genitalia by her therapists can soften the blow.

Psychiatric factors

The major functional psychoses almost invariably cause sexual dysfunction—depression through loss of libido and mania through its excess. Schizophrenia usually leads to a loss of libido, which is contributed to by the libido-blocking effect of the major tranquillizers. Schizophreniform states in old age, such as paraphrenia, are often dominated by sexual delusions, which can seem particularly bizarre when expressed by a lifelong virgin. There is no apparent reason for this, unless one believes the popular notion that preoccupation with the sexual activity of others is a universal human trait. Morbid jealousy also occurs in paraphrenia, though in the elderly it more commonly heralds the onset of dementia.

Case 3

A couple in their seventies were referred when the wife attacked her husband, who was dying of respiratory failure. She was convinced that he was having an affair with a stewardess they had met on a recent flight to Ireland. After she was compulsorily admitted to hospital her husband died, and it was her lack of remorse which revealed her dementia.

Neurotic disorders are not usually associated with sexual difficulties, but individuals with high levels of neuroticism are likely to develop performance anxiety with the onset of declining function due to ageing. The male may respond by trying to insert his penis as soon as it is erect at a time when his partner is far from aroused. The lack of lubrication causes either a failure of penetration, or premature ejaculation in him and dyspareunia and anorgasmia in her. A programme of 'senate focus' (see p. 221) can benefit most patients but should not be regarded as proof that the disorder was psychogenic.

Over- or underweight, often used by younger women to avoid sexual encounters, can reduce libido through a reduction in the levels of LHRH. As a result, patients recovering from depression may take time to recover their libido as their weight returns to normal. Furthermore, most antidepressants reduce sexual function, the newer SSRIs being particularly prone to cause anorgasmia.

Most drugs of addiction reduce sexual function. However, the disinhibiting effect of alcohol may lead the older individual to abuse others. For example, a 60-year-old builder began to make obscene telephone calls when his drinking had deterred his partner from any intimacy.

Cultural factors

Though the anxiety aroused by powerful adolescent sexuality is absent in the elderly, the individual is more subject to social pressures and conflicts because the biological drive to consummate the relationship is weaker. For example, financial considerations may discourage the widow from formalizing her new relationship, yet extramarital sex may incur the wrath of her virtuous children. The growth of sexual imagery in the media is confined to the young, especially women. Older models are dressed in sensible tweeds rather than lingerie or diaphanous ball dresses, whilst naked elderly people are only portrayed as objects of deformity. Though the cessation of coitus is determined by the male, the proceptive sexuality of youth merges into the receptive profile of the female, so that any reluctance of either partner is less likely to be overridden.

The relative lack of attention given in western culture to sex in old age is not typical of the world as a whole. Winn and Newton (1982) looked at such attitudes in 106 traditional societies. They conclude that 'although some decline in the sexual activity of aged males is recorded in a significant proportion of the societies studied, many cultural groups have expectations for continued sexual activity for older men that imply little, if any, loss of their sexual powers until very late in life'. Regarding women, they state: 'Older women frequently express strong sexual desires and interests . . . engage in sexual activity in many instances until extreme old age . . . and may form liaisons with much younger men.'

Cultures which delay marriage often have an age difference of over twenty years between man and wife. The man is under pressure to perform at a time when the sexuality of his spouse is at its height. His death then leaves her bereft of a partner, and this is made worse if she is Muslim by the prohibition on seeking advice from a male doctor.

Case 4

A sixty-year-old Kurdish chief exiled to London sought help when his declining potency failed to satisfy his harem. Confronted with a young female therapist he began to undress, and was quickly ushered out of the hospital by the horrified counsellor. When subsequently seen by a male therapist, he was a most cooperative and pleasant patient.

Institutions

Though only 2.5 per cent of people of pensionable age are in residential homes (Age Concern 1990), this rises to a much higher proportion of those aged over 80 years. Nevertheless, the vast majority of the elderly live in their own homes. Those who enter institutions are too frail to care for themselves, either from dementia, arthritis, or other physical frailty. Not surprisingly, therefore, these homes are not designed to facilitate sexual contact, and sexual behaviour by residents can arouse considerable anxiety. Most surveys show that staff are in fact quite liberal in their attitudes. Damrosch (1984) gave qualified nurses enrolled in a graduate nursing course case vignettes of a 68-year-old woman which differed in one respect: half the vignettes mentioned that she was sexually active, and this client was preferred in all the ten ratings except popularity with the staff. Earlier, Kaas (1978) tested the attitudes to sexuality of 85 nursing-home residents and 207 nursing staff. The staff were more liberal than the residents, except in their agreement with the statement 'Most people over 55 masturbate some of the time.' The statement 'Sexually active elderly are dirty old men and women' provoked definite disagreement from the staff, but residents were nearer neutrality. Statements about sex in the young also elicited more liberal views from the staff, which suggests that these differences are generational. Szasz (1983) gave all grades of nursing staff working in a long-stay unit for elderly men the task of citing two sorts of behaviour that would cause a problem, and one sort that should be encouraged. Most staff were not concerned with sexual behaviour of a patient in private, but not surprisingly they found it difficult to cope with overt sexual approaches.

Most institutions do not provide a place of safety and privacy to enjoy intimacy, either through a lack of individual rooms, or because staff walk into rooms without knocking and waiting for permission to enter. However, there is a narrow line between respecting personal choice, and encouraging sexual exploitation of confused residents. By allowing a relationship to develop, staff can incur the anger of relatives who fear the loss of their inheritance, and resent the implied insult to the other parent. As a result, the success of such relationships depends more often on the attitudes and interventions of others than on the couple themselves. Residents are aware that their ability to remain in the home depends on staff approval.

Homes should provide double rooms, but allow an estranged couple to occupy single ones. Many homes do have such facilities, in marked contrast to long-stay hospital wards, which may still segregate the sexes. The married visitors' flat can expose the resident to ridicule. A policy of liberal leave may be the best way of allowing a couple to continue private coital contact.

MANAGEMENT

Assessment

The first essential of effective management is to establish the nature of the complaint, which is often complicated by both the embarrassment of the patient and their unfamiliarity with sexual jargon. I once spent some time designing a treatment programme for anorgasmia for an elderly Asian gentleman complaining of 'no emission', only to discover that he meant he could not obtain an erection. A full history is essential and should include details about the onset of the condition, its variability, and its relation to circumstances (organic dysfunctions are improved by higher eroticism, unlike most psychogenic ones, causing most organic cases to attribute their problem to the psyche). The sexual history should include information about the length of petting, the effect and fantasies of masturbation, the ages of physical maturation, first date and first coitus, and a list of partners including current ones who may be unknown to the accompanying spouse (an important reason for interviewing each partner on their own, which also gives them the opportunity to describe their true feelings for each other). One must also obtain a detailed medical history, and, if one is likely to be using psychotherapy, information about family and career. A thorough history may take over an hour to compile, but it enables reliable hypotheses to be made about psychogenic causes and also facilitates rapport. Examination includes noting the style of verbal and non-verbal communication of the couple (e.g. one can offer them a choice of chairs to see if they choose to sit close). The extent of the physical examination will obviously depend on the nature of the complaint. Thus a vaginal examination might be insensitive in a woman who developed secondary vaginismus after a rape, but might be offered in case she thought she had incurred physical damage. A male with erectile failure should have the checks itemised in Table 12.7. The intracavernosal papaverine test is used to distinguish between vascular insufficiency where there is little effect, and psychogenic or neurogenic insufficiency where there is. If the injections are too painful, 0.1 mg of phentolamine can be mixed with the papaverine to reduce its acidity and stinging after injection. The papaverine test should only be used if the patient can readily obtain an injection of metaraminol in the following six hours to counteract any priapism that may be induced.

Though there is little place for hormone assays in patients whose libido is well maintained, those with a complaint of lowered libido should have an assay of testosterone, sex-hormone-binding globulin or LH (luteinizing hormone), and prolactin.

Treatment

For a fuller coverage of the treatment of sexual disorders, the reader is referred to manuals such as those by Fairburn *et al.* (1983) and Hawton (1985). Physical remedies are summarized in Table 12.8. The squeeze technique is a method of

Table 12.8. Physical remedies for sexual dysfunctions.

Low libido	Testosterone
	Antidepressants:
	Trazodone
	Viloxazine
	Selegeline
	L-Dopa preparations
Premature ejaculation	Clomipramine
	Clonidine
	Squeeze and stop–start techniques
Erectile failure	Yohimbine
	Auto-intracavernosal injection:
	Papaverine
	Phentolamine
	Prostaglandin E
	Vacuum systems
	Surgical implant
Anorgasmia	Midodrine
Dyspareunia	Lubricants
	Oestrogen creams or tablets

delaying ejaculation by placing firm pressure across the shaft of the penis behind the glans. The 'stop–start' technique uses intermittent stimulation to prolong the erection, usually during masturbation. Vacuum systems employ rigid tubes into which the penis is sucked, and when engorged a band is slipped onto the base of the penis to maintain the erection. If a good erection can be achieved, at least briefly, a band can be slipped on the penis using a simple applicator such as the 'Asset' or 'Rapport'.

The psychological remedies used to treat sexual disorders are summarized in Table 12.9. For most couples, coital failure has led to a discomfort with all sexual contact. Sensate focus exercises are designed to reverse this. At first, a ban is placed on coitus and heavy petting, and the couple are taught to use caressing as a means of relaxation rather than for arousal. The timing, place, and order of type of massage are specified. The couple should avoid distraction, and to seek pleasure primarily for themselves. As relaxation is achieved, in further sessions the massage can become more intimate until finally coitus is allowed. This may throw up problems in communication which can be interpreted with the emphasis on each partner taking responsibility for their feelings. Sexual release by masturbation is allowed until coitus returns. The process works best where the couple are given the task of learning about each other, and a therapist who is seduced into interpretative psychotherapy can retard the process. The arousal circuit is based on a diagram of the brain and genitals to show how the two

Table 12.9. Psychological remedies for sexual dysfunctions.

Education:
  Anatomy
  Age norms
  The guided tour
  The arousal circuit
Sensate focus programme
The ladder concept
Communication patterns
Token systems
Vaginal trainers
Shaping by masturbation
Masturbation prior to penetration for anorgasmia

---

interact. The guided tour can be based on a real examination of the sex organs of each partner, or on a fantasy trip into each other's body.

Briefly, the ladder concept (Stanley 1981) is used to demonstrate how a couple can satisfy each other on different rungs of sexual arousal, without always having to have intercourse. A token system can be used to establish means by which a couple can learn to satisfy each other's needs in their social life together. Thus by bringing his wife tea in bed a husband may earn sufficient tokens for his wife to give him a cuddle before getting up. Vaginal trainers are phallic objects of different sizes which can be used to desensitize the woman to penetration. Masturbatory shaping can be used to reinforce bonding. Thus if the husband is no longer attracted by his wife he can use his most erotic fantasies to initiate masturbation, provided that ejaculation is associated with thoughts or pictures of his wife. Similarly a woman with low self-esteem can masturbate or arouse herself to reflections of herself in a mirror, and regain confidence in her body as an erotic stimulus. The man who ejaculates normally on masturbation but not inside his partner uses masturbation until at the point of ejaculation he inserts his penis. These tools of therapy need to be used flexibly so that a couple who enjoy intercourse but suffer anorgasmia do not necessarily have to go through the whole sensate focus programme.

After the death of a partner, the survivor may wish to remarry but find the process of finding a new partner more difficult than in their youth. They should be encouraged to exploit their interests in order to meet people, and the modern phenomenon of the dating agency is also worth exploring.

The simplicity and effectiveness of many of these techniques has led to a trial comparing treatment with a manual with that carried out by a live therapist, where both were found to be effective (Carney *et al.* 1978). A list of useful self-help books and manuals is given at the end of this chapter.

The boundaries of normal sexual behaviour are defined by society, so that treatment for deviance is often requested by society rather than by the patient. Those whose inclinations break the law find relief in the lower libido of ageing. Others who may have been distressed by their inclinations when young are reconciled to them when older. A few struggle through a form of marriage and welcome the chance to be themselves thereafter by being homosexual or transsexual. Counselling may be necessary to help the person overcome their guilt. Those that do present in old age are usually suffering from some brain damage which is removing their natural inhibitions. Sometimes confused behaviour can be wrongly interpreted as sexual, as, for example, when a demented old lady attempts to undress in public. Patients with Parkinson's disease are prone to a Lewy body dementia, and their dopaminergic treatment may stimulate the libido (Barbeau *et al.* 1969, Harvey 1988). The combination may result in inappropriate sexual behaviour, and such patients may have to be protected from the consequences of their actions.

CONCLUSION

Cyril Connolly in *The Unquiet Grave* (Connolly 1945) has written:

The particular charm of marriage is the duologue, the permanent conversation between two people who talk over everything and everyone till death breaks the record. It is this back-chat which, in the long run, makes a reciprocal equality more intoxicating than any form of servitude or domination.

Such intoxication can lose its power if sexual frustration heightens the tension between partners. The role of the doctor is to provide an ambience where the couple feel free to choose the mode of intimacy that suits them best, whether by vaginal penetration, mutual masturbation, or a face to greet in the morning when emerging from separate bedrooms. The absence of a confidante is a major risk factor for mental illness in old age (Murphy 1982), and there is no better confidante than the one with whom one has shared a bed.

REFERENCES

Age Concern (1990). *Older people in the United Kingdom. Some basic facts*. Age Concern, Mitcham.
Anderson, B., Lachenbruch, P., Andersen, B., and Deprosse, C. (1986). Sexual dysfunction and signs of gynaecologic cancer. *Cancer*, **57**, 1880–6.
Barbeau, L. Bancroft, J., and Mathews, A. (1969). L-Dopa therapy in Parkinson's disease: a critical review of nine years' experience. *Canadian Medical Association Journal*, **101**, 59–68.
Brecher, E. M. (1988). *Love, sex and ageing*. Little Brown, Boston.
Bretschneider, J. G., and McCoy, N. L. (1988). Sexual interest and behaviour in healthy 80 to 102 year olds. *Archives of Sexual Behaviour*, **17**, 109–29.

Carney, A., Bancroft, J., and Mathews, A. (1978). Combination of hormones and psychological treatment for female sexual unresponsiveness: a comparative study. *British Journal of Psychiatry*, **133**, 339–46.

Cartwright, A., and Smith, C. (1988). *Elderly people, their medicines, and their doctors*. Routledge, London.

Connolly C. (1945). *The Uniquiet Grave*. Hamish Hamilton, London.

Cutler, W. B., Garcia, C. R., and McCoy, N. (1987). Perimenopausal sexuality. *Archives of Sexual Behaviour*, **16**, 225–34

Damrosch, S. R. (1984). Graduate nursing students' attitudes toward sexually active older persons. *Gerontologist*, **24**, 299–302.

Davidson, J. M., Chen, J. J., Crapo, L., Gray, G. D, Greenleaf, W. J., and Catania, J. A. (1983). Hormonal changes and sexual function in ageing men. *Journal of Clinical Endocrinology*, **57**, 71–7.

Dow, M. G. T., Hart, D. M., and Forrest, C. A. (1983). Hormonal treatment of sexual unresponsiveness in postmenopausal women: a comparative study. *British Journal of Obstetrics and Gynaecology*, **90**, 361–66.

Fairburn, C. G., McCulluch, D. K., and Wu, F. C. W. (1982). The effects of diabetes on male sexual function. *Clinics of Endocrinology and Metabolism*, **11**, 749–68.

Fairburn, C. G., Dickerson, M. G., and Greenwood J. (1983). *Sexual problems and their management*. Churchill Livingstone, Chichester.

Fallowfield, L., Hall, A., Maguire, G., and Baum, M. (1990). Psychological outcomes of different treatment policies in women with early breast cancer outside a clinical trial. *British Medical Journal*, **301**, 575–80.

Francis, W., and Jeffcoate, T. (1966). Dyspareunia following vaginal operations. *Journal of Obstetrics and Gynaecology of the British Commonwealth*, **68**, 1–10.

George, L. K., and Weiler, S. J. (1981). Sexuality in middle and late life. *Archives of General Psychiatry*, **38**, 919–23.

Gregoire, A. (1990). Physical or psychological: an unhealthy splitting in theory and practice. *Sexual and Marital Therapy*, **5**, 103–4.

Hallstrom, T. (1977). Sexuality in the climacteric. *Clinics in Obstetrics and Gynaecology*, **4**, 227–39.

Hallstrom, T., and Samuelsson, S. (1990). Changes in women's sexual desire in middle life: the longitudinal study of women in Gothenburg. *Archives of Sexual Behaviour*, **19**, 259–68.

Harvey, N. S. (1988). Serial cognitive profiles in levodopa-induced hypersexuality. *British Journal of Psychiatry*, **153**, 833–6.

Hawton, K. (1985). *Sex therapy: a practical guide*. Oxford University Press, Oxford.

Hyppa, M., Rinne, O. K., and Sonnine, V. (1970). The activating effect of L-Dopa treatment on sexual functions and its experimental background. *Acta Neurologica Scandinavica*, **43** (Supp. 46), 232–4.

Jensen, P., Jensen, S. B., Sorensen, P. S., Bjerre, B. D., Rizzi, D. A., Sorensen, A. S., *et al.* (1990). Sexual dysfunction in male and female patients with epilepsy: a study of 86 outpatients. *Archives of Sexual Behaviour*, **19**, 1–14.

Kaas, M. J. (1978). Sexual expression of the elderly in nursing homes. *Gerontologist*, **18**, 372–8.

Kellett, J. M. (1987). Treatment of sexual disorders; a prophylaxis for major pathology? *Journal of the Royal College of Physicians*, **21**, 58–60.

Kellett, J. M. (1990). Physical or psychological: time we bridge the divide. *Sexual and Marital Therapy*, **5**, 101–2.

Kinsey, A. C., Pomeroy, W. B., and Martin, C. E. (1948). *Sexual behaviour in the human male*, pp. 121–53. Saunders, Philadelphia.

Kinsey, A. C., Pomeroy, W. B., Martin, C. E., and Gebhard, P. H. (1953). *Sexual behaviour in the human female*, pp. 66–83. Saunders, Philadelphia.

Masters, W. H., and Johnson, V. E. (1966). *Human sexual response*, pp. 223–60. Little Brown, Boston.

Morgan, K., Dallosso, H., Ebrahim, S., Arie, T., and Fentem, P. (1988). Prevalence, frequency, and duration of hypnotic drug use among the elderly living at home. *British Medical Journal*, **296**, 601–2.

Morris, L. W., Morris, R. G., and Britton, P. G. (1988). The relationship between marital intimacy, personal strain, and depression in spouse care-giver of dementia sufferer. *British Journal of Medical Psychology*, **61**, 231–6.

Murphy, E. (1982). Social origins of depression in old age. *British Journal of Psychiatry*, **141**, 135–42.

O'Brien, I., O'Hare, P., and Corral, R. (1986). Heart rate variability in healthy subjects: effect of age and the derivation of normal ranges for tests of automatic function. *British Heart Journal*, **53**, 348–53.

Office of Population Censuses and Surveys (1994). *Population trends*, No. 75, p. 46. HMSO, London.

Oram, J. J., Edwardson, J., and Millard, P. H. (1981). Investigation of cerebrospinal fluid neuropeptides in idiopathic senile dementia. *Gerontology*, **27**, 216–23.

Osborn, M., Hawton, K., and Gath, D. (1988). Sexual dysfunction among middle-aged women in the community. *British Medical Journal*, **296**, 959–62.

Persson, G. (1980). Sexuality in a 70-year-old urban population. *Journal of Psychosomatic Research*, **24**, 335–42.

Pfeiffer, E., and Davis, G. C. (1972). Determinants of sexual behaviour in middle and old age. *Journal of the American Geriatrics Society*, **20**, 151–8.

Pfeiffer, E., Verwoerdt, A., and Wang, H. (1968). Sexual behaviour in aged men and women. *Archives of General Psychiatry*, **19**, 753–8.

Riley, A. J. (1991). Sexuality and the menopause. *Sexual and Marital Therapy*, **6**, 135–46.

Riley, A., and Riley, E. (1986). The effect of single dose diazepam on female sexual response induced by masturbation. *Sexual and Marital Therapy*, **1**, 49–53.

Sherwin, B. B., and Gelfard, M. M. (1987). The role of androgen in the maintenance of sexual functioning in oopherectomized women. *Psychosomatic Medicine*, **49**, 397–409.

Spark, R. F., Wills, C. A., and Royal, H. (1984). Hypogonadism, hyperprolactinaemia and temporal lobe epilepsy in hyposexual men. *Lancet*, **i**, 413–17.

Stanley, E. (1981). Dealing with fear of failure. *British Medical Journal*, **282**, 1281–4.

Szasz, G. (1983). Sexual incidents in an extended care unit for aged men. *Journal of the American Geriatrics Society*, **31**, 407–11.

Taylor Segraves, R. (1989). Effects of psychotropic drugs on human erection and ejaculation. *Archives of General Psychiatry*, **46**, 275–84.

Vallery Masson, J., Valleron, A., and Poitrenaud, J. (1981). Factors related to sexual intercourse frequency in a group of French pre-retirement managers. *Age and Ageing*, **10**, 53–9.

Winn, R. L., and Newton, N. (1982). Sexuality and ageing: a study of 106 cultures. *Archives of Sexual Behaviour*, **11**, 283–98.

Weizman, R., and Hart, J. (1987). Sexual behaviour in healthy married elderly men. *Archives of Sexual Behaviour*, **16**, 39–44.

Weizman, A., Weizman, R., Hart, J., Maoz, B., Wizjenbeek, H., and Ben, D. M. (1983). The correlation of increased serum prolactin levels with decreased sexual desire and activity in elderly men. *Journal of the American Geriatrics Society*, **31**, 485–8.

Zeiss, A. M., Davies, H. D., Wood, M., and Tinklenberg, J. R. (1990). The incidence and correlates of erectile problems in patients with Alzheimer's disease. *Archives of Sexual Behaviour*, **19**, 325–33.

USEFUL SOURCES OF INFORMATION

Gibson, H. B. (1992). *The emotional and sexual lives of older people*. Chapman and Hall, London.

Greengross, W., and Greengross, S. (1989). *Living, loving and ageing: sexual and personal relationships in later life*. Age Concern, Mitcham.

Heiman, J., LoPiccolo, L., and LoPiccolo, J. (1976). *Becoming orgasmic: a sexual growth programme for women*. Prentice Hall, London.

Jaffe, M., and Fenwick, E. (1986). *Sexual happiness for men*. Dorling Kindersley, London.

Jaffe, M., and Fenwick, E. (1986). *Sexual happiness for women*. Dorling Kindersley, London.

Zilbergeld, B. (1980). *Men and sex*. Fontana, London.

Educational videotapes available from: Focus Therapy Co., Ltd., Dept MO, PO Box 12, Chertsey, Surrey KT16 8YA.

Help for the disabled: SPOD, 286 Camden Road, London N7 0BJ.

13

Sleep and its disorders
DAVID BRAMBLE

INTRODUCTION

It is now well established that disordered sleep is common at all ages (Kripke *et al.* 1983; National Institute of Mental Health 1984). Each stage of human development is characterized by different types of sleep problems: the young child who won't settle and who wakes repeatedly during the night demanding parental attention; the excessively sleepy adolescent; the insomniac young adult; and the elderly person who lies awake at night and naps during the day. The prevalence rates of the most common sleep problems—insomnia, snoring, leg movements, night waking, etc.—tend to increase with age (Kripke *et al.* 1983). Several large population surveys have revealed that nearly one third of elderly people have significant sleep problems. Furthermore, there are closer links between these problems (mostly various forms of insomnia) and both psychiatric and chronic medical conditions than are seen in younger people. Sleep disorders are generally more prevalent in elderly women than elderly men (Kales *et al.* 1979, Ford and Kamarrow 1989).

The past twenty years have seen an explosion of scientific interest in sleep and its disorders, and this has led in turn to the emergence of a new medical specialty, sleep-disorder medicine, which has yielded important information and several new treatment techniques. Unfortunately, dissemination of this information into the consulting rooms of clinicians has not yet been very successful, particularly in the United Kingdom where currently only three medical schools (to the author's knowledge) provide any undergraduate instruction in the assessment and treatment of common sleep problems. As a result, most doctors, psychiatrists included, are not trained to take a sleep history, nor are they able to address in a systematic manner common disorders such as insomnia, excessive daytime sleepiness and nightmares. Insomniac patients are still more likely to receive a prescription for a hypnotic drug, or take an untested non-prescription nostrum, than to receive helpful advice concerning how and where they should sleep. This is unfortunate, because sleep difficulties are among the most common presenting problems in primary-care clinics (Coleman 1982); indeed, it is unusual to encounter a major illness that does not disturb sleep to a greater or lesser extent. Sleep disturbances, together with their common daytime sequelae, namely excessive sleepiness, reduce quality of life, and can cause substantial and prolonged individual suffering which may well contribute to the development of physical and psychiatric disorders. Recently it has been recognized that sleep disorders also exact a very high economic toll through impaired work efficiency and absenteeism; they are also a significant cause of accidents – in the workplace, on the road, and in the home (Saario and Linnoila 1976). Elderly people are more likely to have domestic accidents, and this is particularly the case when they are also taking regular night sedation agents for sleep problems (Fancourt and Castleden 1986).

The growing health awareness and expectations of older people require that medicine delivers a better service to this group. Sleep problems in the elderly need to be treated seriously and efficiently in order to reduce sufferers' distress and disability, and ultimately improve the quality of their lives. This chapter reviews the assessment and treatment of the sleep disorders that present characteristically in older people; however, many of the treatment techniques described are also applicable to sleep disorders presenting at any age.

NORMAL CHANGES IN SLEEP PATTERN WITH AGE

Sleep is a reversible behavioural state characterized by profound, alternating shifts in levels of arousal. As with most other vital physiological processes, it changes in both its quantity and to a lesser degree its quality throughout life. It is not known why we sleep, although there are several competing theories, among the most compelling of which is that proposed by Horne (1988), who suggests that human adults require only a few (4 or 5) hours sleep per day to perform optimally. He refers to this as 'core' sleep; the additional sleep time that most people obtain is determined circumstantially or societally (referred to as 'optional' sleep). Horne uses the analogy of food: we require a certain amount to survive, and the rest we eat for a variety of reasons. Horne speculates that only core sleep, comprising a high proportion of 'deep', slow-wave (SWS) sleep, is required for optimal brain function, specifically in the prefrontal areas of the cerebral cortex.

Newborn babies sleep most of the day, waking every hour or so to feed and/or eliminate. A cycle of sleep and wakefulness is quickly established, and by 3 months of age the infant is sleeping for 4 hours at a stretch, extending gradually to 12 hours at 6 months with regular daytime naps totalling about 3 hours. From the end of the first year to mid-toddlerhood, daytime napping declines, and the night sleep period slowly reduces to 9 hours by late childhood and 8 hours by early adolescence. Children wake very briefly during the night, but this is rarely remembered unless it is associated with a specific sleep disorder such as a nightmare. Early adulthood sees a reduction in the total sleep period down to an average of 7.5 hours with a standard deviation of 1 hour; this figure remains remarkably constant into old age.

Qualitative changes in the relative proportions of light and deep sleep occur during the normal ageing process. Infant sleep initially comprises high levels of rapid-eye-movement (REM) sleep and, later, deep sleep appears, which probably reflects rapid growth and development of the central nervous system (Denenberg and Thomas 1981). From late infancy, SWS (stages 3 and 4) predominates in the first half of the night, the lighter sleep stages (stages 1, 2, and REM) in the latter half. Deep and light sleep stages alternate every 90 minutes or so throughout the sleep period in adulthood. As individuals age there is a marked tendency for sleep to become progressively lighter, a consequence of this in old age being an increased tendency to wake at night and be unable to fall asleep again (i.e. maintain sleep). With advancing age, waking at night becomes more frequent and is also more likely to be remembered, and this is particularly the case after the mid-forties (Reynolds *et al.* 1985). Pathological significance is often attributed to this normal change in sleep by elderly insomniacs. During the day, sustained wakefulness is difficult to maintain, which results in the daytime napping so characteristic of old age (Morgan *et al.* 1989). Deterioration of the normal circadian pacemaker control of the sleep–wake cycle with age has been described (Czeisler *et al.* 1992), and this may be the cause of sleep problems arising *de novo* in old age.

CLASSIFICATION OF SLEEP DISORDERS

There are currently three major classification schemes for sleep disorders: the International Classification of Sleep Disorders (ICSD) (Thorpy 1990), the *Diagnostic and statistical manual of mental disorders*, fourth edition (DSM-IV) (American Psychiatric Association 1994) and the *International classification of diseases*, tenth edition (ICD-10) (World Health Organization 1992). These schemes are mostly compatible with one another, although sleep researchers tend to prefer the ICSD for diagnostic and epidemiological use because its operational diagnostic criteria are more exhaustive than the other schemes. In the ICSD, sleep disorders are divided into four major categories: *dyssomnias*, which are the disorders of initiating and maintaining sleep (the 'insomnias') as well as the disorders of hypersomnolence (eg. those caused by shift work and jet lag); *parasomnias*, those sleep disorders that do not involve insomnia or hypersomnolence (e.g. nightmares and somnambulism); *sleep disorders associated with medical/psychiatric disorders* (e.g. obstructive sleep apnoea and dementia); and *proposed sleep disorders*, a category for conditions as yet not accorded full nosological status owing to insufficient validatory information, such as 'sleep-choking syndrome'.

INVESTIGATION OF SLEEP DISORDERS

Sleep history

In order to diagnose accurately any particular type of sleep disorder, it is necessary to take a comprehensive *sleep history* in addition to a routine medical and psychiatric history. A concise scheme for such a history is as follows:

1. Establish whether the problem involves difficulty falling asleep, staying asleep, waking too early, and/or feeling sleepy and unrefreshed the following morning or at specific times during the day. It is important to differentiate between *sleepiness*, which is a propensity to fall asleep quickly, and *tiredness* resulting from stress or exertion.

2. Ask the patient to describe the routine of a typical night. What time do they usually go to bed? How long does it take to get to sleep? What do they do if they cannot get to sleep? Do they wake up during the night, and if so, when, and how often? What do they do once awake? Do they do anything unusual during sleep, such as have recurrent disturbing dreams, sleepwalk, snore excessively and also appear to stop breathing for longer than 30 seconds, or experience excessive and/or painful leg or body movements? What time do they eventually wake up? In what precise ways do they consider their sleep to be unsatisfactory? It is particularly important to discover who else is affected by the sleep problem, such as the spouse, other members of the family, professional carers—even the doctor! Their perceptions can be invaluable in accurate assessment, and an acknowledgement of their involvement can facilitate their participation in any treatment programme. It may well be that the index patient is actually presenting with a sleep disorder induced by a snoring, kicking, wandering, or repeatedly nocturic spouse.

3. Enquire about the sleeper's physical environment. Do they sleep with a partner? Do other individuals or pets share the bed or bedroom? Are the temperature, humidity, and noise levels satisfactory? Is the bed sufficiently comfortable?

4. Establish the duration of the current problem and whether or not there have been similar or different sleep problems in the past. Have they had previous treatment for these problems, and, if so, was it successful?

5. Is there a relationship and/or sexual problem with the patient's partner which is disturbing their sleep?

6. Screen for physical causes. Table 13.1 lists common symptoms, disorders, and drugs that can contribute to sleep disturbance in the elderly.

7. Conduct a current mental state examination with particular reference to affective and neurotic psychopathology that may be underlying the disturbed

Table 13.1. Common physical causes of sleep disturbance.

Cardiovascular
Orthopnoea resulting from congestive cardiac failure
Nocturnal angina

Respiratory
Chronic cough
Dyspnoea
Pleuritic or costochondrial pain
Asthma
Obstructive sleep apnoea

Genitourinary
Nocturia resulting from obstructive uropathy

Musculoskeletal
Arthritic pain

Neurological
Headache
Nocturnal myoclonus
Akathisia

Drugs
Caffeine
Alcohol
Antihistamines
Nicotine
Benzodiazepines
Beta blockers
Methyldopa
Thyroxine
Phenytoin

---

sleep. This examination should include an assessment of cognitive function if the history suggests a picture of emergent dementia. Psychiatric disorders that commonly disturb sleep in old age include depressive illness, neuroses, late-onset schizophrenia, dementia, and acute reactions to stress (see p. 237 *et seq.*).

Most sleep disorders and their causes can be usually identified from the history alone. Nevertheless, a small minority of conditions (in particular, suspected sleep apnoea and nocturnal myoclonus) require laboratory investigation, and the traditional setting for this is in the sleep laboratory, where full polysomnological studies can be conducted (Kales *et al.* 1982). This allows whole-sleep-period real-time monitoring of electroencephalography (EEG), electromyography (EOG), oximetry, and other physiological variables. The diagnosis of obstructive sleep apnoea, for example, can be confirmed by observing the characteristic dips in oxygen saturation by oximetry.

Insomnia

Not surprisingly, the largest category of sleep disorders encountered in old age is also the same as that which obtains in younger adults, namely the various manifestations of insomnia. Insomnia is not a diagnostic category but a subjective appraisal of the sleep period by the patient, concerning both the quantity and the quality of their night's sleep. The principal components of this problem are: difficulty falling asleep (prolonged sleep latency), difficulty maintaining sleep, and feeling unrefreshed upon waking in the morning. There are several broad subtypes of sleep disorder which can comprise any combination of these symptoms: among the most common is 'psycho-physiological insomnia' (Thorpy 1990), which results from tension and habitual thoughts and behaviours at bedtime which induce physiological and psychological arousal incompatible with sleep onset. This can be a lifelong problem or can arise for the first time in old age.

For practical purposes the severity of insomnia may be divided into *transient*, *short-term* and *long-term* types. By definition, transient insomnias last a few days and occur in relation to minor stressful life events such as brief hospitalization or jet lag; short-term insomnias, of a few weeks duration, result from more serious stresses and life events (such as moving house or bereavement). Long-term insomnias, of several months, years, or even lifelong duration, can result from chronic physical illness (eg. arthritic pain) or long-term psychological problems (eg. affective disorders (Tan *et al.* 1984)). A full sleep history (see p. 230) will usually reveal the underlying causes of patients' complaints of insomnia. Grief and mourning, and fear of being alone or even dying whilst asleep may be particularly important factors operating in patients presenting with insomnia for the first time in old age.

Treatment

The choice of treatment depends upon the nature of the insomnia revealed by the history and any additional investigations. There follows a description of the general therapeutic approaches currently regarded as being effective in the management of insomnia in the elderly.

Sleep hygiene

The term 'sleep hygiene' refers to a system of advice which consists of a package of educative and behavioural measures which can help the insomniac to achieve a healthy sleep habit (Morin and Rapp 1987). The following scheme is appropriate for elderly sufferers:

1. Education of the sleep-disordered patient is paramount, and this should include an explanation of the normal changes of sleep associated with age. Any unrealistic expectations regarding sleep requirements need to be

identified, since misattribution of pathological significance to the normal changes of sleep experienced in old age may be a strong aetiological or maintaining factor in some cases.

2. Help the patient develop a daily bedtime routine involving a regular settling and waking time, with the proviso that the sufferer should not attempt to catch up lost sleep from the previous night by going to bed early.

3. The bedroom environment needs to be relaxing and unstimulating, and should as far as possible be used only for sleep, quiet and relaxing activities, and sex. Stimulating factors, be they physical or psychological, should be removed from the bedroom environment. The physical environment of the bedroom should promote sleep and restfulness. Temperature, humidity, noise, and light should be controlled and, most importantly, the patient should endeavour to acquire as comfortable a bed and mattress as possible.

4. Daily physical exercise will help promote sleep; however, it is best that this is done during the day, or at the latest, the early evening, at least three hours before the regular bedtime. Vigorous exercise taken shortly before bedtime can delay sleep onset significantly through physiological over-arousal.

5. Large meals taken immediately prior to bedtime are best avoided. However, snacks and milky drinks may help to sustain sleep in the latter part of the night (Hartmann and Spinweber 1979). Caffeine, nicotine, and excessive alcohol ingestion should be avoided in the evenings. Advising alcohol as a routine hypnotic in established chronic insomniacs is never justified clinically (Consumers' Association 1990).

6. Immediately prior to sleep, pleasant relaxing activities should be engaged in in order to promote sleep and to associate the bedroom with relaxation and quiet wakefulness.

If this advice is followed, and sleep onset is still delayed for more than 20 minutes, then the following suggestions may help:

1. The patient should get out of bed and engage in a relaxing activity (reading, listening to music, etc.) in another room.

2. When the patient feels sleepy again, they should return to the bedroom and try to get to sleep. However, if sleep onset does not occur quickly then the previous exercise should be repeated as often as necessary.

3. Psychological techniques such as paradoxical intention ('try to stay awake') and thought stopping can break obsessional thoughts concerning the inability to get to sleep.

4. Pre-sleep relaxation programmes (using audio tapes) can sometimes be beneficial, as can setting aside a time removed from bedtime for worrying about daily issues. It is helpful to give patients the injunction that they must make every effort not to take worries to bed—because they require an undisturbed night's sleep to face the challenges of the day effectively.

In those with marked sleep fragmentation who routinely wake after only two or three hours' sleep despite all the above measures, it can be helpful to have a brief mid-evening nap followed by a period of 4 or 5 hours of wakefulness whilst the house is still warm and there are television programmes to watch, and then go to bed again around 2 or 3 o'clock in the morning.

In cases where there is a fixed advance of the normal sleep circadian rhythm, and there is late onset of sleep with consequential and disturbing persistent morning hypersomnolence, the patient can sometimes be helped by advancing the usual settling time by three hours each successive day until a desired settling time is achieved. Exposure to artificial sunlight in the late evening can also entrain insomniacs' circadian pacemakers (Campbell and Dawson, 1991)

Pharmacotherapy

Drugs are the traditional first line of treatment for the various forms of insomnia; in a recent survey it was estimated that between 10 and 15 per cent of elderly people in Great Britain (0.8–1.0 million people) take hypnotic medication each night (Morgan *et al.* 1988). Nowadays, non-pharmacological approaches should always be tried (see p. 232) before a hypnotic is considered. Hypnotics should not be prescribed routinely, particularly to elderly patients who are prone to accumulation problems which may result in accidents and falls (Lader and Lawson 1987).

The ideal hypnotic should promote sleep quickly, sustain this state until the morning and also allow a full day of wakefulness without intrusive sleepiness or tiredness resulting from residual drug activity ('hangover' effects). There is currently a bewildering choice of hypnotic agents available to the physician. Older drugs such as the barbiturates, chloral hydrate, glutethamide and chlormethiazole are still generally available but are now outmoded because they have the potential to be abused, can be potentiated by alcohol and other CNS (central nervous system) depressants, and may prove fatal in overdose (particularly the barbiturates). Currently the most popular hypnotic agents are the short-acting benzodiazepines such as temazepam. Although the benzodiazepines have in recent years received much adverse publicity, their safety and efficiency as hypnotics are unparalleled when they are used correctly. However, benzodiazepines can be dangerous when combined with other CNS depressants, particularly in patients with coexisting respiratory problems. Also, like all sedative agents, they have abuse potential.

Physiological changes that occur in old age influence the choice and dose of hypnotic agent. In particular, the fat:water ratio of the body tissues tends to increase with age, so for a given dose of a lipophilic benzodiazepine (particularly lorazepam and diazepam) there is a greater risk of accumulation with consequent day time hangover effects which can cause impaired psychomotor performance. There are also less important pharmacokinetic effects; therefore a low dose of a short-acting sedative with low lipophilicity would be the ideal for an older person. The benzodiazepines are conjugated in the liver and excreted in the urine, therefore caution is required when contemplating prescription for a patient with either hepatic or renal impairment.

As a rule, hypnotics should only be prescribed in elderly patients suffering from transient or short-term forms of insomnia (see p. 232), and then only when non-pharmacological approaches have failed. A drug should be selected that not only promotes and maintains sleep but also does not impair subsequent daytime cognitive functioning (memory and concentration particularly). A minimum dose should be used for the shortest possible time, for example, temazepam, 10–20 mg *nocte* for 10 days, or, as an alternative, zopiclone, 7.5 mg *nocte* for 10 days. The dosage of any hypnotic should be tailed off towards the end of the course to reduce the possibility of rebound insomnia (Consumers' Association 1990). Any elderly patient prescribed hypnotics should be reviewed during the course of treatment in order to gauge efficacy and also to detect any emergent side-effects (daytime sedation). The possibility of hypnotic abuse also needs to be considered; for example, is the patient running out of tablets before the prescription suggests they should? Patients should be reviewed about a month after the conclusion of a course of hypnotic pharmacotherapy in order to detect whether there has been any return of disturbed sleep or emergence of symptoms suggestive of significant psychopathology (especially depressive symptoms).

A very small minority of chronic insomniacs will continue to demand long-term prescription of an hypnotic, rejecting or failing to respond to any other help. It is up to prescribing clinicians to decide whether or not they are prepared to accept the responsibility for this type of prescription. It needs to be borne in mind that withdrawal of modern hypnotic agents from this group may result in their seeking relief by use of over-the-counter nostrums, folk remedies, or alcohol, which may represent a far greater long-term threat to their health.

OTHER SLEEP DISORDERS IN OLD AGE

Narcolepsy

Narcolepsy is a genetically based neurological condition whose cardinal symptoms are sudden-onset REM sleep, cataplexy (sudden loss of muscle tone), sleep paralysis (waking up whilst in REM paralysis), and hypnagogic hallucinations (pre-sleep dreaming). The condition is often lifelong with a peak age of onset in the teens and early adulthood, but occasionally it first presents in old age. In addition to patient education and counselling, the pharmacological treatment of hypersomnolence in this disorder is usually by means of psychostimulants (e.g. methylphenidate) and of the cataplexy by tricyclic antidepressants. As a rule, these patients should be reviewed by an interested sleep specialist or neurologist (Parkes 1985).

Periodic leg movements syndrome and restless legs syndrome (PLMS and RLS)

Involuntary or irresistible uncomfortable jerky or akathisic movements of the legs occurring repeatedly during the night and disrupting sleep are a common complaint in elderly people. Although normally discrete from one another the two forms may coexist. It is estimated that nearly 44 per cent of the over-sixties suffer from PLMS (Rosenthal *et al.* 1984). The incidence of this condition increases with age, with between 16 per cent and 33 per cent of elderly insomniacs reporting this problem (Dement 1982). It is important to take a full medical history in these cases, as these symptoms can be a manifestation of underlying metabolic disorders, such as uraemia, and neurological disorders, such as narcolepsy. PLMS should always be suspected in elderly insomniacs who also present with daytime hypersomnolence, since this activity is severely disruptive of sleep and can also be a major source of tension between the sufferer and their bedtime partner. Other important differential diagnoses to consider are: Parkinson's disease, myoclonic epilepsy, drug withdrawal, and akathisia as a side effect of maintenance neuroleptics. There is no specific treatment for PLMS, but benzodiazepines, in particular clonazepam, at a dose of 0.5 to 2.0 mg *nocte*, can benefit some sufferers (Mitler *et al.* 1986). These drugs may not actually reduce the movements, but they can improve the continuity of sleep. Other drugs which have been shown to benefit some patients with PLMS are L-dopa and some synthetic opioids (Akpinar 1987; Hening *et al.* 1986).

The sleep apnoea syndromes

In any patient presenting with a sleep problem, the cardinal symptoms of the sleep apnoea need to be enquired about: excessive loud snoring, repeated periods of apnoea (sometimes several hundred times a night) lasting from between a few seconds to a couple of minutes, night-time restlessness and confusional arousals, excessive daytime irritability, reduced libido, and morning headaches and sleepiness. By far the most common form of sleep apnoea is the *obstructive* type. This is most commonly encountered in obese males, particularly those with very thick necks (Halperin *et al.* 1979). The symptoms of the sleep apnoea syndrome are due to the relative hypotonia of sleep (particularly REM sleep) combined with the additional burden of excessively bulky soft nasopharyngeal tissues, which results in collapse of the normally patent oropharyngeal airway. Diaphragmatic and chest muscles move during these periods of apnoea, but there is no oronasal airflow. Increasing involuntary respiratory efforts to overcome this obstruction result in the 'jackhammer' loud snoring so characteristic of the syndrome. These periods of apnoea result in marked transient hypercapnia and hypoxemia, and it may well be that this mild respiratory failure may ultimately result in death for the affected sufferer in a proportion of cases who have the often coexisting medical conditions of ischaemic heart disease and hypertension (Guilleminault 1989). The rarer condition of *central* sleep apnoea, occuring in about 10 per cent of cases, is thought to be caused by pathology of the brainstem respiratory drive centres, resulting in sleep apnoea without compensatory respiratory movements. The two forms may coexist (the *mixed* type). Accurate diagnosis of sleep apnoea is best achieved in a sleep laboratory where polysomnographic evidence of repeated respiratory malfunction may be obtained.

The treatment of obstructive sleep apnoea involves an explanation of the disorder and its attendant risks, and the necessity for the patient to consider major lifestyle changes, such as reducing weight, taking more exercise, and avoiding alcohol, cigarettes and other sedatives. These measures may be all that is required in milder cases but more severe cases merit more specialist treatment methods. Direct treatment of the obstructive sleep apnoea aims at removal, prevention, or by-pass of the obstruction. A surgical technique known as uvulopalato-pharyngoplasty, which essentially clears away all of the unnecessary soft tissue in the oropharynx, has been reported to have been successful in severe cases (Silvestri *et al.* 1983). Laser excision of soft tissue is a more recent development. A less drastic alternative is continuous nasal positive airways pressure (C-PAP), which provides effectively a pneumatic splint that keeps the airway patent. This technique has been developed for home use. Management over and beyond lifestyle change and weight reduction should be the responsibility of a sleep-disorder, respiratory, or ENT specialist.

PSYCHIATRIC DISORDERS AND SLEEP DISTURBANCE IN OLD AGE

Depression

At all ages, the most important differential diagnosis to make in the patient presenting with disordered sleep is an affective disorder, since these conditions have the closest link with disturbed sleep patterns. Studies have shown that nearly 90 per cent of sufferers of major depression have sleep disturbances that can be confirmed by polysomnography (Reynolds *et al.* 1985). Given that the prevalences of both affective disorders and sleep disorders increase with age and are known to be closely associated, it is important that clinicians can differentiate between them and treat accordingly.

In major depression the most sensitive change of sleep pattern is disturbance of sleep continuity, i.e. prolonged sleep latency, increased nocturnal waking, and, most specifically in severe depression, early-morning waking with an inability to return to sleep thereafter. A minority of sufferers report hypersomnolence. There can also be changes in the objective quality of depressed patients' sleep, with shortened REM latency (earlier onset of the first REM period of the night with more total REM sleep), and reduced non-REM activity in the first third of the night.

A small minority of even severely depressed people do not report disturbed sleep, nor is their sleep abnormal upon testing. Whether or not the sleep abnormalities observed in depressed individuals are the result of the depressed state or are in some way related to their aetiology remains in question. One of the most sensitive predictors of impending relapse in manic–depressive disorder is reduced total sleep time as well as over-activity during the day; however, it should be emphasized that no specific changes in sleep patterns are entirely pathognomonic of any psychiatric disorder.

Between one-third to one half of patients of all ages with chronic insomnia have an underlying psychiatric disorder; affective disorders comprise the largest subgroup (Addy 1988). Naturally, the treatment of any sleep disorder associated with depression is treatment of the underlying affective disorder; there is currently some dispute as to whether agitated elderly people who have severe sleep problems should also be prescribed a hypnotic agent in addition to standard antidepressant therapy. There are claims that the serotonin re-uptake inhibitors actually improve sleep architecture and promote normal sleep. However, it is not clear whether this is a symptomatic change in the underlying depressive state or a specific effect on sleep quality. Given that the sleep of depressed patients has usually been disturbed for several months before presentation, most patients would accept a couple of weeks' further disruption before an antidepressant agent starts to work, and hence avoid the additional prescription of an hypnotic drug with its attendant risks.

Finally, issues related to grief and loss generally are more common with elderly patients, and should be enquired about and the appropriate treatment given. Grief counselling and focused brief psychotherapy are the first lines of treatment in these cases, rather than hypnotics or antidepressants.

Dementia

It is now generally appreciated that the major forms of dementia (Alzheimer's and multi-infarct types) are often associated with marked disturbances of the sleep–wake cycle. Indeed, it is often these disturbances that ultimately exhaust carers and lead to admission to residential care. The major components of sleep disturbance linked to established dementia are: agitation, worsening confusion, nocturnal wandering, and frequent night waking and restlessness. While many of these problems can occur in the daytime, they are often exacerbated at night-time or during the individual's main sleep period. This general picture is referred to as 'sundowning' in the United States. This habitual pattern of sleep-related exacerbations of confusion differentiates sundowning from other conditions which may transiently impair cognition (transient ischaemic attacks, respiratory infections, etc.).

Various theories have been proposed to explain sleep disturbance in dementia, but none can fully explain all the features. Deterioration of the suprachaismatic nucleus of the hypothalamus, which maintains endogenous circadian control of sleep and wakefulness, may be associated with the late general cerebral and midbrain deterioration found in Alzheimer's disease. However, it has not been shown to be associated consistently with this clinical state. Sleep apnoea has also been shown to be associated with severe night-time behavioural problems in demented subjects (Smallwood *et al.* 1983). Other possible explanations are: increased disorientation at night due to the lack of light; concurrent use of hypnotics; prostatism (in males); bodily discomfort as a result of joint or muscular pain; environmental factors such as extraneous noise; and even an exaggeration of the normal age-related changes in sleep architecture in the context of cognitive impairment.

When assessing a demented patient with disturbed sleep, full physical, psychiatric, and sleep histories should be obtained in order to characterize the precise form, intensity, and frequency of the problem behaviours. Corroborative information should always be obtained from a spouse or principal carer. Special attention should be paid to metabolic, cardiorespiratory, urological, and pharmacological factors which may be potentially reversible. The possibility of a depressive pseudodementia must also be considered: the in-patient can be totally sleep-deprived for 24 hours and this often results in an improvement in the mental state of depressed patients but not with demented individuals; indeed, the latter frequently become worse.

These problems pose a major therapeutic challenge to clinicians involved in the care of dementing individuals and their families. As with non-demented patients with disturbed sleep, it is important to treat any reversible causes, and to ensure good sleep hygiene before having recourse to pharmacotherapy. The aim of sleep hygiene strategies with demented individuals should be to promote activity and exercise during the day and a quiet unstimulating environment which encourages sleep at night. Carers should be encouraged to be generally firm with these patients, particularly at night, and to provide a fixed bedtime routine in order to help cue the sufferer into sleep. Reduction of excessive daytime napping in severely affected individuals may also be helpful.

Pharmacotherapy remains a mainstay of treatment of sleep disturbance in dementia. As a general rule, sedative hypnotic medication is best avoided in this patient group because of its lack of effectiveness and also its propensity paradoxically to worsen both sleep disturbance and daytime functioning. A low dose of a neuroleptic agent such as thioridazine, 10–50 mg in the early evening, is a standard initial treatment. Other agents and regimes have been suggested, although none to date has been subjected to systematic research trial scrutiny. The sensitivity of elderly patients, and particularly those with coexistent parkinsonism and other movement disorders, to neuroleptic agents requires that they are reviewed regularly for evidence of exacerbation of these conditions or emergence of other movement disorders.

The need for carers to obtain a restorative night's sleep is also of paramount importance, and must be attended to in its own right. Their own habits may have been altered substantially as a result of caring for their dementing relative often for several years and, despite effective treatment of their charge's sleep disturbance, may continue with a disturbed sleep pattern. Sleep-hygiene advice (see p. 232) may also benefit these individuals.

Anxiety

As can be seen from the rest of this book, neurotic disorders are not uncommonly encountered in the elderly population, and disturbed sleep often forms part of the clinical picture. Generalized anxiety is associated with daytime tiredness, initial insomnia, and less frequently with repeated nocturnal waking and night-mares. In phobic states, sleep is generally only affected in cases when the feared stimulus is associated with bedtime (the dark, fear of death during sleep, etc.), and in obsessive–compulsive disorder, ruminations and rituals may interfere with sleep routines. An additional problem in this group is chronic hypnotic and sedative abuse, which can compound the sleep problem. Treatment of the underlying neurotic disorder as described elsewhere in this book is the initial step. Residual sleep-onset or maintenance insomnia can be treated along the lines already described in this chapter.

SLEEP PROBLEMS IN SPECIFIC POPULATIONS

Institutionalized elderly people

In addition to the majority of severely dependent elderly people who are cared for at home, many are cared for in a range of non-domestic settings and, more often than not, these are not geriatric or psychogeriatric hospital wards but community-based private, statutory, or voluntary sector-run residential units. A valuable contribution can be made by a psychiatrist or physician with a special interest in sleep disorders in terms of consulting with care staff to prevent or reduce the likelihood of sleep problems developing by establishing bedtime routines and generally providing an environment that promotes sleep at bedtime and wakefulness during the day. These clinicians can also help reduce the likelihood of residents being maintained on long-term hypnotics and major tranquillizers with their attendant problems. In residential care settings, a viable alternative to imposing a regime on severely sleep-disturbed individuals might be to adapt the routines of the unit to their sleep–wake cycles by providing activities, meals and companionship at all times of the day and night.

Mentally handicapped elderly people

Increasing numbers of people with all degrees of mental handicaps are living into old age. Elderly people with severe disabilities have been found to have high prevalences of psychiatric disorders (Cooper 1992), so it is likely (although not proven) that they will also suffer from associated sleep problems. Behavioural sleep problems (i.e. those resulting from poor sleep habits) in this population tend to decline with age, but in individual cases they may continue to be extremely burdensome to carers. It is important when dealing with a sleep problem presenting in a patient from this group to take a developmental perspective, discovering how and when it emerged in the patient's life, and, having accurately characterized the problem, work closely with the principal carers when implementing a treatment package. As a rule, firm setting of limits and stimulus-control techniques which help the patient associate the bedroom and night-time with sleep rather than wakefulness are helpful with night-settling and night-waking problems. Sometimes, major life events can provoke both transient and long-term insomnias in elderly mentally handicapped individuals; in such cases, however, the sleep disturbance is usually associated with other behavioural problems.

Elderly acute in-patients

Elderly people admitted to hospital as a result of sudden illness are likely to develop reactive sleep problems (transient insomnias). It is beholden upon medical and nursing staff to be aware that the illness, the stress of admission and the impact of medication can lead to confusion and night-time disturbance. Awareness of this, and practice in the management of these problems will reduce the likelihood of the sufferer becoming distressed and, most importantly, taking a sleep problem (or a prescription for an hypnotic) home with them upon discharge.

Elderly motorists

One-third of fatal road traffic accidents are thought to be the result of drivers falling asleep at the wheel (Horne 1992). Consequently, it is important to enquire whether an elderly sleep-disordered patient drives, and to find out if they have ever been excessively drowsy or even fallen transiently asleep at the wheel. If daytime somnolence is severe, and particularly if it is associated with a significant degree of general cognitive impairment, the clinician should take steps to ensure that the patient stops driving. In less severe cases, the patient should be advised to take regular naps and to avoid sleep-inducing practices whilst at the wheel, such as having the heating turned up too high, or listening to monotonous music. As soon as drivers find themselves becoming drowsy, they should pull off the road and take a refreshing nap before resuming their journeys.

CONCLUSIONS

Although sleep disorders in the elderly are many and various, a consistent approach to both their diagnosis and management can reduce their impact on patients' quality of life. The current low profile of sleep disorders within medicine in the United Kingdom is regrettable, given the high prevalence of sleep disorders within the community and their associated high morbidity in both physical and psychological terms. In this era of health promotion, all elderly patients should be asked routinely about the quality of their sleep and also about daytime sleepiness, and be given suitable advice and treatment if necessary. The cardinal aim of sleep-disorder medicine is to prevent the pathological intrusion of sleep into wakefulness and wakefulness into sleep, thus optimizing the quality of both states.

REFERENCES

Addy, R. O. (1988). The causes and management of chronic insomnia. *Clinical Advances in the Treatment of Psychiatric Disorders.* **99**, July/August 1–3.

Akpinar, S. (1987). Treatment of restless legs syndrome with dopaminergic drugs. *Clinical Neuropharmacology*, **10**, 69–79.

American Psychiatric Association (1994). *Diagnostic and statistical manual of mental disorders* (4th edn). American Psychiatric Association, Washington.

Bixler, E. O., Kales, A., Soldatos, C. R., Kales, J. D., and Healey, S. (1979). Prevalence of sleep disorders in the Los Angeles metropolitan area. *American Journal of Psychiatry*, **136**, 1257–63.

Campbell, S. S., and Dawson, D. (1991). Bright light treatment of sleep disturbance in older subjects. *Sleep Research*, **20**, 448.

Coleman, R. M., Roffwarg, H. P., Kennedy, S. J., Cuillaminault, C., Cohn, M. A., and Karacan, I. (1982). Sleep-wake disorders based on a polysomnographic diagnosis. A national cooperative study. *Journal of the American Medical Association*, **247**, 997–1003.

Consumer's Association (1990). The treatment of insomnia. *Drug and Therapeutics Bulletin*, **28** (25), 97–9.

Cooper, S. A. (1992). The psychiatry of elderly people with mental handicaps. *International Journal of Geriatric Psychiatry*, **7**, 865–74.

Czeisler, C. A., Dumont, M. Duffy, J. F., Steinberg, J. D., Richardson, G. S., Brown, E. N., *et al.* (1992). Association of sleep–wake habits in older people with changes in output of circadian pacemaker. *Lancet*, **340**, 933–6.

Dement, W. C., Miles, L. E., and Carskadon, M. A. (1982). 'White Paper' on sleep and aging. *Journal of the American Geriatrics Society*, **30**, 25–50.

Denenberg, V. H., and Thomas, E. B. (1981). Evidence for a functional role for active (REM) sleep in infancy. *Sleep*, **4**, 185–92.

Fancourt, G., and Castleden, M. (1986). The use of benzodiazepines with particular reference to the elderly. *British Journal of Hospital Medicine*, **35**, 13–26.

Ford, D. E., and Kamarrow, D. B. (1989). Epidemiological studies of sleep disturbance and psychiatric disturbance: an opportunity for prevention? *Journal of the American Medical Association*, **262**, 1479–84.

Guilleminault, C. (1989). Clinical features and evaluation of obstructive sleep apnoea. In *Principles and practice of sleep medicine* (ed. M. Kryger, T. Roth, and W. Dement), pp. 552–8. W. B. Saunders Company, New York.

Halperin, E., Lavie, P., Alroy, G., Eliashar, I., and Gordon, C. (1979). The hypersomnia–sleep–apnea syndrome (HSAS): ENT findings. *Sleep Research*, **8**, 188.

Hartmann, E., and Spinweber, C. L. (1979). Sleep induced by L-tryptophan: effect of dosage within the normal dietary intake. *Journal of Nervous and Mental Disorders*, **167**, 497–9.

Hening, W. A., Walters, A., Kavay, N., Giprō-Frank, S., Côté, L., and Fahn, S. (1986). Dyskinesias while awake and periodic movements in sleep in restless legs syndrome: treatment with opioids. *Neurology*, **36**, 1363–6.

Horne, J. A. (1988). *Why we sleep: the function of sleep in humans and other mammals*, pp. 180–21. Oxford University Press, Oxford.

Horne, J. A. (1992). Stay awake, stay alive. *New Scientist*, **133**, 20–4.

Kales, A., Kales, J. D., and Soldatos, C. R. (1982). Insomnia and other sleep disorders. *Medical Clinics of North America*, **66**, 971–91.

Kales, J. D., Kales, A., Bixler, E. O., and Soldatos, C. R. (1979). Resources for managing sleep disorders. *Journal of the American Medical Association*, **24**, 2413–6.

Kripke, D. F., Ancoli-Israel, S., Mason, M., and Messin, S. (1983). Sleep-related mortality and morbidity in the aged. In *Sleep disorders: basic and clinical research* (ed. M. H. Chase and E. D. Weitzman), pp. 415–44. Spectrum, New York.

Lader, M., and Lawson, C. (1987). Sleep studies and rebound insomnia: methodology and problems, laboratory findings and clinical implications. *Clinical Neuropharmacology*, **10**, 291–312.

Mitler, M. M. Browman, C. P., Menn, S. J., Gujavarti, K., and Timms, R. M. (1986). Nocturnal myoclonus: treatment efficacy of clonazepam and temazepam. *Sleep*, **9**, 385–92.

Morgan, K., Dallasso, H., Ebrahim, S., Arie, T., and Fentem, P. H. (1988). Prevalence, frequency and duration of hypnotic use among the elderly living at home. *British Medical Journal*, **296**, 601–2.

Morgan, K., Healey, D. W., and Healey, P. J. (1989). Factors influencing persistent subjective insomnia in old age: a follow-up study of good and poor sleepers aged 65–74. *Age and Ageing*, **18**, 117–22.

Morin, C., and Rapp, S. R. (1987). Behavioural management of geriatric insomnia. *Clinical Gerontology*, **6**, 15–23.

National Institute of Mental Health (1984). Consensus Development Conference: Drugs and insomnia- the use of medications to promote sleep. *Journal of the American Medical Association*, **251**, 2410–4.

Parkes, D. (1985). Sleep apnoea and respiratory disorders during sleep. In *Sleep and its disorders: major problems in neurology* (Ed. J. Walton). W. B. Saunders Company, New York.

Reynolds, C. F., Kupfer, D. J., Taska, L. S., Hoch, C. C., Spiker, D. G., Sewitch, D. E., *et al.* (1985). EEG sleep in elderly depressed, demented and healthy subjects. *Biological Psychiatry*, **20**, 431–42.

Rosenthal, L., Roehrs, T., Sicklesteel, J., Zorick, F., Wittig, R., and Roth, T. (1984). Periodic movements during sleep, sleep fragmentation and sleep–wake complaints. *Sleep*, **7**, 326–30.

Saario, I., and Linnoila, M. (1976) Effect of subacute treatment with hypnotics alone or in combination with alcohol on psychomotor skills related to driving. *Acta Pharmacologica Toxicologica*, **38**, 382–92.

Silvestri, R., Guilleminault, C., and Simmons, F. B. (1983). Palatopharyngoplasty in the treatment of obstructive sleep apnea. In *Sleep/wake disorders: natural history, epidemiology and long-term evolution* (ed. C. Guilleminault and E. Lugaresi). Raven Press, New York.

Smallwood, R. G, Vitiello, M. V., Giblin, E. C, and Prinz, P. N. (1983). Sleep apnea: relationship to age, sex and Alzheimer's dementia. *Sleep*, **6**, 16–22.

Tan, T. L., Kales, J. D., Kales, A., Soldatos, C. R., and Bixler, E. O. (1984). Biopsychobehavioural correlates of insomnia. IV: diagnosis based on DSM III. *American Journal of Psychiatry*, **141**, 357–63.

Thorpy, M. J. (ed.) 1990). *International classification of sleep disorders: diagnostic and coding manual*. Diagnostic Classification Steering Committee, American Sleep Disorder Association, Rochester, Minnesota.

World Health Organization (1992). *International Classification of diseases* (10th revision). World Health Organization, Geneva.

Index